AUG -- 2007

Advance Praise for

## *Cancer: 101 Solutions to a Preventable Epidemic*

Any sane person will want to know the information set out in this highly readable, powerful primer on how to stop the cancer epidemic engulfing us.

— Linda McQuaig, author and journalist

The authors of *Cancer* have taken up where most doctors, public health officials, scientists, businesspeople and regulators have left off. They have assembled and digested a vast array of information from a wide variety of sources, and turned it into a "handbook" for arresting the tide of unnecessary, premature death from exposure to the carcinogens we still produce in untold quantities. This book is wonderful tool for enhancing your own health — and the health of our planetary home.

— Dr. Warren Bell, MD, from the Preface

*Cancer: 101 Solutions to a Preventable Epidemic* delivers on the promise of its title. It is a well researched and comprehensive analysis of today's cancer epidemic. It's practical recommendations are illustrated by encouraging examples of successful initiatives that will surely inspire readers to action.

— Ruth Grier, former Minister of Environment and Minister of Health for Ontario, current volunteer with the Toronto Cancer Prevention Coalition and the Provincial Cancer Prevention and Screening Council

One of most overlooked reasons for high cancer rates in North America is the continued toleration of toxic substances in so many workplaces. Blue-collar workers, especially, have been virtually expendable in numerous occupations and — if we want to end the cancer epidemic — we must take action to stop this travesty. This is one of the few books that fully grasps the links between workplace hazards and cancer, and suggests many useful solutions to this sadly neglected problem.

— Jim Brophy, PhD, Executive Director, Occupational Health Clinic for Ontario Workers, Sarnia, Ontario

D1472320

Despite a large scientific literature documenting possible links between chemicals and cancer, there has been insufficient effort made to put chemicals on the cancer agenda. This important and comprehensive book with its focus on practical solutions will help put environmental causes and solutions centre stage. Canada is taking a world lead in this area and other countries including the UK need to replicate what is happening there.

— Jamie D. Page, The Cancer Prevention and Education Society


*Cancer: 101 Solutions to a Preventable Epidemic* puts key elements of environmental risk and protective opportunities in a meaningful systems perspective. To learn about what science has to say about how to strongly reduce the risk of getting cancer, and improve on life-quality in general from doing so, should appeal to most readers who want to learn from facts that are put in purposeful, tangible, and hopeful contexts.

— Karl-Henrik Robèrt, MD, PhD, Founder of The Natural Step International, Adjunct Professor of Sustainable Product Development at Blekinge Institute of Technology


In my 40+ years of activism, I have rarely seen a book filled with so much valuable information that focuses on solutions and not just the difficult problems that confront us. Bravo for *Cancer: 101 Solutions to a Preventable Epidemic.* With it, there are no more excuses for not taking action.

— Dr. Dorothy Goldin Rosenberg, MES, PhD, environmental health educator, University of Toronto; principal research consultant and associate producer of *Exposure: Environmental Links to Breast Cancer* (1997); executive producer, *Toxic Trespass, a film about children's health and the environment* (2007)

The Solutions Project

# CANCER

## 101 SOLUTIONS
### TO A PREVENTABLE EPIDEMIC

LIZ ARMSTRONG, GUY DAUNCEY and ANNE WORDSWORTH

NEW SOCIETY PUBLISHERS

**Cataloging in Publication Data:**
A catalog record for this publication is available from the National Library of Canada.

**Copyright © 2007 by Liz Armstrong, Guy Dauncey and Anne Wordsworth
All rights reserved.**

Cover design by Diane McIntosh. Images: iStock

Printed in Canada.
First printing April 2007.

New Society Publishers acknowledges the support of the Government of Canada through the Book Publishing Industry Development Program (BPIDP) for our publishing activities.

Paperback ISBN: 978-0-86571-542-4

Inquiries regarding requests to reprint all or part of *Cancer* should be addressed to New Society Publishers at the address below.

To order directly from the publishers, please call toll-free (North America) 1-800-567-6772, or order online at www.newsociety.com

Any other inquiries can be directed by mail to:

New Society Publishers
P.O. Box 189, Gabriola Island, BC V0R 1X0, Canada
1-800-567-6772

New Society Publishers' missing is to publish books that contribute in fundamental ways to building an ecologically sustainable and just society, and to do so with the least possible impact on the environment, in a manner that models this vision. We are committed to doing this not just through education, but through action. This book is one step toward ending globla deforestation and climate change. It is printed on acid-free paper that is **100% post-consumer recycled** (old-growth forest-free), processed chlorine-free, and printed with vegetable-based, low-VOC inks, with covers produced using Forest Stewardship Council-certified stock. Additionall, New Society purchases carbon offsets annually, operating with a carbon-neutral footprint. For further information, or to browse our full list of books and purchase securely, visit our website at newsociety.com

NEW SOCIETY PUBLISHERS                                                    www.newsociety.com

To special friends, family members and others we "met" while working on this book who died too soon from cancer. "Statistics are people with the tears washed off." Thank you for being our inspiration.

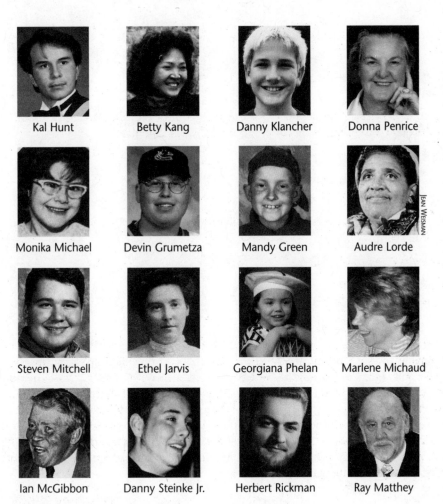

Kal Hunt     Betty Kang     Danny Klancher     Donna Penrice

Monika Michael     Devin Grumetza     Mandy Green     Audre Lorde

Steven Mitchell     Ethel Jarvis     Georgiana Phelan     Marlene Michaud

Ian McGibbon     Danny Steinke Jr.     Herbert Rickman     Ray Matthey

# Contents

# Author's Preface

by Guy Dauncey

I came to write this book because I am pursuing something larger called The Solutions Project, animated by the understanding that in spite of the hopelessness many people feel about the state of the world, there are really only two problems that we have to solve.

The first is the total of all our social, health, environmental, economic, political and religious problems, which need not appear so numerous if we each become engaged in one small part of the puzzle. The second is the belief that we cannot solve our problems.

If we succumb to this despairing belief, whether regarding the break-up of our marriages, the corruption of American democracy, or the way we are destroying our environment, we become part of the problem.

We can never achieve a goal if we believe deep down that it's a hopeless quest, for one of the keys to success is a firm belief in the possibility of success. That key, once turned, opens up a wellspring of creativity, engagement and persistence that can deliver previously unimaginable results, and inspire us to further action.

Success also needs sound understanding, working examples, and solid information. The Solutions Project therefore takes our problems one at a time and gathers the best examples of success, laying them out so that readers can find reason to believe and the courage to get involved.

So why cancer?

Because it is such an enormous problem that is in dire need of a solution — a permanent solution built around prevention. To work for a cure is clearly important — but it is equally important prevent cancer before it starts.

The exciting news is that when we look with an open mind at the many factors which we know contribute to the causes of cancer, many solutions begin to appear.

Many of these solutions ask us to change the way we eat, live and work. They also ask us to change the way we travel, farm, and generate energy; the way we make things; the way we regulate our industries; and the way we allow corporations to corrupt both governments and democracy.

As well as reducing the epidemic of cancer, however, and all the suffering it brings, these changes will also help us to build a peaceful, healthy, sustainable society. They make such eminent sense above and beyond the need to stop the scourge of cancer. They will save us all money as the health care costs of treating cancer fall, and they will save companies money as they substitute less toxic ways of making things. It's a no-brainer. Why would we not want to do this?

As our children learn about this world they live in, they are increasingly looking at us with concern in their eyes.

"What kind of a world are you handing over to us?" they ask us. "What did you do to tackle these problems, and make our world a better place?"

If we tackle these problems, this will be our legacy. They will say of us:

"Your actions gave us hope."

There are many who have helped us with this project, who we thank collectively below.

I especially want to thank my co-authors, Liz Armstrong and Anne Wordsworth, without whose skill, encouragement and persistence this project would never have been completed. With support from others, Liz and I also founded a Canadian non-profit society, Prevent Cancer Now, which we hope all our Canadian readers will join (www.preventcancernow.ca). US readers can find similar encouragement in the Collaborative for Health and the Environment (www.healthandenvironment.org), and British readers in the Cancer Prevention and Education Society (www.cancerpreventionsociety.org).

All three of us — Liz Anne and I — want to thank Judith and Chris Plant, our publishers, Judith Brand and Ingrid Witwoet, our eagle-eyed editors, and the whole team at New Society Publishers for your deep commitment to a more just, sustainable world.

I want to thank Carolyn Herriot, my wife and partner of 17 years, for her support and encouragement while I engage in my various projects. During the years while I was working on Cancer she too became an author with A Year on the Garden Path: A 52-Week Guide to Organic Gardening (Earthfuture/New Society Publishers) which won her the ultimate accolade when her readers said they enjoyed it so much they were staying up all night to read it. Gardeners, take note! (www.earthfuture.com/gardenpath)

Finally, I want to thank the silent, miraculous spirit of life that inspires me to take on my various projects, supports me in all that I do, and fills me with gratefulness for this life, this beautiful world, and all the possibilities that we hold in our hands.

— Guy Dauncey, December 2006

- **The Solutions Project** www.earthfuture.com
- *Stormy Weather: 101 Solutions to Global Climate Change* by Guy Dauncey with Patrick Mazza (New Society Publishers 2001).
- *Enough Blood Shed: 101 Solutions to Violence, Terror and War* by Mary-Wynne Ashford with Guy Dauncey (New Society Publishers 2006)
- *Building an Ark: 101 Solutions to Animal Suffering* by Ethan Smith with Guy Dauncey (New Society Publishers 2007)
- *A Room Somewhere: 101 Solutions to Homelessness* (coming soon)
- *The Great Climate Challenge: 101 Solutions to Global Warming* by Guy Dauncey (coming soon)

# Author's Preface

by Liz Armstrong

I am writing this on January 5, 2007, the day after our beautiful friend Donna Penrice died following an anguishing struggle with leukemia. This creative, caring, witty, wonderful woman did not want to die at age 63. All of us who loved her did not want her to die either, although those last unsettled days before the morphine eased her gently out of this world made us pray the end would come quickly.

The love will never die.

Most people believe the cancer epidemic now upon us is simply impossible to rein in and stop. We know this is not true, and through the 101 Solutions format so cleverly fashioned by Guy, we are able to share scores — in fact, many hundreds — of practical ways each of us can take action for cancer prevention on our own, and with others — and it's all under one book cover.

We are not cancer experts, but Anne, Guy and I have all focused on scientific data and trends long enough to observe that cancer is clearly connected to the larger world of environmental health. Nature's gifts of pure air, water, soil and food are indispensable life supports, and we need to hold up our end of the bargain by restoring their integrity. As Jane Houlihan of the Environmental Working Group said, "Babies aren't supposed to be born pre-polluted." We have it in our hands to cleanse our toxic world — not just for kids, but for all life on Earth.

While there *is* a great deal of cancer prevention information in this book — each segment could be a book in itself — we have deliberately chosen not to tackle several issues. There is nothing about the possible role of stress and emotions, or alternative and complementary cancer treatments, or special diets or vitamin therapies. Yes, these and other topics are important, but we want our readers to focus on the opportunities most overlooked in the big picture — occupational and environmental links to cancer.

In many ways, this is very much a work in progress. Every day a flood of new information surfaces on the environmental health front. Much of it is discouraging, but there are usually some victories to celebrate. As authors of *Cancer: 101 Solutions to a Preventable Epidemic*, here's our stand: that copies of this book gets so thumbed and underlined and bookmarked and *used* by so many people that they become a vital part of the tipping point that ends the cancer epidemic.

Huge thanks to many wonderful friends and family members who have cheered this project on over the past four years — especially to Linda Rosier, for her relentlessly positive outlook and encouragement, and to Zorro the dog, who provides daily lessons in the fine art of total relaxation (and not taking oneself too seriously) as he gently snores at his post next to my computer.

— Liz Armstrong, January 2007

# Author's Preface

by Anne Wordsworth

On Earth Day 1970, my best friend, Kat McCarthy, conscripted me to educate teachers about garbage and our wasteful society. I had no idea about it, but I learned quickly and remember pulling Styrofoam cups out of a green garbage bag and talking about biodegradability. Little did I know that, from that day on, I would be involved in a lifelong engagement with environmental and health issues. In fact, I have come at it from almost every angle — first, as an activist calling on government to do the environmental right thing, then as an advocacy journalist trying to inspire television viewers and, finally, for one glorious moment, working in the Environment Ministry itself.

It became clear to me a long time ago that environmental and occupational problems were directly and intimately linked with our health. It isn't possible to poison waterways, the air, fish and the other living beings with which we share the planet without it ricocheting back on ourselves. I've always called it my "chickens come home to roost" theory. It seems obvious that cancer, autism, learning disorders, asthma and other chronic illnesses are, if not rooted, at least connected to the environmental and occupational contaminants to which we are all exposed. I think almost everyone at some fundamental level knows this now, and the question is what can we do about it.

What I am doing about it, and what many others I know are doing about it, is this — demanding that carcinogens be removed from our daily life. How surprising can it be that cancer is on the rise when for 50 years we have accepted shampoos, pans, foods, building materials and packaging made of materials of questionable safety. Sadly, the more things we buy, use and stuff into our houses, the higher the levels of toxins around us and the higher our overall risk. If there's anything people should take away from this book, I think it is to simplify and detoxify your life. It is the best chance for a healthy and happy future. And once your own house is in order, help your community refocus on respecting and restoring the local environment. Then, send the message up to the next level of government. It's an awesome task, but it's one that becomes inevitable once you know what the stakes are. Like my job on that first Earth Day, I didn't really choose to be concerned about the environment and our health but once I did it for Kat, I just had to keep doing it.

— Anne Wordsworth, January 2007

# Acknowledgments

As authors of this book, we would like to thank the many people who have helped us along the way. For their advice, ideas, and critiquing of the manuscript, we would like to thank Devra Lee Davis, PhD, Director of the Centre for Environmental Oncology at the University of Pittsburgh Center Institute; Maryann Donovan, PhD, Scientific Director at the same; and Dr Peter Carter, MD, past President of Canadian Association of Physicians for the Environment.

And for their many and various contributions, we would like to thank the following. Our appreciation is immense, and the responsibility for any errors or omissions is entirely ours: Rita Arditti, Mary-Wynne Ashford, Mary Bachran, Jen Baker, Thomas Bierma, Judy Brady, Warren Bell, Dave Bennett, Madeleine Bird, Jim Brophy, Mae Burrows, Moni Campbell, Morag Carter, Theo Colborn Kathleen Cooper, Sylvain De Guise, Karen DeKoning, Fe DeLeon, Lissa Donner, Vern Edwards, Donna Ell, Suzanne Elston, Nancy Evans, Marian Feinberg, Helke Ferrie, Robert Ferrie, David Gerratt, Michael Gilbertson, Dorothy Goldin Rosenberg, Tim Grant, William Grant, Ruth Grier, Magda Havas, Mandy Hawes, Genevieve Howe, Rhonda Hustler, Molly Jacobs, Sat Dharam Kaur, Margaret Keith, Marjorie Lamb, Elizabeth Lamb, Sue Larsh, Michael Lerner, Rick Lindgren, Helen Lynn, Joe Mangano, Elizabeth May, Janet May, Janet McNeill, Loretta Michaud, Brian Milani, Katrina Miller, Sarah Miller, Joe Odie, Jamie Page, Ian Panton, Michael Perley, Leo Petrilli , Gerry Potter, Barbara Reid, Angela Rickman, Karl-Henrik Robert, Karen Robinson, Anne Rochon Ford, Cheryl Rook, Sara Rosenthal, Nicola Ross, Norm Rubin, Patricia Running-Horan, Cindy Sage, Brian Schaeffer, Janette Sherman, Sandra Steingraber, Elisabeth Sterken, Larry Stoffman, Laura Telford, Beverley Thorpe, Joel Tickner, Joan Vincent, Cathy Walker, Laura Weinberg, Rich Whate, Mark Winfield, Marilyn Wolfe and Miriam Wyman.

We thank the families of the people included on the Dedication page for permission to use their photos.

We would also like to thank all those who encouraged us while we worked on the book, knowing how important this work is. To quote the Roman author, lawyer and statesman Cicero:

*Salus populi suprema est lex*
The welfare of the people is the highest law

For our modern context, we need to add:

*Salus mondi suprema est lex*
The welfare of the planet is the highest law

# Preface

by Warren Bell

Let me tell you why this book is important and valuable.

When I completed my family medicine residency at McGill in 1976, there was a final exam. It included interviews with simulated patients. One such person was a woman in her fifties who, I was told, had just been confirmed to have terminal cancer. It was my task to tell her this fact.

It was an emotional encounter. I had already completed an elective in palliative care, and was not at all uncomfortable talking about death. But the woman — even though she was simply an actress playing a role — somehow connected deeply to the experience of having cancer and being close to death. Afterwards, she wept, and told me about the overwhelmingly sense of loss she had felt while we were speaking.

Over the decades, I have had many encounters with people with terminal cancer. Death is not the problem — every dawn is followed by a sunset. But premature, preventable disease and death — that's another matter. When I meet someone sick with a cancer that could clearly have been prevented, I feel a sense of disquiet, and even frustration. In particular, I am deeply concerned about the rising toll of cancer that comes from *involuntary* exposures to carcinogens.

While many cancers are caused by personal behaviours (e.g. smoking) or "bad genes" (about 5% of breast and bowel cancer), there are a rapidly growing number that are caused by man-made contaminants in the environment. Exposure to them is leading to steadily rising cancer rates, especially in children.

And that's why this book is important and valuable.

The authors of *Cancer: 101 Solutions to a Preventable Epidemic* have taken up where most doctors, public health officials, scientists, businesspeople and regulators have left off. They have assembled and digested a vast array of information from a wide variety of sources, and turned it into a "handbook" for arresting the tide of unnecessary, premature death from exposure to the carcinogens we still produce in untold quantities. They have laid out, for every reader, a series of practical steps to prevent exposure, reduce risk, and ultimately restore Planet Earth.

In this well-organized volume, you will find a road map out of the morass of what oncologist Karl-Henrik Robert, founder of **The Natural Step**, has called "molecular garbage".

This book is wonderful tool for enhancing your own health – and the health of our planetary home.

— Dr. Warren Bell, M.D.
Family physician. President of Medical Staff and Active Staff member, Shuswap Lake General Hospital. President of the Association of Complementary and Integrative Physicians of BC. Past Founding President, Canadian Association of Physicians for the Environment (CAPE).

# foreword

by Devra Davis

I'm a cancer orphan. Both my parents died from the disease that now affects almost one out of every two men and more than one in every three women in North America today.

I know what cancer looks and feels like. I have also come to know that much of the disease could have been prevented, if only we had paid attention to what some people have been warning for years.

In this book, Liz Armstrong, Guy Dauncey and Anne Wordsworth turn the dominant paradigm about cancer upside down. In North America, for years, the debate on the environmental causes of cancer has been whether there is sufficient proof to declare that any given substance causes our cancers. Risks are generally assessed one substance at a time, and only a small percentage of the hazardous substances that are part and parcel of our daily lives are tested. Obscure models using animals exposed to these substances are used to estimate their likely impact on humans.

The authors show us that this approach has not worked. They confirm the tragic and continuing saga of individuals, workers and communities whose continuing exposure to the risks of cancer has endangered their lives and those of their families, and killed far too many humans — and other living creatures.

The world is changing, and Canadians are at the center in two major roles. Prompted by engaged citizens, the provincial governments of Alberta, Quebec and Ontario have begun efforts to get rid of cancerous agents, and businesses are emerging to create greener, more efficient and less polluting products of all kinds.

The Canadian Cancer Society has spoken out against the use of 'cosmetic' pesticides and adopted the precautionary principle. California has produced a major report on Green Chemistry, linking the health impacts of toxic chemicals to the urgent need to develop a new approach.

Massachusetts has shown the way with toxics use reduction legislation that has helped hundreds of companies not just to clean up their act, but to prosper financially. Sweden has made a commitment to phase out all hazardous chemicals by 2020. President Jacques Chirac has called for candidates for the French national presidency to make public declarations of their intent to reduce the environmental burden on cancer.

This book sends an urgent wake-up call. It exposes some troubling episodes in public health where people have been denied the fundamental human right to know about the dangers that exist in their everyday world, and it provides copious evidence of policies, practices and principles that offer us the possibility of a far safer, healthier world, if we are willing to embrace them.

Some may be challenged by the passion of this book. Some may be uncomfortable with its tone, but no one can dispute the solid grounds on which it rests.

— Devra Davis, Ph.D., MPH
Director of the Center for Environmental Oncology at the University of Pittsburgh Cancer Institute, and Professor, Department of Epidemiology, Graduate School of Public Health. Author of *When Smoke Ran Like Water* (Basic Books, 2002) and *The Secret History of the War on Cancer* (Basic Books, Fall 2007).

# Part I
## The Global Epidemic

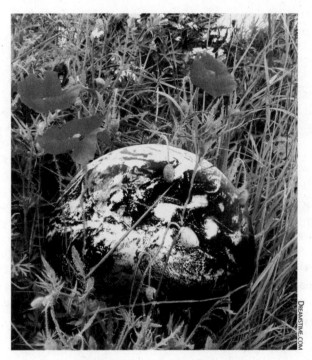

Beauty discarded, or beauty found?

**It is time to start pursuing alternative paths. From the right to know and the duty to inquire follows the obligation to act.**

**— Sandra Steingraber**

# The Global Cancer Crisis

The most determined effort should be made to eliminate those carcinogens that now contaminate our food, our water supplies and our atmosphere, because these provide the most dangerous type of contact — minute exposures, repeated over and over throughout the years.[1]

— Rachel Carson

We first saw it pinned on the sweater of a breast cancer survivor in Boston — a small, round, pink button with just four words printed in black type: "Rachel Carson was right."[2]

For most people under 50, the button begs two questions: who is Rachel Carson, and why was she right?

1. Rachel Carson was a marine biologist, and author of three best-selling books about the mystery and magic of life in the oceans.[3] Her final book, *Silent Spring*, published in 1962, was a major departure, a scrupulously researched exposé about the health hazards of modern pesticides and nuclear radiation. Cancer was a prominent theme.

2. Rachel Carson died from breast cancer in 1964. Because she identified man-made chemicals and radiation as major causes of cancer and other illnesses, she became the target of a fierce industry campaign to destroy her reputation and credibility. In *Silent Spring* she issued this clarion call: To prevent cancer, we must rid society of man-made substances causing the disease.[4]

In 1964 Wilhelm Heuper and W.C. Conway of the National Cancer Institute described cancer as "an epidemic in slow motion" and predicted a future catastrophe resulting from "reckless" chemical contamination.[5]

All three were right.

In the early 1960s cancer struck one of every four Americans and Canadians and killed one in five. In 2007 cancer strikes nearly one in two males and over a third of all females, and one in four will die. Cancer recently overtook heart disease as the leading cause of death in both the US and Canada and is head and shoulders above the rest in the category "potential years of life lost."

Is cancer primarily connected to aging? According to *Canadian Cancer Statistics 2006*, 43% of all new cancer cases and 60% of deaths occur in people 70 years and older.[6] As more of us live longer, the total burden of cancer in Canada and the US will grow accordingly. But some of the increases have nothing to do with age; more people in *all* age groups are developing certain types of cancer than in the past.[7]

The incidence rates of breast, prostate, brain, non-Hodgkins lymphoma, thyroid, melanoma and multiple myeloma are continuing to climb, while only a few, such as stomach cancer in both men and women, lung cancer in men and cervical cancer in women are declining. Several escalating cancers have clear links to environmental hazards.[8]

In Canada from 1975 to 2000, the age-standardized incidence of cancer among females increased by 19.5% (from 290.2 to 346.5 per 100,000 population) and among males by 29.2% (from 357.7 to 462.0 per 100,000 population). The increase is higher for men and lower for women when lung cancer is excluded, as Canadian smoking rates dropped for males and rose for females.[9]

In the US cancer incidence in children under 15 years of age climbed 27% between 1975 and

2002,[10]. Worrisome increases are also evident among young adults aged 20 to 44.[11]

In 1998 the National Cancer Institute and the American Cancer Society claimed with some relief that the rates of many common cancers had stabilized during the 1990s and were finally on the decline. But in a 2002 research paper, NCI's scientists reported that the apparent downturns were due to a delay in reporting new cases. Once corrected, the data showed that breast cancer was still rising by 0.6% a year, melanoma in white men by 4.1% a year and that prostate cancer in black men was 14% higher in 1998 than originally reported.[12]

Worldwide the burden of cancer is rising. In 2002 there were 10.9 million new cases and 6.7 million deaths. Lung cancer led the way, followed by breast and colorectal cancer. The World Health Organization has warned that this will rise by 50% to 15 million new cases a year by 2020 unless major public health and prevention programs are aggressively pursued.[13]

The most common cancers in developed countries are of the colon and rectum, breast, prostate, brain, nervous system and testes. In developing countries, cancers of the liver, stomach and esophagus are more common.[14] As developing nations adopt Western ways of life, the rates of many of "our" cancers are increasing, including lung cancer, caused by an explosion in the number of smokers.

This brings us to our book's main theme: the cancer epidemic is being fueled by carcinogens in our air, water and food; by poor-quality processed food stripped of its protective nutrients and loaded with additives; and by an assault on our immune systems by toxic substances.

The latest science is proving that Rachel Carson was right about this, too.

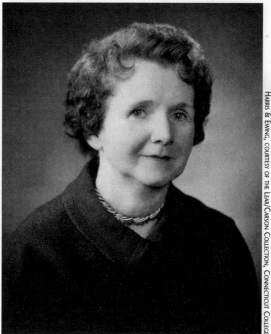

HARRIS & EWING, COURTESY OF THE LEAR/CARSON COLLECTION, CONNECTICUT COLLEGE

Born in 1907, Rachel Carson, author of *Silent Spring*, died from breast cancer at age 56 in 1964. "There is so much more I want to do," she wrote her closest friend in November 1963, "and it is hard to accept that in all probability, I must leave most of it undone."

# Our Body Burden

**If ever we had proof that our nation's pollution laws aren't working, it's reading the list of industrial chemicals in the bodies of babies who have not yet lived outside the womb.**

— Congresswoman Louise Slaughter

Our bodies are truly amazing. The fact that you are alive today means you have inherited an unbroken chain of being that stretches right back to the first single-celled organisms, 4,000 million years ago — that's 4 billion years.

Your body contains between 50 and 75 trillion cells, and each cellular nucleus contains up to 25,000 genes. You breathe in and out 23,000 times a day from the same air that was breathed by the dinosaurs, and your body is 60% water, from the same ever-recycling water that is shared by every being in the world.[1]

When you consider this amazing complexity, it is remarkable how healthy most of us are. When your body receives the nutrients it needs, breathes clean air, drinks pure water and gets the exercise needed to keep your oxygen pumping and your muscles fit, it should last a hundred years.

It is very disturbing, therefore, to learn that our bodies are being contaminated with a burden of toxic chemicals. In 2003 the Mount Sinai School of Medicine in New York conducted a study with the Environmental Working Group (EWG) in which nine healthy volunteers, none of whom worked with chemicals, had their blood and urine tested.[2] They found 167 industrial chemicals, including:

- 76 chemicals linked to cancer in humans or animals (average 53 per person)
- 94 chemicals that are toxic to the brain and nervous system (average 62)
- 86 chemicals that interfere with the hormone system (average 58)
- 79 chemicals associated with birth defects or abnormal development (average 55)
- 77 chemicals that are toxic to the reproductive system (average 55)
- 77 chemicals that are toxic to the immune system (average 53)

The chemicals came from everyday things such as adhesives, pesticides, food additives, fire-retardants, hair sprays, perfumes, lubricants, brake fluid, varnishes, paints, dyes and cleaning products. A Canadian study came up with similar results,[3] as did a European study including 47 Members of the EU Parliament from 17 nations.[4]

When the EWG examined the breast milk of 20 nursing mothers, it found levels of brominated fire-retardants (PDBEs) from furniture foam, computers and televisions that were 75 times higher than the average found in recent

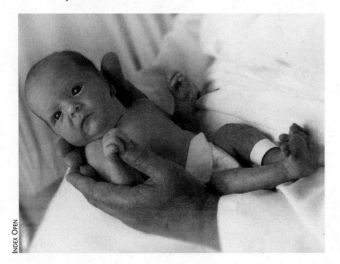

INDEX OPEN

European studies. The PDBEs accumulate in the food chain and human tissues and adversely affect brain development and the thyroid.[5]

In 2004 when they looked at the umbilical cord blood of ten newborn babies, they found that 287 chemicals had passed through their mothers' placentas, averaging 230 contaminants.[6]

The US Centers for Disease Control is also monitoring environmental chemicals in our bodies. In 2005, as well as finding similar results to the other studies, they found that children had higher levels than adults for residues from second-hand smoke, for some pesticides and for chemicals such as phthalates that leach from plastics.

The good news is that they observed a steep decline in lead in the children's blood, following regulations to remove it from gasoline and paint, and in second-hand smoke residues, following smoking bans. The bad news is that these studies do not include the effects of ionizing radiation, a known carcinogen that is adding to our body burden.

When the chemicals are not removed, however, they often contribute to cancer. In 2003 a Belgian study found that women with breast cancer were 5 times more likely than healthy women to have residues of the pesticide DDT in their blood.[7] In 2006 a US study found that men whose bodies were contaminated with PCB 153 were 30 times more likely to have prostate cancer than those who were not contaminated.[8]

Why is this being allowed? A lack of regulatory oversight and constant pressure from

- Body Burden: The Pollution in Newborns: www.ewg.org/reports/bodyburden2
- California's Body Burden Campaign: www.calbbc.org
- CDC National Report on Human Exposure to Environmental Chemicals: www.cdc.gov/exposurereport
- Chemical Body Burden: www.chemicalbodyburden.org
- Environmental Defence Canada: www.ToxicNation.ca
- Environmental Working Group: www.ewg.org
- WWF: www.worldwildlife.org/toxics

industry not to interfere have combined to allow over 100,000 novel chemicals to be used, most of which have never been examined for their health impacts (see p. 30). When chemicals *are* studied, they are almost never studied in combination with other chemicals, and rarely at the minute levels of contamination that can undermine the body's exquisitely sensitive hormonal systems.

We should be outraged that this is being allowed. Hazardous substances linked to cancer and other health problems are being found in the tissue of almost every living creature on Earth, and it is up to us to do something to stop this toxic trespass.

> For too long, policy-makers have retrospectively pleaded, "if only we had known earlier what we know now." I believe that what we do know now must guide us in our review and approval processes, and should become the basis of a bold new precautionary approach that puts the burden of evidence on safety first.
>
> — Dr. Roberto Bertollini,
> World Health Organization

# The Cost of Cancer

There is just no way to control the cost.
The manufacturers have zero incentive to
reduce their prices.

— Tom Baker, drug-cost expert
with Zitter Group, San Francisco[1]

## The Personal Cost

First, there's the emotional cost. Most of us fear dying. We are afraid that we will not live to see our children get married, or our grandchildren grow up. We dread the anguish of watching helplessly as a small child or teenager dies from cancer.

Then there's the pain: the nausea and vomiting that are experienced by 70% to 80% of those who receive chemotherapy, and 70% to 90% of those who go through radiation. And the fatigue, hair-loss, blood disorders and bone pain that often accompany cancer treatments, in spite of a fall in the incidence of side effects, and their treatment.

We celebrate the survivors of cancer — as we should — but we must never forget those who lose the most precious gift of all, whose loved ones are left weeping and bereft. Look around you. One in four of the people you see will die from cancer. On average each one loses 15 precious years of life that could have been filled with love, adventure, family and music.

## The Financial Cost

People with cancer live longer today than in the past, but the cost of treatments has risen enormously. In 1994 doctors could extend the life of a patient for a year by using a combination of drugs worth $500 in today's dollars. By 2004 they could extend a life by almost two years, but the cost had escalated to $250,000.[2]

The wholesale price for Avastin, a colon cancer drug that extends patients' lives by five months, is $46,000 a year. Tarceva, a lung cancer drug that increases survival by two months,

costs $6,500 to $9,000 a year. Herceptin, which increases the survival for certain breast cancer patients by five months, costs $22,500 a year.[3] The cost of these drugs can be two to five times higher in the US than in Canada.

## Going Bankrupt for Cancer

Who can afford this? In America only 27% of the population is covered by government health care programs — Medicare for the elderly and Medicaid for those with very low incomes.

Thirty-five million Americans have private health insurance that comes with restrictions, high deductibles and caps. You think your insurance will cover your treatment, until you discover the cost of chemotherapy may reach $6,000 a day but your plan only allows for $1,000. There are other costs, too, such as the loss of income when you take time off for sickness, or to look after a spouse or child, and the need for transport, daycare and home health care. Even with the much touted US drug benefits, people needing cancer treatment will still have to pay more than $1,500 a year out of their own pocket.

A quarter of all Americans cannot afford the cost of cancer. For many the only solution is bankruptcy. A study in 2005 by the Harvard Medical School found that illness and medical bills contributed to half of all bankruptcy filings, representing two million Americans a year, a 2,200% increase since 1981. Three quarters had medical insurance at the start of their illness, but illness led to job loss and the loss of insurance. In 2001 Americans with cancer had average medical debts of $35,878.[4]

Whichever way US citizens are covered, the cost of cancer is huge, and a financial collapse of the system is a real possibility. For the 48 million Americans — including 9 million children[5] — who are not covered at all — a single health crisis may spell disaster.

In Canada, the public health care system pays for the cost of treatment, which is an enormous blessing, but once a drug has been approved by the federal government, if a province does not approve of its use, or if a doctor fails to do the necessary paperwork, cancer patients either have to go without or pay for it themselves, creating a two-tiered system for rich and poor.[6]

### Where Will This Lead?

In 1990 the direct cost of cancer treatment to the US health care system was $35 billion, representing 10% of national health expenditures.[7] By 2003 it had risen to $64 billion, representing 20% of expenditures.[8] The total cost of cancer, including financial losses from premature death and reduced productivity, was over $171 billion. In Canada the total cost of cancer in 1998 was $14 billion.[9]

With survival rates rising, there is expected to be a 50% increase in the number of people living with cancer by 2015, leading to a vast new demand for drugs and treatments.

To the drug companies, this represents an enormous opportunity. In 2005 the worldwide cost of cancer drugs was estimated at $24 billion, of which $15 billion was spent in the US. If effective cancer drugs emerge, the market could reach $300 billion by 2025 as pharmaceutical companies seek to make cancer a chronic, controllable illness

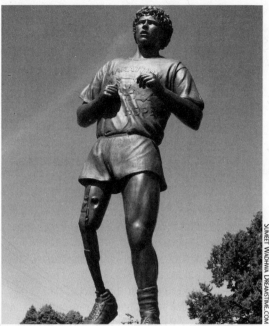

The Terry Fox statue in Victoria, BC. In 1977, Terry Fox ran 3,107 miles across Canada in The Marathon of Hope, to raise funds for cancer research. He was forced to stop when his own osteosarcoma cancer spread to his lungs. He died on June 28, 1981, aged 22. By 2007, the annual Terry Fox Run had raised more than $400 million. www.terryfoxrun.org.

similar to diabetes. To some drug companies, it is a "vast healthcare and commercial opportunity."[10]

Regarding the social and economic costs of cancer — the work days lost, the agonies of families torn apart by illness — the true costs are incalculable but could well run to nearly half a trillion dollars in the US.

### Prevention: The Only Answer

There is only one possible way out of this mess. We have to stop cancer at its source by focusing on eliminating the preventable carcinogens from our lives and by maximizing our natural abilities to fight cancer.

# What Causes Cancer?

Scientific research has made it clear that preventable environmental and occupational exposures are fueling excess cancers cases and deaths.[1]

— Richard Clapp

Cancer is a general term for over 200 similar diseases that are characterized by a process of abnormal, uncontrolled cell division. Cancers evolve through a complicated web of multiple causes that interact with each other.[2]

Most cancers begin when something damages a healthy cell, followed by further injuries that accumulate over time. It might be exposure to one of the 69 carcinogens in cigarette smoke, to ionizing radiation, to one of over 80,000 modern chemicals that are used in products and processes, or to a natural carcinogen such as arsenic.

The injuries may damage the DNA strands that govern reproduction, causing genes to become deranged, natural repair mechanisms to fail and cancerous cells to multiply out of control. Some pollutants also damage the immune system, rendering it less able to protect us.

Cancers can start without damage to the DNA. When a toxic substance mimics human hormones, as some pesticides, plastics and pharmaceuticals do (see p. 32), it can fool the body's endocrine system by latching onto receptors that are meant for natural hormones, unleashing a cascade of mistaken outcomes including cancers of the breast, prostate and testicle.

There is also an epigenetic factor. The epigenome is the chemical and physical code that governs a gene sequence, acting as a messenger between the genes and their environment. When it encounters a novel chemical, it can wrongly tell a tumor suppressor gene to turn itself off. There is evidence that damage to a mother's or father's epigenome may trigger cancer in the next generation.

Then there is diet. Our bodies evolved on a diet of healthy plants that develop natural disease-fighting compounds when attacked by fungi or pests. When modern farming sprays crops with pesticides and fungicides, the plants are no longer exposed, so they no longer generate these compounds.

There are also genetic traits that make some people more susceptible to cancer than others. A study of children's leukemia in Quebec showed that the cancer risk was higher in children who carried a certain genetic mutation, who had also been exposed to pesticides in the womb.[3]

These factors accumulate, and some substances only become carcinogenic in the presence of others. The evidence seems to show that most cancers have a multi-factorial origin.

## The Conventional Response

The conventional explanation focuses almost exclusively on the role of tobacco, alcohol, poor diet, lack of exercise, exposure to the sun, infectious agents and drugs. It also says that cancer is increasing because we live longer, even though close to 60% of new cancers appear in people under 70.[4] The danger from novel chemicals and radiation is minimized.

Conventional prevention programs urge us to stop smoking, eat more fruits and vegetables and so on. This is good advice, but it is very limited.

Why? Here's your principal clue: *Doll and Peto*.

Sir Richard Doll was a British scientist of high renown who, with Richard Peto, laid out his assessment of the causes of deaths from cancer in 1981,[5] followed by similar reports by the

Harvard Center for Cancer Prevention in 1996[6] and again by Doll in 1998.[7]

In their 1981 analysis, Doll and Peto concluded that no more than 2% to 4% of cancers were caused by occupational exposure, and 1% to 5% by pollution. The rest were attributed to tobacco, diet, solar UV, infections and lack of exercise. By 2004 their work had been cited in 441 scientific articles and had become the foundation for the conventional "lifestyle" explanation of the causes of cancer.

Doll and Peto's analysis was very limited, however. They looked only at deaths, not the incidence of cancer. In their analysis of occupational cancers, they excluded anyone over 65 due to the non-availability of systematically collected data, even though more than 70% of cancers were occurring after 65. They excluded African-Americans, who were more likely than whites to work in dirtier, dustier workplaces, and they ignored the steady increase in cancer among children and young people. They paid no attention to cancer vulnerability pre-conceptually, in the womb or during puberty. Their work, based chiefly on epidemiologic evidence, ignored animal and other laboratory studies that would have demonstrated likely harm, and did not address the multi-factorial manner in which carcinogens and other risk factors combine.[8]

As a result, they seriously underestimated the role of environmental pollution. They based their 1981 research on just 16 known carcinogens, whereas in 2006 the International Agency for Research on Cancer listed 414 known or suspected carcinogens. (See Appendix 1)

In summary, Doll and Peto's work should no longer be used as an explanation of the causes of cancer.

In 2006 it was disclosed that Doll had a long-term financial relationship between 1970 and 1990 with Monsanto. While he was reviewing the cancer risks of vinyl chloride, dioxin and phenoxy herbicides, he received payments from the American Chemical Council and the chemical companies ICI and Dow.[9] He (and Green College, Oxford, that he founded) also received payments from the asbestos industry and General Motors.[10]

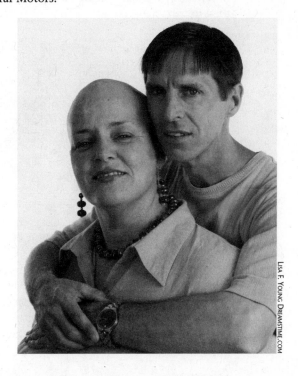

LISA F. YOUNG DREAMSTIME.COM

# What About Aging, Genetics and Lifestyle?

The number of people getting cancer is wrong. Our failure to do better fighting this disease is wrong. I just think we need to be wiser about the world we are creating.[1]

— Wendy Mesley

"Cancer is primarily a disease of the elderly."

We've heard this statement from cancer agencies for so long that we rarely question it.

But let's look again. According to the 2006 edition of *Canadian Cancer Statistics*, 57% of the 153,100 new cancer cases are predicted to occur in Canadians less than 69 years old, not in the elderly population. We know from the age-adjusted statistics — which take into account shifting ratios of young to old in our population over time — that more Canadians and Americans in *every* age group are diagnosed with cancer than decades ago.

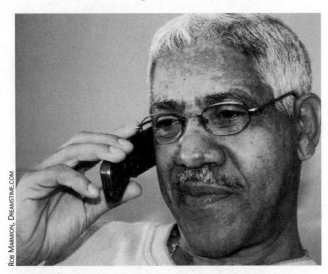

It's important for cancer prevention to adopt and keep good personal habits, but our Western 'lifestyle' is more than the sum of diet, smoking, drinking alcohol, exercise and avoiding the midday sun.

Still when we take away the age-adjustment factor, the cancer situation becomes more chilling at this time in history. The explosion we're experiencing is definitely more pronounced because the average North American is older now than 20 years ago. The baby boomers — that enormous batch of infants born between 1946 and 1964 and now moving through middle age — will soon reach Prime Cancer Time.

Even the Canadian Cancer Control Strategy calls what lies ahead a "looming cancer catastrophe." Over the next three decades, almost 6 million Canadians will get some type of cancer, with more than 38 million "potential years of life lost."[2]

Yes, there are more cancers as we age. Of all new diagnoses, 25% occur in the 60 to 69 age group; less than 1% of cancers affect kids aged 20 and younger.[3] But age does not "cause" cancer. It is environmental factors such as smoking, toxic chemicals, radiation, infections and empty junk food, often in combination with "internal" factors such as inherited genes and immune deficiencies, that cause cancer.[4]

What about genetics? The number of hereditary cancers, passed via damaged genes from our parents, is very small. "About 5% to 10% of all cancers are strongly hereditary," ... the American Cancer Society explains. "However, most cancers do not result from inherited genes, but rather are the result of damage (mutations) to genes that occurs during one's lifetime."[5] We all vary in our genetic susceptibility to cancer: that's a fact of life.

And then there's "lifestyle." Wendy Mesley, co-host of the CBC television show *Marketplace*,

- American Cancer Statistics: www.cancer.org
- Canadian Cancer Statistics: www.cancer.ca
- The Green Guide: www.thegreenguide.com
- *Green Living, The E Magazine Handbook for Living Lightly on the Earth*: www.emagazine.com

said she thought she was doing everything right according to the Canadian Cancer Society's guidelines. "Don't smoke. Eat your veggies. Exercise. Stay out of the sun." Like many Canadians, she did all these things and was still diagnosed with breast cancer in 2004. Her documentary "Chasing the Cancer Answer" chose to focus on "what else" in our lives might cause cancer. It attracted a record audience and was subsequently aired many more times in Spring 2006.[6]

What is this thing called "lifestyle"? As defined by cancer agencies, lifestyle is about smoking, diet, exercise, alcohol and avoiding the midday sun. Yet we are all children of a toxic industrial age, and how we live is more than the sum of personal habits.

A typical "day in the life" might unfold something like this:

7 am: Shut off the alarm on the clock radio (exposure to electromagnetic fields). Hit the synthetic carpet (too many off-gassing chemicals to list) running. Take a shower in hot chlorinated water (chloroform, etc.) using an anti-bacterial body wash (triclosan). Apply several personal care products including underarm deodorant/antiperspirant (parabens), lipstick (coal tar dyes) and blusher (main ingredient, talc, possibly contaminated with asbestos). Step into a freshly dry-cleaned (perchlorethylene), perma-pressed (formaldehyde-finished) business suit. Fry eggs

for breakfast in a Teflon-coated pan, burn the toast a little but eat it anyway (PAHs, acrylamide), heat coffee made from city tap water (chlorine by-products, trace toxins). Drive to the office in the brand new car (plastics and glues off-gassing formaldehyde) in heavy traffic (diesel particulates, benzene). Turn on the computer and copier (EMFs, cadmium), breathe copious amounts of indoor office air (too many chemicals to list). Eat lunch with fatty foods that are non-organic (deprived of antioxidants). Keep hydrated with water from polycarbonate plastic bottles (bisphenol-A). Home again at 6 pm to relax with glass of red wine (pesticide residues) and a scented candle (too many chemicals to name). Poach some farmed salmon (mercury and PCBs); serve with non-organic spinach, potatoes, sweet bell peppers and celery (veggies most likely to be contaminated with pesticides).[7] Go to sleep on a mattress made with petrochemicals and flame retardants.[8]

Yes, of course, it's important to cultivate good personal habits, but — at the same time — let's acknowledge that "lifestyle" is way more than diet, smoking, alcohol, physical exercise and staying out of the sun. Transforming the toxic lives we lead is an exciting challenge — and unquestionably possible.

# The Environmental Links

> For most people, cancer comes not from preprogrammed genes, but from conditions and exposures that are encountered throughout their life.
>
> — Devra Lee Davis

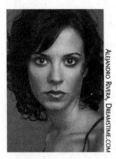

Permanent dark hair dyes: one of the most suspected causes of cancer.

For years the traditional analysis of the causes of cancer has played down or ignored environmental factors. This is convenient, since it means we do not have to make troublesome changes to the way we live, eat and run our society.

The reality is very different, with a growing understanding that cancer is tragically connected to environmental pollution.

Some of the known environmental causes of cancer are shown in the chart opposite, drawn from a detailed survey of scientific studies done for the Collaborative on Health and the Environment in 2005. For every reference (pesticides linked to brain cancer, solvents linked to cancer of the kidney), there is a peer-reviewed study of humans that reflects careful scientific work.

It is wrong to assert that "1% to 5% of cancers are caused by pollution," as epidemiologists Doll and Peto did in 1981 and the Harvard Center for Cancer Prevention did in 1996. Cancer is a complex disease that involves at least six different

- Breast Cancer Environmental Risk Factors: www.envirocancer.cornell.edu
- CHE Toxicant and Disease Database: http://database.healthandenvironment.org
- Collaborative on Health and the Environment: www.healthandenvironment.org
- *Environmental and Occupational Causes of Cancer*: www.sustainableproduction.org/pres.shtml

alterations before it succeeds in overwhelming the body's defenses and producing cancerous cells. At any one of these stages, multiple factors are involved, any or all of which may need external carcinogens to promote the cancer.

We need to remember that it took almost 50 years for society to accept that smoking caused lung cancer and to bring in anti-smoking rules. The evidence was clear in 1950, when several different studies in England and America were published showing that lung cancer patients smoked, while those without the disease did so rarely.

In 1958 a Harley Street physician objected to the Medical Research Council's link between smoking and cancer as "a staggering and most unscientific claim ... They will be blaming mother's milk next."[1] The tobacco industry paid a number of highly respected scientists in America, England and elsewhere to confuse us, delaying for five decades the measures needed to discourage and prevent smoking. During that time, 5 million people died prematurely in North America from smoking.[2]

Today we are seeing the same resistance to environmental pollution and radiation as contributing causes of cancer. We cannot afford to wait another 50 years.

It is not necessary to propose a hierarchy, or play one component off against another. Preventing carcinogenic exposures wherever possible should be the goal, and comprehensive cancer prevention programs should aim to reduce exposures from all avoidable sources, including environmental and occupational sources.

| Cancer of the: | Pollutants that are known to be contributing factors:[3] |
|---|---|
| Bladder | Arsenic in drinking water, chlorination by-products, solvents (e.g., among dry-cleaning workers), hair dyes, petrochemicals, coal tars, metalworking fluids, ionizing radiation |
| Bone | Ionizing radiation from X-rays, CT scans, nuclear exposure, medical experiments |
| Brain & nervous system | Solvents, paints, inks, ionizing radiation, low-frequency non-ionizing EMF radiation, pesticides, maternal consumption of cured meats during pregnancy (N-nitriso) |
| Breast | Ionizing radiation; endocrine disruptors that mimic the actions of estrogens, found in many pesticides, fuels, plastics, detergents and prescription drugs, the drug diethylstilbestrol (DES), solvents (e.g., among electronics, metals, furniture, printing, chemical, textiles and clothing industries workers), pesticides, benzene, and more |
| Cervix | Solvents (e.g., dry cleaners) |
| Colon | Limited and inconsistent evidence: ionizing radiation, chlorination by-products |
| Esophagus | Solvents (e.g., dry cleaners and dye-house workers), metalworking fluids and oils |
| Kidney | Solvents (e.g., trichloroethylene TCE), pesticides, metals |
| Larynx | Metalworking fluids, asbestos, wood dust, reactive chemicals |
| Leukemia | Solvents, benzene, reactive chemicals, ionizing radiation (e.g., diagnostic X-rays during pregnancy), pesticides (including while pregnant) |
| Liver | Metals (especially arsenic), solvents, ionizing radiation, reactive chemicals, PCBs |
| Lymph (Hodgkin's & Non-Hodgkin's) | Solvents, pesticides, hair dyes |
| Lung | Tobacco smoke, environmental (second-hand) tobacco smoke, outdoor air pollution, indoor air pollution, petrochemical by-products, metalworking fluid, natural fibers (silica, wood dust, asbestos, mineral fibers), radon |
| Mesothelioma | Asbestos |
| Multiple myeloma | Solvents, ionizing radiation, pesticides, occupational exposure to hair dyes |
| Nasal & Pharynx | Solvents, reactive chemicals, metalworking fluids, ionizing radiation |
| Ovary | Pesticides, ionizing radiation, talc powder, products used by hairdressers and beauticians |
| Pancreas | Solvents, metals (cadmium, nickel), reactive chemicals, pesticides, metalworking fluids, mineral oils |
| Prostate | Pesticides, endocrine disrupting chemicals such as Bisphenol-A, metallic dusts, metalworking fluids, polyaromatic hydrocarbons (PAH), fuel combustion products, aromatic amines (from cooked red meat), metals |
| Rectum | Solvents, chlorination by-products, metalworking fluids, mineral oils |
| Soft Tissue | Metals, reactive chemicals, ionizing radiation, pesticides |
| Skin | Ionizing radiation (UV radiation), metals, metalworking fluids, mineral oils, creosotes, coal tars |
| Stomach | Metals (e.g., lead), ionizing radiation, pesticides, metalworking fluids, mineral oils, asbestos |
| Testes | Endocrine disrupting chemicals, PCBs, especially in the womb, work in agriculture, tanning, mechanical painting, mining, plastics and metalworking industries |
| Thyroid | Ionizing radiation (nuclear fallout, medical X-rays, workers at nuclear facilities) |

Dr. Richard Clapp, et al., *Environmental and Occupational Causes of Cancer*

# Cancer in Children

**Babies aren't supposed to be born pre-polluted.**
**— Jane Houlihan, Environmental Working Group**

It's a sure sign that something is very wrong when children get cancer. Some infants are even born with the disease.

As Sandra Steingraber wrote in her landmark book, *Living Downstream*, children don't smoke, drink or hold stressful jobs. And yet in Europe[1] and the US[2] from the 1970s to the 1990s there was a steady 1% annual rise in childhood cancers, and a slightly smaller rise in Canada.[3] There were 9,500 new cases in the US in 2005, representing 15 children per 100,000.

The main childhood cancers are leukemias, which are cancers of the blood (30% of the total), and cancers of the brain and nervous system (21%).[4]

While the number of children with cancer has stabilized or fallen since the 1990s, and the number of children dying has been cut by half since the 1950s as treatments have improved,[5] this is little comfort if a child you know has cancer.

Why is this happening? There are some strong environmental clues:

- The human embryo is especially vulnerable to chemicals. Recent data from hormone disruptor pioneer Theo Colborn indicates that several adult and childhood cancers are programmed before birth, making the fetal origins of cancer a troubling new frontier.[6]

- The developing fetus is also more susceptible to DNA damage from vehicle pollution and second-hand smoke than its mother, despite the protection of the placenta.[7] One study concluded that the children of fathers who worked with benzene or alcohols in industry prior to conception are nearly six times more likely to develop leukemia.[8]

- The average newborn has 230 industrial chemicals in its blood at birth, 180 of which are known to cause cancer in humans or animals.[9] That's surely not a healthy way to start life on Earth.

- Children are also exposed to chemicals in breast milk from consumer products such as plastics and carpets and from the air, water and food, many of which disrupt biological processes. The US Environmental Protection Agency (EPA) says infants and young children are ten times more vulnerable to cancer-causing substances than adults because they live longer after the time of exposure and they eat, drink and breathe more than adults relative to their weight.[10]

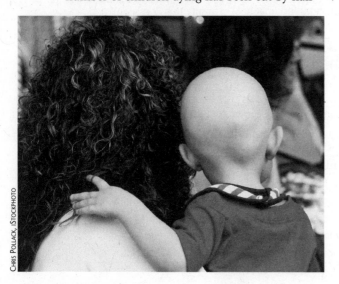

CHRIS POLLACK, ISTOCKPHOTO

- Exposure to pesticides is also linked to childhood cancer. Children whose yards are treated with pesticides are four times more likely to have soft-tissue sarcomas.[11] A Los Angeles study linked the parents' use of pesticides during pregnancy to a 3- to 9-fold increase in leukemia.[12]

- In the 1950s Dr. Alice Stewart carried out a landmark study that showed that a single fetal X-ray doubled the risk of childhood leukemia, which is why pregnant women should avoid them.[13]

- Exposure to electromagnetic fields is also a risk. A large seven-year British study showed that children who lived in homes within 200 meters of high-voltage power lines when they were born are almost twice as likely to get leukemia as those who lived more than 600 meters away.[14] This has been supported by other British, Swedish and Canadian studies.

- In 2001 the World Health Organization concluded that power-frequency magnetic fields are possible human carcinogens, based on a consistent association between childhood leukemia and residential exposure to extremely low-frequency electromagnetic fields. Children who live in homes with high magnetic fields (> 0.4 µT) have twice the risk of getting leukemia.

Enough is enough! We need strong, decisive action to keep toxic substances out of our children's bodies and to protect them from as many risks of childhood cancer as possible.

---

- Cancer Incidence and Survival Among US Children & Adolescents: www.seer.cancer.gov/publications/childhood
- Center for Children's Environmental Health: www.ccceh.org
- Center for Children's Health and the Environment: www.childenvironment.org
- Child Health and the Environment: www.healthyenvironmentforkids.ca
- Childhood Cancer Research Group, Oxford: www.ccrg.ox.ac.uk
- Children's Environmental Health Network: www.cehn.org
- Families Against Cancer and Toxics: www.familiesagainstcancer.org
- Health Effects of Pesticides: www.kidsforsavingearth.org/mnchec/articles/pesticides.htm
- Kids with Cancer: www.kidswithcancer.ca
- Making Our Milk Safe (MOMS): www.safemilk.org
- Preventing Harm: www.preventingharm.org

---

Jean-Dominic Lévesque-René of Île Bizard near Montreal was ten when he found a lump on his neck in 1994. A biopsy led to the diagnosis of non-Hodgkin's lymphoma, and he was told he had a 50% chance of surviving. While in hospital, he met other children with cancer and discovered that half the area of Île Bizard had golf courses sprayed with pesticides. He posted a map of Quebec in his hospital room, and each time a child with cancer was admitted, he asked where they lived. Twenty-two were from Île Bizard, out of a population of 4,000 children — 37 times higher than the normal rate.[15] He also learned that the herbicide 2,4-D, linked to non-Hodgkin's lymphoma, had been sprayed on the grass at home every summer since he was a toddler. Since leaving hospital, Jean-Dominic has been a persistent activist and campaigner for bylaws to ban the cosmetic use of pesticides.[16]

# Cancer in Animals and Fish

It's not only humans. The beluga whales in Canada's St. Lawrence estuary are getting cancer, while those in the less-polluted Arctic waters are not. Fish in contaminated waters have tumors, but not those in clean water. Dogs that are exposed to herbicides from chemically treated lawns have more cancers than those that are not. In her book detailing the global reach of environmental pollution, Devra Davis reported that polar bears in the Arctic have major body burdens of carcinogens, and that 1 out of 100 of the Arctic's largest land-based mammals is reported to be a hermaphrodite.

It can't get much clearer.

The belugas have survived in the world's northern waters for millions of years, eating octopus, crabs and fish. Now one in four of the St. Lawrence whales is dying from cancer, mostly intestinal.[1] They are also having trouble reproducing. When scientists examined their bodies, the autopsies revealed high levels of polycyclic aromatic hydrocarbons (PAHs), which almost certainly came from an upstream aluminum smelter.

- Cancer Registry for Companion Animals: http://envirocancer.cornell.edu/Research/AnimalReg
- Registry of Tumors in Lower Animals: www.pathology-registry.org
- Sprecher Institute for Comparative Cancer: www.vet.cornell.edu/cancer
- *Tainted Catch: Toxic Fire Retardants in San Francisco Bay Fish — and People*: www.ewg.org/reports/taintedcatch

Does the St. Lawrence beluga drink too much alcohol? Does the St. Lawrence beluga smoke too much? Does the St. Lawrence beluga have a bad diet? Is that why the beluga whales are ill? Do you think you are somehow immune and that it is only the beluga whale that is being affected?
— Leone Pippard, Canadian Ecology Advocates

## Cancer in Wildlife and Fish

In Washington DC, four blocks from the White House, the Registry of Tumors in Lower Animals has almost 4,000 specimens of cancer in fish, amphibians, reptiles and invertebrates collected by the Smithsonian and the National Cancer Institute. Epidemics of liver cancer have been found in 16 species of fish in 25 different polluted freshwater and saltwater locations, while in non-polluted waters, fish with cancer are almost non-existent.[2] The same tumors have been found in bottom-feeding fish in industrialized and urbanized areas along the Atlantic and Pacific coasts of Canada.[3]

## Cancer in Sea Lions

During the 1960s and 1970s, persistent organic pollutants were dumped in California's coastal waters, where they bio-accumulated through the food chain. Twenty years later, people started noticing dead and stranded California sea lions. When examined, 20% of the sea lions were found to have cancer of the urinary and genital tracts and toxic chemicals in their blubber that had accumulated through the anchovies, squid, salmon and mussels they ate.[4]

## Cancer in Dogs

A study of more than 8,000 dogs showed that canine bladder cancer was associated with their living in industrialized counties, mimicking the distribution of bladder cancer among humans.[5]

The Sprecher Institute for Animal Cancer Research estimated that in New York State 15,000 dogs and 9,000 cats develop cancer each year and that the number of companion animals in the state with cancer at any given time is between 1 and 2 million.

Between 1975 and 1995 the incidence of bladder cancer in dogs examined at veterinary teaching schools in North America increased six-fold. Scottish terriers, Shetland sheepdogs, wirehaired fox terriers and West Highland white terriers had a higher risk than mixed breeds, suggesting a genetic susceptibility to cancer among the terriers, but not a reason for the increase.

When the researchers interviewed the owners of Scottish terriers with bladder cancer, they found that dogs whose owners had used phenoxy acid herbicides on their lawns were 4 to 7 times more likely to have cancer than dogs whose owners had not.[6] Phenoxy acid is an active ingredient in 2,4-D, a widely used herbicide that has been linked to cancers, neurological impairment and reproductive problems.[7]

The "cancer in dogs" studies reveal the multifactorial nature of cancer. Their cancer is linked to the use of insecticidal flea and tick dips, but more so if the dogs were obese and lived near another source of pesticides.[8] In the terrier study, the researchers found that when the Scotties ate green leafy vegetables three times a week, there was a 90% reduction in their risk of cancer.

## Danger Ahead

We need to ring all the alarm bells about the accumulation of chemical wastes in the bodies

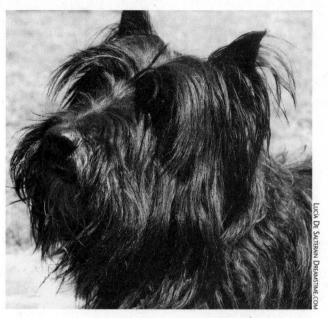

Why me?

of wildlife. The fire-retardant chemicals known as PDBEs have been found in every fish sampled in San Francisco Bay. They are similar to PCBs in their chemical structure, and the levels found in breast, blood and breast-milk samples of US women are the highest in the world. Is it a coincidence that women in San Francisco also have the highest levels of breast cancer anywhere?

PDBEs have been linked to an array of adverse health effects, including the possibility of cancer. When Sweden noticed a 60-fold increase of PDBEs in human breast milk between 1972 and 1997, it led to a ban throughout the European Union. In the San Francisco Bay area, the level in breast milk is 12 to 300 times higher than it was in Sweden, but the chemical industry has blocked California's attempts to legislate.[9]

We have to fight back, if we want to regain our health and the health of the world's wildlife.

LUCIA DE SALTERAIN DREAMSTIME.COM

# Cancer: The Bigger Picture

The elite of our nation have failed to internalize the ecological principle that every poison we put out into the environment comes right back to us in our air, water and food.

— Anil Agarwal

What causes cancer? Far more than "lifestyle and diet." This diagram does not claim to represent a complete list of the contributing factors; but it is an indication that are many more factors than we usually think about. The good news is that most are avoidable.

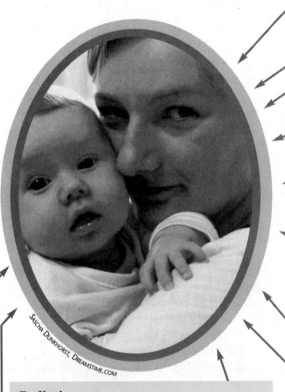

Sascha Dunkhorst, Dreamstime.com

## Lifestyle and Diet Factors

- Smoking, and second-hand smoke
- Diet — too much meat, not enough fruits and vegetables
- Suntanning
- Absence of UV sunlight in some regions, reducing cancer-protecting vitamin D
- Obesity, and lack of regular exercise

## Other Food Factors

- Processed foods such as nitrosamines, aspartame, some food colorants
- Bovine growth hormone in milk
- Some salt-cured, pickled and smoked food
- Charred meat, processed meat, red meat
- Sugar and alcohol consumption
- Absence of cancer-protecting compounds in food not grown organically
- Food contaminated with pesticides and herbicides

## Occupational Factors

- Workplace exposure to carcinogens, including solvents, heavy metals, radiation, pesticides, diesel fuel, benzene, asbestos. For full list, see www.cdc.gov/niosh/npotocca.html

## Radiation

- Solar UV radiation from ozone depletion
- Ionizing radiation from diagnostic x-rays, especially CT scans and mammograms; nuclear medicine, radiation therapy
- Electromagnetic radiation from power lines, cell towers, cellphones, electronic devices (both wired and wireless)
- Ionizing radiation from uranium mining, nuclear power plants, atomic bomb tests, depleted uranium.

### Air Pollution

- Carcinogens such as benzene, diesel, vehicle exhaust, coal-fired power emissions, asbestos fibres, industrial chemicals, incinerators, pesticides, soot, wood dust, indoor air pollutants

### Water Pollution

- Carcinogens such as chlorine by-products, industrial chemicals, heavy metals, pesticide residues, fluoride, arsenic, hormone-disrupting chemicals, coal-fired power wastes

### Toxic Products

- Toxic chemicals in household products such as cosmetics, fire-retardants, non-stick agents, solvents, cleaning products, building products
- Plasticizers such as bisphenol A and phthalates in various plastic food containers, water coolers and bottles, baby bottles, children's toys, teethers, dental sealants, canned foods
- Some drugs, including immuno-suppressants, birth control pills, hormone pills, hormone replacement therapy, androgenic steroids, anti-depressants, proton pump inhibitors, behavior modifying drugs and drugs used to treat cancer
- Some surgical implants

### Natural Carcinogens

- Foods contaminated with fungal aflatoxins
- Various phytochemicals in foods
- Chewing betel nuts
- Radon gas leaking into buildings
- Cosmic and solar radiation

### Infectious Agents

- Infectious agents such as hepatitis B and C, HIV, human papilloma virus

### Reduced Immunity

- Toxic substances that weaken the immune system's ability to fight cancer

### Endocrine/Hormone Disruptors

- Endocrine disrupting chemicals in air, water, consumer products
- Increased exposure to a woman's own (endogenous) estrogens
- Loss of darkness related to rotating shift work, reducing cancer-protecting hormone melatonin

### Other Factors

- Windows of vulnerability: exposure to toxic substances pre-conceptually, in utero, during infancy, during puberty
- Family history of cancer — shared habits, shared pollution, shared genes
- Parental and grandparental exposure to contaminants, causing faulty epigenetic expression
- Poverty
- Living near toxic sources
- Genetic variability — some people are more vulnerable than others

# Risk Assessment and the Precautionary Principle

> Risk assessment always asks the wrong question: it asks how much damage is safe instead of asking how little damage is possible.
> — Peter Montague

Risk-taking is a matter of pride in most "developed" countries. But the price of leaping before looking long, hard and carefully can deliver some truly calamitous side effects.

Think of the drugs thalidomide and Vioxx. Think of Agent Orange, leaded gasoline and asbestos. The atom bomb. Chernobyl. CFCs and our tattered ozone layer. In all these cases, we began using technologies or products without asking if there were hidden risks, only to experience disastrous impacts years later.

DDT, the "miracle" pesticide, is a perfect example. It boldly charged into a world wracked by insect-borne diseases and global warfare during the early 1940s. "DDT quickly became the atomic bomb of insecticides," John Wargo explained in his excellent book, *Our Children's Toxic Legacy*.[1] But along with killing insects very effectively (and cheaply), DDT served up many "unpleasant surprises," including the ability to climb the food chain and accumulate in the fatty tissues of wildlife, where it sabotaged the reproduction of many species, including America's iconic bald eagle.

- Critiques of Risk Assessment, *Rachel's Democracy & Health News*: www.rachel.org
- *Making Better Environmental Decisions: An Alternative to Risk Assessment*, by Mary O'Brien, MIT Press, 2000: www.healthcoalition.ca/MaryObrien.pdf
- The Precautionary Principle: www.sehn.org/precaution.html

Why has science, which has created so many brilliant innovations, failed to keep us safe? There is much more to the answer than just science, because politics and corporate profits play enormous roles too (see p. 54). But the scientific disciplines themselves have serious limitations, especially when human health is at stake.

Examples such as DDT clearly show there were no long-term health and safety studies for novel products and technologies when the chemical and nuclear industries hit full throttle after World War II. Pesticides and plastics, solvents and pharmaceuticals were all marketed as "better living through chemistry" to a trusting public. A brand new generation of ionizing radiation applications followed right behind, including treatments for acne and mastitis, and x-ray machines to measure customers' feet at shoe stores.[2]

In 1962 Rachel Carson's *Silent Spring* called for a halt to the recklessness. The book galvanized people everywhere — especially women — to demand more caution and better protection.

Then along came risk assessment, something akin to the Emperor's new clothes. One historian generously described it as "a distinct discipline which uses toxicology data collected from animal studies and human epidemiology, combined with information about the degree of exposure, to quantitatively predict the likelihood that a particular adverse response will be seen in a specific human population."[3]

It sounds impressive, but risk assessment does not and cannot mirror the real world. It studies new chemicals one at a time, measures

## Looking Before We Leap: The Precautionary Principle

"When an activity raises threats of harm to human health or the environment, precautionary measures should be taken even if some cause and effect relationships are not fully established scientifically. In this context the proponent of an activity, rather than the public, should bear the burden of proof. The process of applying the precautionary principle must be open, informed and democratic and must include potentially affected parties. It must also involve an examination of the full range of alternatives, including no action. "

Wingspread Statement on the
Precautionary Principle, January 1998

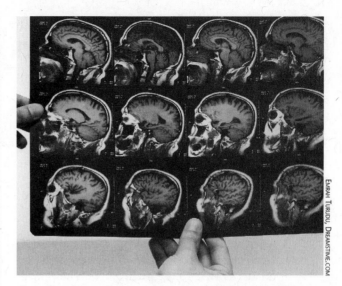

EMRAH TURUDU, DREAMSTIME.COM

Over time, X-rays have proven to be a good example of the need to apply the precautionary principle. Doctors in the early 20th century mistakenly thought radiation was totally safe, and many people died unnecessarily. Even now, computed tomography (aka 'CAT' scans) and similar diagnostic instruments need to be calibrated with care, as they have been linked to higher rates of cancer, especially in children.

their impact on healthy adult males weighing 70 kilograms and most often describes an "acceptable risk" as one cancer in a million over a lifetime of exposure, which is truly impossible to gauge or predict (see "Reference Man," p. 131). Recently the EPA developed a more appropriate tool for children that is far more sensitive than the conventional model, but it still hails from the "how much damage is safe" school.

Ironically, toxicology and epidemiology are confounded by the tens of thousands of novel substances that are now in use. Toxicologists face the nearly impossible task of testing mixtures and combinations (see p. 61). Epidemiologists are confronted with the equally forbidding challenge of comparing one contaminated group of human beings with another. No wonder so many studies are inconclusive and wind up calling for "more research," a state of affairs that serves polluters far better than it serves the public.

Recent scientific studies have revealed that vanishingly small doses of hormone disruptors

cause adverse health effects, challenging the once invincible belief that "the dose makes the poison." *The Wall Street Journal* reported in 2005: "It appears that some substances [such as the widely used plasticizer bisphenol-A] may have biological effects at the very lowest exposures that are absent at higher levels."[4] More studies and more fearless journalists may finally expose risk assessment as the pretender it is.

It is well past time that we adopted the precautionary principle as the foundation of public health and cancer prevention. We also need a practical, effective "alternatives assessment" approach, such as the one described by Dr. Mary O'Brien in *Making Better Environmental Decisions*, based on the premise that it is simply not acceptable to damage health or the environment if there are reasonable alternatives.

# Changing the Cancer Paradigm

> The historian of science may be tempted to exclaim that when paradigms change, the world itself changes with them.
>
> — Thomas Kuhn

"Paradigm" is a useful word that describes a predominant theory and the assumptions that underpin it. Paradigms are a bit like the gospels — they are believed and rarely questioned.

In the medieval world, everyone assumed that the Sun revolved around the Earth. This was seen to be obvious, and all astronomy worked on this basis. When Copernicus and Galileo challenged the paradigm with new evidence, their ideas caused a furor, but over time they opened up a whole new approach to science and astronomy.

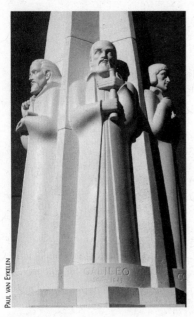

One of the points in Thomas Kuhn's seminal book, *The Structure of Scientific Revolutions*, is that paradigms never shift easily, since their believers hold onto them in spite of evidence that ought to make them crumble. When paradigms *do* shift, however, a flood of creativity is released, and changes occur with great speed.

As authors, we believe that a paradigm shift is long overdue in our understanding of cancer.

PAUL VAN EYKELEN

Nicolaus Copernicus (1473-1543), whose new paradigm opened up a whole new world of understanding.

The conventional cancer paradigm claims as its foundation a 1981 report, commissioned by the US Congress and written by two British scientists, Richard Doll and Richard Peto, called "The Causes of Cancer: Quantitative Estimate of Avoidable Risks of Cancer in the United States Today."[1] This attributed about 65% of all cancers to tobacco smoking and diet and virtually dismissed environmental and occupational threats. The report was enthusiastically embraced by many, including the conservative cancer establishment of the time, and went on to become the gospel of cancer causation in epidemiology textbooks, public health and medical schools nearly everywhere.

The political context is important. Doll and Peto's report was released early in President Ronald Reagan's first term, when deregulation was the new creed and environmental protection was coming under fierce attack. Sparks that had been kindled during Jimmy Carter's presidency to regulate workplace carcinogens were snuffed out early in Reagan's pro-business regime.[2] Much of the energetic cancer prevention activism of the 1960s and 70s — epitomized in books such as *Silent Spring* and Dr. Samuel Epstein's *Politics of Cancer* — faded to near oblivion.

Doll and Peto's document, and others that fall into the "cancer is a lifestyle disease" genre — including the industry-funded Harvard Center for Cancer Prevention reports published in the late 1990s[3] — fail to consider many new factors. If we are to come to grips with the cancer epidemic, it is time to embrace a new paradigm, incorporating the latest knowledge.

| THE OLD PARADIGM SAYS... | THE NEW PARADIGM SAYS... |
|---|---|
| 1. The 20th century increase in cancer is mostly caused by our lifestyles and only a very little by environmental and workplace carcinogens. | 1. The 20th century increase in cancer is caused by many interacting factors, including toxic chemicals, radiation and health-deficient food.[4] |
| 2. Doll and Peto's 1981 report laid down the causes of cancer: smoking 30%, diet 20%-50%, pollution 1%-5%, occupational exposures 2%-4%. | 2. Doll and Peto's report contained key research flaws and no longer reflects current evidence. Much was not known at the time, and they also had doubts of their own. |
| 3. Poor diet is a major cause of cancer. Pesticide residues pose negligible risks. Organic food is left out of the equation. | 3. Poor diet, including processed foods, is a major risk for cancer. Pesticide residues contribute to more cancers. Organic food needs to be included in all studies. |
| 4. Historically, chemicals have been assumed safe until proven harmful. In the US 60,000 pre-1976 chemicals have been allowed to remain in use without health and safety testing.[5] | 4. All novel chemicals should be assumed harmful until proven safe. All suspect chemicals and hazardous substances must be tested. |
| 5. When chemicals are tested, they are nearly always tested one substance at a time. | 5. Chemicals need to be tested in combination, since mixtures may be more toxic than single substances. |
| 6. The process of risk assessment gives a valid measure of acceptable risk, e.g., that a chemical will cause one additional cancer per million people, or one per 100,000. | 6. Where there is indication of harm to human health and the environment, the precautionary principle should be applied to preclude that risk. |
| 7. The process of risk assessment looks for health impacts on a 155lb (70kg) adult male. | 7. Risk assessment should look for impacts during "windows of vulnerability": pre-conception, during pregnancy, infancy, childhood, puberty and old age. |
| 8. Paracelsus's 16th century theory "the dose makes the poison" is the cornerstone of toxicology. Very small doses pose negligible risks. | 8. Very small doses of some substances sometimes have a more harmful effect than larger doses (e.g., hormone disruptors such as bisphenol-A). |
| 9. Environmentally triggered hormone disruption and epigenetic disturbances are not important as causes of cancer. | 9. Emerging science points to environmentally triggered hormone disruption and epigenetic disturbances as contributing causes of cancer. |
| 10. The solution to cancer involves pursuing more research for the cure. | 10. The solution to cancer involves paying more attention to prevention. |

# It's Not Just Cancer

**Exposure to chemical contaminants on the job, at home, in the outdoors, and even in utero are increasingly recognized as important contributors to human disease.**

**— Ted Schettler, MD, Boston Medical Center**

During the millions of years when our ances-tors evolved, humans were always vulnerable to infections and diseases caused by malnutrition. During the last 100 years, how-ever, and particularly since the 1970s, people in the developed world have become vulnerable to unusual and rare diseases such as Alzheimer's, Parkinson's and chronic fatigue syndrome, as well as familiar ones that are becoming more widespread.

In 2004 doctors at the Boston Medical Center showed that there were strong links

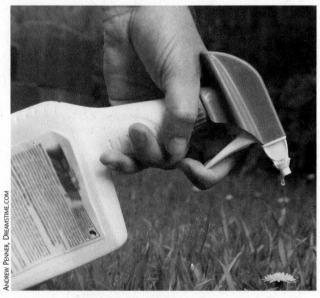

Exposure to pesticides and herbicides has been linked to asthma, Alzheimer's disease, chronic fatigue syndrome, infertility, learning disorders, reproductive problems and auto-immune disorders.

ANDREW PENNER, DREAMSTIME.COM

between environmental contamination and 120 different diseases.[1] It's not just cancer. Our exposure to hazardous chemicals combined with the depleted food we are eating is causing a wide array of health problems.

## Asthma

There have always been people who suffered from asthma, including Beethoven and Peter the Great of Russia, but now it is on the rise world-wide. The number of sufferers in the US has doubled since 1980, and its intensity is getting worse. In Canada childhood asthma jumped by 35% between 1994 and 1999.

Asthma can be triggered by natural factors such as pollen and dust, but they have always been with us. So what has changed? Studies shows causal links to off-gassing from chemical solvents in our bedrooms, homes and places of work; proximity to air pollution from busy traf-fic (a two-fold increased risk); the presence of phthalate chemicals from plastics and PVC floor-ing in the dust in children's bedrooms (a two- to three-fold increased risk); fumes from domestic products such as air fresheners, furniture polish and household cleaners (a four-fold increased risk); and exposure to herbicides and pesticides (a ten-fold increased risk).

## Brain Diseases

Since 1980 the number of people suffering from brain diseases such as Alzheimer's, Parkinson's and Lou Gehrig's Disease has tripled all across the developed world.[2] In the West the increase in neurological deaths mirrors the rise of cancer rates.

• Collaborative on Health and the Environment:
www.healthandenvironment.org

Genetic causes can be ruled out because changes in DNA need hundreds of years to take effect.

There is clear evidence that Parkinson's is linked to exposure to pesticides and combined exposures that work together to decimate brain cells. When mice were exposed to the pesticide maneb as fetuses and then to paraquat as adults, their motor activity declined by 90% and their dopamine neurons by 80%. Chemical testing is almost never done for the effect of chemical combinations.[3] The evidence for Alzheimer's is more sketchy, but it points to an association with exposure to glues, fertilizers and pesticides.[4]

## Chronic Fatigue Syndrome

In Britain chronic fatigue syndrome affects around one person in every thousand, yet it has often been treated as "the illness that doesn't exist." It is still a mystery, but evidence point towards exposure to organochlorine pesticides placing stress on the sympathetic nervous system and overloading the lymph ducts.[5] Multiple chemical sensitivity, an associated disorder, is related to exposure to pesticides, solvents, cleaning agents, fragrances and vehicle exhaust.

## Infertility

Something disturbing is also going on with our reproductive systems. In 1992 a survey showed that between 1938 and 1990 there was an overall decline in the male sperm count in various countries from 113 million sperms per milliliter to 66 million. A 2005 study of Danish military recruits showed that 40% of the recruits had sperm counts below 40 million, a level that is associated with infertility. Infertility affects one in ten couples in the US; one in six in Britain, especially among young women aged 15 to 24. Testicular cancer has increased by 200% to 400% in some US, Canadian and European populations in the last 20 years. Why is this happening?

In Italy a study of tollbooth workers linked their decreased sperm quality to exposure to vehicle exhaust.[6] A study in Missouri that found that men in rural and semi-rural areas had poorer sperm concentration and motility than men in more urban regions suggested the probable culprit was agricultural pesticides.[7] In Wisconsin a study found that infertile women were 27 times more likely to have mixed or applied herbicides in the two years prior to attempting conception than women who were fertile.[8] There is also evidence that reproductive damage is being caused by brominated flame-retardants, lawn care chemicals, smoking during pregnancy, and exposure to phthalate chemicals such as bisphenol A.

## Other Diseases

Evidence also links environmental contaminants to a growing number of auto-immune disorders[9] and to developmental disorders such as ADHD, behavioral problems and autism that make life truly difficult for millions of children and their families.[10]

These diseases are causing enormous grief and suffering. The solution is straightforward: we need to clear these hazardous chemicals out of our lives, out of our cities and farmlands and out of our world.

# Prevention, Early Detection and Screening

> Economic and political interests have interfered substantially with priorities in the defense of public health.[1]
>
> — Dr. Lorenzo Tomatis

This is a book about preventing cancer before it starts, so we have not focused on screening and early detection, a.k.a. "secondary prevention," that aims to discover cancers when they are small and readily treatable. Since many cancer agencies have proclaimed that "early detection is the best protection," however, a few words are in order.

Cancer screening programs test large groups of people who appear to be healthy, in order to discover who has or does not have the particular cancer being investigated. Screening can play a useful role in early detection, especially when precancerous conditions flag the disease itself.

For **cervical cancer**, the Pap test, involving early detection of the human papilloma virus (HPV), however, has led to a sharp reduction in both incidence and death.[2] (The new vaccine to combat HPV, however, does not protect against all cervical cancers, so it is still critical for women to have regular Pap tests.[3])

For **colorectal cancer**, the fairly simple fecal occult blood test (FOTB) can identify precancerous polyps early, enabling them to be removed before malignancies develop. Studies show that use of FOTB has led to reductions in mortality between 15% and 33%,[4] and even larger decreases appear to be possible with regular colonoscopies or sigmoidoscopies.

**Breast cancer** is altogether another matter. Population-wide screening has fallen well short of its highly touted promise ("breast cancer found early is almost 100% curable") and may put some women at risk for the disease, given that a mammogram, which utilizes ionizing radiation, is a key part of the protocol. This is especially an issue in the United States, where regular screening mammography is recommended to begin at age 40.

"This emphasis on breast cancer screening has perpetuated the belief that all breast cancers can be cured if found early," stated Dr. Susan Love.[5] The reality, she added, is quite different. Several types of breast cancer are now recognized. Some tumors are localized and will never spread, so timing of detection doesn't matter. Others are so aggressive that they will be lethal no matter how early they are found. For a third group, about 30% of all diagnosed breast cancers, screening is important, because this type can spread and eventually kill, but will also respond to currently available treatments. *Breast Cancer Action* provides an excellent commentary on this issue (www.bcaction.org).[6]

The shortcomings of the breast cancer screening program, in our opinion, ought to turn public health efforts back to the critical importance of *primary* prevention — identifying and eliminating the root causes of cancer. The Doll and Peto paradigm (see p. 22) essentially sidelined environmental and occupational causes, concluding that most cancers are caused by personal "lifestyle" and diet, and stripped primary prevention of many possibilities.

In this weakened form, primary prevention could never achieve much. Meanwhile, the American Society of Clinical Oncology has filled the void: "A wave of new technology (e.g., multiplex gene expression/protein arrays, laser-capture microdissection, high-resolution endoscopy and molecular imaging) is rapidly refining the definition of carcinogenesis and transformation. These important molecular advances, coupled with others in our understanding of cancer susceptibility, create opportunities for developing novel, multidisciplinary approaches for preventing cancer."[7] Impressive, but not "primary."

As Dr. Lorenzo Tomatis, director of the International Agency for Research on Cancer (IARC) from 1982 to 1993, stated in the 2005 Ramazzini Lecture, "It might appear unnecessary to recall the distinction between primary and secondary prevention, but a look at the current scientific literature indicates some sort of oblivion."[8] An ardent primary prevention advocate, Tomatis has paid a price for his stand, as he is no longer welcome at IARC after publishing an article in 2002 accusing the agency of soft-pedaling the risks of several "economically important" industrial substances and chemicals.[9]

It has been eye-opening to discover while writing this book that most cancer agencies focus so little attention on carcinogens identified by IARC. Even for agents known to cause cancer in humans (IARC Group 1), there are no universal approaches to controlling or limiting their use.

Then there are the "possible carcinogens." Tomatis lamented that these 246 substances (IARC Group 2B) represent "a large parking lot" which may become "the official perpetuation of risk conditions" because it is very difficult to design studies demonstrating a cancer risk at lower exposure levels. Some of these agents, he argued, such as gasoline (which contains known

IARC carcinogens such as benzene and cadmium), bitumen and carbon tetrachloride, should undergo in-depth review immediately.[10]

Much prevention research funding today focuses on unraveling the complexities of gene-environment interactions, with the goal of developing new therapies. Even anticipating substantial progress on this front, Tomatis remains firm: "We should never forget that ... a key role in the protection of public health will be played by actions aimed at banning or sharply decreasing the presence of noxious chemicals in our environment."[11]

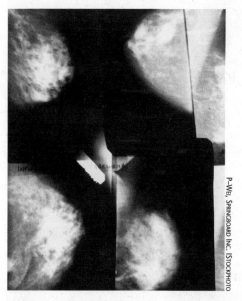

P-WE, SPRINGBOARD INC. ISTOCKPHOTO

These mammogram plates show cases of breast carcinomas viewed on a lightbox. Screening mammography, especially beginning at age 40, is a highly controversial issue.

# Our Weakened Immunity

A woman's body is the first environment. Whatever contaminants are in a woman's body find their way into the next generation. And I think there is no better argument for the precautionary principle than that.

— Sandra Steingraber

The very fact that you are alive today means that all your direct ancestors lived long enough to mate and produce offspring, right back into the mists of time.

We are the living, breathing evidence of Darwin's "survival of the fittest," but that unbroken record of successful reproduction couldn't have happened without an equally long line of healthy immune systems. Whenever our predecessors' bodies sensed an invader, or a DNA duplication error, their immune systems responded with leucocytes and lymphocytes,

Stranded baby beluga whale from the contaminated St. Lawrence River, Canada.

ROBERT MICHAUD, MARINE ENVIRONMENT RESEARCH AND EDUCATION GROUP

macrophages, tumor suppressor genes and other repair responses that scientists are still discovering. According to Nobel laureate J. Michael Bishop, every gene in our DNA is damaged some 10 billion times in a lifetime, so under normal circumstances, a healthy immune system is conducting an astounding amount of routine repair work all the time.[1]

The world that our ancestors evolved in, however, did not include fire-retardants, pesticides, plastics and man-made radiation:

- Exposure to dioxins can damage the effectiveness of immune cells for 20 years after exposure.[2]
- In agricultural districts of central Moldova where pesticides were used heavily, 80% of the children have suppressed immunity and are up to five times more likely to have infectious diseases of the digestive and respiratory tracts.[3]
- In lab studies, a wide range of pollutants has been shown to harm the immune system, including heavy metals, air pollutants such as ozone and nitrogen dioxide, and polycyclic aromatic hydrocarbons that form during the incomplete burning of fossil fuels, garbage, tobacco and charbroiled meat.[4]
- Our bodies did not evolve with processed food lacking vitamins, minerals and phytonutrients and stuffed instead with sugar, colors, flavors and preservatives.

The Pottenger Cat experiments illustrated the importance of real, whole foods appropriate for each species, in this case, cats. During the 1940s a medical doctor, Francis Pottenger, created an experiment using 900 cats to determine what effects processed, cooked foods have on the body. The cats were divided into five groups. Two of the groups were fed whole foods ideally suited to cats — raw milk and raw meat. The other three groups were given denatured foods, including pasteurized, evaporated and condensed milk. The cats were subsequently observed over a four-generation period. The results were illuminating. The kittens and adult cats fed raw food lived healthy, normal lives, but the first generation fed processed food developed chronic diseases later in life; the second generation got sick in mid-life; and the third generation encountered the same chronic ailments early in life, with many dying before six months. There was no fourth generation in the processed food group, as these weakling "junk food" eaters simply could not reproduce.[5]

The American physician Dr. Andrew Weil has said that cancer represents a failure of the healing system.[7] Is it any wonder we have an epidemic of cancer when our immune systems are being damaged by toxic substances and malnourished by industrial food?

There are several other pieces to this puzzle. First, there is rarely any testing of chemicals for their potential impact on the immune system.

Second, on the rare occasion when chemicals *are* tested, they are tested in isolation, not in combination — yet we know we are being exposed to many chemicals simultaneously.

Third, when a chemical is an endocrine disruptor, toxic effects are being observed at extremely low doses, far below the recognized health thresholds. This confounds the standard assumption and calls for a completely new approach to testing. (See p. 61)

A healthy immune system is critical for good health. If we want to keep our immune systems strong, we must eliminate the pollutants and bad diets that undermine them.

Outside the sterile environment of the womb, a human infant immediately encounters roving gangs of bacteria, viruses and fungi, many of which cause disease. But a newborn is armed with only a rudimentary immune system that won't completely mature for at least two years ... Essentially, an infant is born with most, but not all, of its essential life-support systems up and running. Within a few minutes of birth, it can breathe on its own. Within a few days, it can eat on its own. [Yet] it takes a year or more to fight off infections on its own and learn to distinguish between truly harmful invaders and benign ones, between self and non-self. During this time of transition, the breast is perfectly prepared to take over from the placenta the role of nurturer and teacher.[6]

— Sandra Steingraber, *Having Faith: An Ecologist's Journey to Motherhood*

# The Chemical Deluge

We have chemicals linked to cancer, both known carcinogens and suspected carcinogens, inside all the bodies of people who live in North America.

— Sandra Steingraber

Ahh, those "spring-fresh" fragrances wafting from our soaps, shower gels and a thousand other personal products...

They may seem — and smell — innocent enough, but don't breathe too deeply. "There can be as many as 100 chemicals in a single fragrance," reported the Environmental Health Association of Nova Scotia in its *Guide to Less Toxic Products*.[1] In 1989, the guide said, the US National Institute of Occupational Safety and Health evaluated 2,983 fragrance chemicals for health effects and identified 884 as toxic

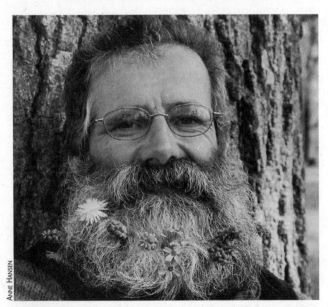

"From age 14-28, I did the pesticide applications on our family farm. Almost every pesticide I used then is now banned as carcinogenic." Henry Kock, pesticide-free activist, born in 1952, died of brain cancer on Christmas Day 2005.

substances. You will probably never see the ingredient list for these fragrances on a product container — they're exempt from disclosure as trade secrets.[2]

Fragrances are just one small slice of a huge chemical industry that contributes considerably to our burden of chronic disease, including many cancers.

Statistics about the raw chemicals that become part and parcel of our daily lives are almost unfathomable. Every day, the United States produces or imports 42 billion pounds of chemicals, with 90% procured from non-renewable fossil fuels. This is the equivalent of 623,000 gasoline tanker trucks — each carrying 8,000 gallons — stretching from San Francisco to Washington DC and back if placed end to end.[3] Global chemical production is expected to double every 25 years for the foreseeable future (California's 2006 *Green Chemistry Report).*

And now add these facts: the majority of the 100,000 chemicals in commercial use did not exist before World War II. Every year another 1,800 new compounds are created in laboratories. Nature, which has evolved slowly over millions of years, has little capacity to accommodate these novelties.

And more: over the next three decades, 600 new hazardous waste sites will appear *every month* in the United States, adding 216,000 new sites to the 77,000 already on the map in early 2006.[4]

The air, water and our food are also dumping grounds for chemical wastes. We know from scores of body burden tests that hundreds of chemicals released into the environment end up in humans and other living creatures. The California *Green Chemistry Report* concluded that workers pay the highest price of all. Every month 1,900 workers in California alone are diagnosed with deadly chronic diseases, including cancers that are linked to chemical exposures in occupational settings.[5] Nearly all are preventable.

And yet some prominent cancer experts, such as professors Bruce Ames, at the University of California, Berkeley, and Stephen Safe, at Texas A&M University, reject the idea that man-made chemicals play much of a role in cancer incidence. Safe has worked directly for industry in a number of instances. Both contend we have chemophobia and that natural carcinogens play a far larger role in causing cancer than most imagine.

Natural carcinogens are not rarities — we encounter hundreds of them in our daily lives. Cosmic radiation, radon gas and certain substances in plants and food are carcinogenic, such as aflatoxins in moldy corn, cheese and nuts.[6] We also know that some biologic agents can cause cancer, such as the Epstein-Barr and Hepatitis B and C viruses.[7] And when we dig down under the Earth's green mantle, substances such as asbestos, uranium, arsenic, silica and beryllium are exposed that cause cancer when they are extracted, refined and used in society.

The debate should not be about natural versus synthetic carcinogens. It should be about reducing our uses of and exposures to all cancer-causing agents. Humans have evolved to cope with many natural carcinogens at levels they are commonly encountered; it is the new synthetic

## But aren't they tested for health and safety? Think again!

Studies by Environmental Defense and the US Environmental Protection Agency have found that the vast majority of chemicals in widespread commercial use lack basic toxicity data in the public record. There are close to 3,000 chemicals (excluding polymers and inorganic chemicals) that the US produces or imports in quantities of over 1 million pounds per year. The EPA has reviewed the publicly available data on these chemicals and concluded that most may have never been tested to determine how toxic they are to humans or the environment. When the EPA evaluated all 2,863 of the "high production volume" chemicals, they found that only 7% had publicly available results for all eight of the standard, basic screening tests. Almost half (43%) had no data in any test category.[9]

ones that are more problematic. How we have increased exposures to natural cancer-causing materials, such as asbestos and radon, also affects our risk.

Professor John Wargo of Yale University wrote:

**If anything, an awareness of our exposure to natural carcinogens (especially in plants) should generate greater urgency toward eliminating the avoidable synthetic ones. Unlike their synthetic counterparts, plant-generated chemicals do not spill into waterways, pollute groundwater, contaminate sport fish, waft up from dump-sites or drift into other continents. Presumably, natural carcinogens have not skyrocketed in production over the past half century. They cannot explain the coincident rise in cancer rates.[8]**

The big question: When will the human experiment with man-made carcinogens stop?

# Gender Benders

These chemicals are working at a concentration of 1/10 of a trillionth of a gram. That is all it takes for a hormone to make a change in how an individual develops in the womb.

— Theo Colborn

Call them endocrine disruptors, hormone mimics — even "gender benders." But no matter what you call them, pay close attention because they are almost certainly a significant contributor to cancer.

Synthetic hormone disruptors can cause harmful effects even in microscopic amounts by imitating the body's own hormones, blocking them from carrying out their usual tasks or acting in numerous other ways which we are only beginning to understand.

Researchers at the University of London, England, studied a mixture of 11 chemicals that can mimic estrogen. "Alone, each was very weak," Peter Waldman reported in *The Wall Street Journal*. "But when scientists mixed low doses of all 11 in a solution with natural estrogen — thus simulating the chemical cocktail that's inside the human body today — they found the hormonal strength of natural estrogen was doubled. Such an effect inside the body could disrupt hormonal action."[1]

"The most insidious endocrine disruptors are man-made synthetic chemicals. We are routinely exposed to them in most areas of our daily lives ... The list includes cosmetics, sunscreens, perfumes and soaps; several pharmaceuticals; dental sealants; solvents; surfactants; pesticides; and PVC, polystyrene and other plastics," said Paul Goettlich.[2]

On the pharmaceutical front, long-term use by post-menopausal women of estrogen-progestin hormone replacement therapy (HRT) doubles the risk of breast cancer.[3]

It has long been known that hormonal drugs can have a profound effect on human biology — the birth control pill and hormone replacement therapy are good examples. But it is only over the past two decades that we have come to understand how infinitesimal amounts of man-made chemicals leaching into the air, water and soil can acutely affect both wildlife and humans.

It was the environmental health analyst Theo Colborn who found the wildlife piece of the endocrine disruptor puzzle. Working in the Great Lakes region during the late 1980s, she was looking for cancer, expecting to find evidence that fish malignancies mirrored human cancers in polluted regions of the lakes. She was confused when she found no parallels. She then reviewed the reams of research data she had collected, documenting bizarre physical problems affecting local wildlife such as unhatched eggs, birth deformities and whole populations of animals such as mink disappearing from their traditional habitats.

In their groundbreaking 1996 book, *Our Stolen Future*, Colborn, Dianne Dumanoski and J. Peterson Myers explained what came next for Colborn. "Moving beyond cancer proved to be the most important step in her journey, for as she looked at the same material with new eyes, she gradually began to recognize important clues and follow where they led."[4] They led her slowly but surely to solve much of the mystery of the chemical substances now known as endocrine disruptors.

Colborn's work has brought her full circle back to cancer. In 2005 her organization, The Endocrine Disruption Exchange (TEDX), a

- Endocrine Disruptors:
  www.nrdc.org/health/effects/qendoc.asp
- Fetal Origins of Cancer Database:
  www.healthandenvironment.org/wg_cancer_news/365
- Our Stolen Future: www.ourstolenfuture.org

clearinghouse for scientific papers on hormone disruptors, published a groundbreaking database called *Fetal Origins of Cancer* that provides the evidence that some adult, child and infant cancers might be determined *before* birth. Colborn and her colleague Mary Bachran were stunned at the clues coming out of their project. The evidence indicates that many kinds of cancers seem to be "programmed" before birth, pointing to the exceptional vulnerability of the embryo and fetus. "We don't know if this is the tip of the iceberg or not," the scientists commented, "but it surely demonstrates the need for better protection of the unborn."

While many causes of breast cancer have yet to be established, it *is* clear is that the higher a woman's lifetime exposure to her own (endogenous) estrogens, the greater her risk for breast cancer. Women who have several children, and who breastfeed, start their periods late and reach menopause early — all of which decrease estrogen levels — are at less risk than women who have no children and who experience early puberty and late menopause. Is something adding to a woman's natural estrogen exposure that may explain the steep rise in breast cancer? One widely supported theory is that "exogenous" estrogens (*xeno-estrogens*) from man-made hormone disruptors and perhaps isoflavones in soy foods are increasing a woman's lifetime exposure to estrogen, contributing to more breast cancer, especially the type known as "estrogen receptor positive" that has escalated significantly over the past few decades.[5] Several other hormone-related

malignancies have also increased, including prostate and testicular cancers.

Is it mere coincidence that the widely reported 12% decrease from 2002 to 2003 of new breast cancer cases in post-menopausal American women corresponded with a 30% reduction in the use of hormone replacement therapy in 2002, following warnings about its dangers?[6] As this decline was not shared by African-American women, only time will tell if the correlation stands, but the speculation is intriguing.

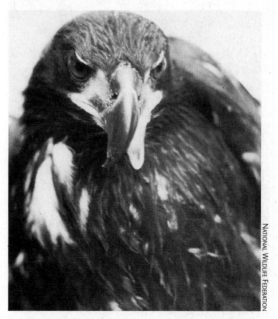

An eagle chick born with a crossed bill. During the 1980s, zoologist Theo Colborn began solving the puzzle of endocrine disruptors with copious wildlife evidence from around the Great Lakes region.

# Cancer Where You Work

> If you poison your boss a little each day it's called murder; if your boss poisons you a little each day, it's called Threshold Limit Value.
>
> — James P. Keogh, MD

Simple arithmetic tells a grim story of work-related cancers. As Canadian labor leader Larry Stoffman said, "No single number is going to provide an accurate estimate of risks from so many hazardous substances linked to dozens of different types of cancer across all occupations."[1] However, a realistic calculation puts the number of Canadians and Americans dying from work-related cancers between 60,000 to 80,000 every year.

Nearly all are preventable.

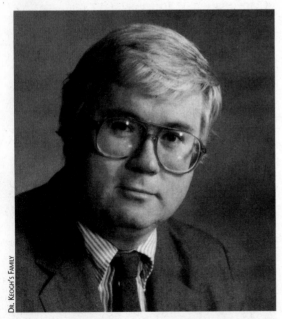

Dr. James P. Keogh was a tireless advocate for worker health and safety in the US who exposed cases of asbestosis and lung cancer in steel and construction workers. He died from liver cancer in June 1999, at the age of 49.

Workers in at least 60 occupations have higher death rates from cancer than the general population. "The auto industry is producing laryngeal, stomach and colorectal cancers along with its cars. Aluminum smelter workers are contracting bladder cancer. Firefighters contract brain and blood-related cancers at many times the expected levels. Women in the plastics industry are at greater risk for uterine and possibly breast cancer," according to the Canadian Labour Congress. The list goes on and on. Blue-collar workers bear the brunt, but many others, such as chemotherapy nurses, chemists and dentists, also experience higher rates of cancer.

Identifying cancers linked to workplaces is over 200 years old. In 1775 the British physician Sir Percivall Pott reported that chimney sweeps suffered an excess of scrotal cancers from their continual exposure to soot and coal tar. In 1879 two German physicians identified "mountain sickness" afflicting silver and uranium miners as lung cancer. As the industrial revolution gathered steam, so did work-related cancers.

In 2007 workers still operate at the front lines of exposure to carcinogens with little concern for their well-being. "Who cares?" asked Dr. Peter Infante in 1995. "Blue-collar workers appear to be the canaries in our society for identifying human chemical carcinogens in the general environment."[2] Aside from tobacco, 21 of 22 chemicals recognized as lung carcinogens by the International Agency for Research on Cancer were first identified in the workplace.

The Louisville Charter for Safer Chemicals pointed out that 26 *million* chemicals and

- *Hazards Magazine*: www.hazards.org
- Louisville Charter for Safer Chemicals, *Take Immediate Action to Protect Communities and Workers*: www.louisvillecharter.org

chemical compounds registered with the Chemical Abstract Service have been assigned a number. Our creativity in the laboratory knows no bounds. Some 100,000 synthetic chemicals are used commercially, but only about 500 chemicals have legally enforceable worker exposure limits, many which are well above the levels known to cause harm.[3] Nuclear workers also have a higher risk of cancer from job-related ionizing radiation.

Rory O'Neill of *Hazards Magazine* charges governments and regulators with careless indifference: "While smoking cessation has become a major public health priority and has spurred an entire prevention industry, no similar campaign has been waged to address the carcinogens encountered and inhaled by millions at work. Primary prevention — removing the risks — could prevent all occupational cancers."[4]

"'Not enough evidence of cancer risk' has been used by governments to evade their obligation for worker safety. This is often a red herring," said Larry Stoffman. "We refuse to collect data on occupational exposures and histories, we do not monitor for environmental exposures, we do not enforce regulations, nor do we carry out much research in Canada on environmentally induced chronic disease. Not bothering to gather the evidence, we then ask, 'Where is the evidence?'"

Fettered by politics and overmatched by industry, the US Occupational Safety and Health Administration has tightened standards for only 26 of an estimated 650,000 chemicals and mixtures to which US workers are exposed. Some on the list are known to be dangerous; others have never been studied.

Industry challenges to proposed limits, backed by industry-funded science, are the norm. They always demand proof, then more proof. Years, sometimes decades, pass.[5]

There are also major differences between the standards for workplace and environmental exposure. In California 68 chemicals that are known to cause cancer or reproductive harm are totally unregulated in state workplaces, except for non-cancer effects. Even when exposure standards are adequate, enforcement is often lax or negligent.

Peter Infante has calculated that the cancer risk among workers exposed to known International Agency for Research on Cancer (IARC) carcinogens is up to 12 excess cases per 1,000 workers exposed at the current exposure limits. This is 12 times higher than the "acceptable risk" as defined by the National Institute for Occupational Safety and Health in the US.

There is enormous work to do to defeat occupational cancer, and no shortage of solutions.

> The government didn't care at Holmes Foundry that workers were exposed to thousands of times over the legal limit of asbestos. That wasn't in the equation. They didn't care at Holmes Corning. They don't care today that workers are exposed to diesel exhaust and metal working fluids, to electro-magnetic fields. They still don't care....
>
> — Jim Brophy, in the documentary film, *Never Walk Alone*

# Cancer Where You Live

**If you catch the metro train in downtown Washington DC, to the suburbs in Maryland, life expectancy is 57 years at beginning of the journey. At the end of the journey, it is 77 years.**[1]
— UN Commission on Social Determinants of Health

There is a 20-year difference in the average lifespan of poor, mostly African-American citizens living in older, decaying city cores, and the richer, mostly white residents in leafy suburbs. Cancer alone isn't responsible for this major discrepancy, but it's certainly part of the picture.

What are the root causes? Many cancer agencies see "lifestyle" choices deeply embedded in poverty, as this *Scientific American* paper reported in 1996:

> **Underprivileged people have higher rates of cancers of the mouth, stomach, lung, cervix and liver, and a type of esophageal cancer. Poverty may be thought of as the underlying cause, because it is almost universally associated with the higher rates of tobacco smoking, alcohol consumption, poor nutrition, and exposure to certain infectious agents which, together, can explain most of these cancer risks.**[2]

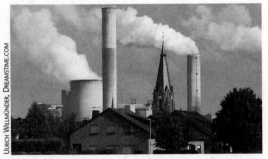

The poorer your neighborhood, the shorter your life expectancy, but virtually all urban communities experience toxic exposures. Indoor air, to the surprise of many, is often more toxic than the most polluted city air.

Distressed, unstable social environments need to be in this equation. Poor neighborhoods are disadvantaged compared to wealthier ones in several ways:

- They have inferior schools, and second- or third-rate support services.
- They are deliberately targeted with more tobacco, liquor and junk food outlets than richer communities.
- They lack tree-lined parks, safe recreational facilities, lively, walkable streets and stores with healthy foods.
- They are far more likely to experience the continual stress of low wages, poverty and racism that can depress human immunity.[3]

Low-income communities are also exposed to higher levels of hazardous waste, landfills and incinerators, as well as vehicle and industrial pollution, factors often denied or neglected in traditional lifestyle analyses,[4] stated *Rachel's Democracy and Health News* in 2003.

> **People with low income, no matter what their race, are much more likely to be exposed to contaminants in their daily lives — like diesel fumes, smog and strong chemicals at work — and they are much more likely to suffer from chronic diseases like asthma, diabetes, cancer, high blood pressure and stroke.**[5]

It's not just cities. This pattern is repeated many times over in rural communities across Canada and the US. They may be downwind or

- Cabinet Confidential — Toxic Products in the Home: www.net.org/health/cabcon_report.vtml
- Disease Cluster and Hotspot Map: www.healthyamericans.org/state/clusters
- Fallon Cancer Crisis: www.falloncancercrisis.org
- HealtheHouse Tour: www.healthychild.org/HealtheHouse
- Tox Town: www.toxtown.nlm.nih.gov

downstream of toxic industries, or on the fenceline adjacent to a petrochemical complex. People on First Nations reserves, tribal Indian lands and hardscrabble farms near highways and industrial parks often pay a high price for exposure to pollutants with poorer health and shorter life expectancy.

Some communities have "cancer clusters." Sometimes this is a matter of perception: with rates so high, it's not hard to find other neighbors with cancer. In other places, however, such as Fallon, Nevada, there are definite problems. There, 17 children were diagnosed with leukemia, and three died. After many studies, and frequent denial, Mark Witten, a University of Arizona professor of pediatrics, showed that exposure to tungsten and cobalt, from a local heavy metals firm and military releases, is likely to play a role in the development of these cancers.

**Home, Toxic Home**
Whether you live in the poorest city 'hood or the wealthiest country estate, your home probably shelters numerous cancer hazards. There's no discrimination here.

Entire books have been written about building healthy houses and "'fixing" the toxic ones. As a start, we recommend *Homes That Heal (and Those That Don't)* by Athena Thompson (New Society Publishers, 2004). We also invite you to take a virtual house tour to get a sense of the perils that may lurk in your home. The HealtheHouse Tour, created by the California group, Healthy Child, Healthy World, includes information on electromagnetic fields (EMF),

teflon-coated pans and safe alternatives to toxic arts and crafts supplies, as well as more well-known hazards.

We discuss building products in Solution 6 and household cleaning products in 7, but here's just a quick look at three common home purchases:

- Synthetic carpeting may off-gas up to 120 volatile chemicals, especially in the first few months after installation, including the carcinogens formaldehyde, butadiene and styrene. Dyes, binders and stain-resistant treatments are also hazardous.

- Most mattresses contain more synthetic chemicals than a barrel of crude oil,[6] including toluene, formaldehyde, benzene and fire-retardants such as PBDEs, classified as a possible human carcinogen, neurotoxin and suspected hormone disrupter. Even bed frames and other furniture made from wood — generally thought to be "natural" and therefore safe — may contain toxic glues, and chemical stains and finishes.

- Many curtains, tablecloths and designer fabrics are finished with formaldehyde as a perma-press agent, dyed with fixing compounds that include heavy metals, and coated with brominated fire-retardants.

Your home sweet home may be a very dangerous place, unless you swap all the toxic products for healthier alternatives.

# Cancer from Cars, Trucks and Buses

Across the state, cancer risk is driven greatly by benzene, and a large source of benzene emissions is automobiles.

— Paul Dubenetsky,
Indiana Office of Air Quality

We are a car-loving world, driving over 600 million passenger vehicles. Our cars represent wealth, pride and fun, while giving us comfort and convenience, so we have a blind spot when it comes to their downside. A *big* blind spot.

Globally, cars kill 1.2 million people a year — over 3,000 a day — and injure a further 50 million.[1] For anyone who has been impacted by a car crash, it is horribly real.

Cars also fuel the fires of global warming, since they burn fossil fuels. Our concern here, however, is the link with cancer. There are 225 different toxic pollutants in petroleum products — and they all end up somewhere.[2]

In his superb book *Lives Per Gallon*, Terry Tamminen (past Secretary of the California Environmental Protection Agency and Special Advisor to California Governor Arnold Schwarzenegger) laid out the true cost of our addiction to oil. We have grown so used to filling up at the pump that we rarely think what happens to the fuel when it's burnt.

### The First Villain: Particulate Matter (PM)

These are the tiny particles of black soot that get belched out of tailpipes when vehicles accelerate. The smallest (2.5 microns) are the most dangerous because they penetrate deep into our lungs (a human hair is 100 microns thick). A 2002 study that examined the impact of air pollution over 16 years found that deaths from lung cancer increased by 8% for every 10 micrograms of fine particulate matter per cubic meter.[3] In 2000 the average in New York was 16 micrograms per cubic meter, so New Yorkers faced a 16% increased risk of lung cancer from air pollution. It was 20 in Los Angeles, 18 in Chicago and 15 in Washington DC.

"The risk of dying from lung cancer as well as heart disease in the most polluted cities was comparable to the risk associated with non-smokers being exposed to second-hand smoke over a long period of time," the study reported. The tiny particles also cause many other ailments, including asthma.

### The Second Villain: Volatile Organic Compounds (VOCs)

That smell of diesel or gasoline fumes is not the healthy smell of fresh flowers. What you smell are compounds within fuels that evaporate, which is why they are called "volatile." They include the highly toxic benzene, 1,3-butadiene and polycyclic aromatic hydrocarbons — all of which are known to cause cancer, as well as birth defects and lung diseases.[4] Benzene is particularly harmful, even at very low levels.[5] In California, gas stations are obliged to post a warning that the fumes can cause cancer.

### The Third Villain: Diesel Exhaust

The villains work together, but it's important to line up diesel exhaust separately in the identity

- California Diesel Activities: www.arb.ca.gov/diesel
- Diesel's Cancer Risk: www.rag.org.au/buc/cancerrisk.htm
- *Lives Per Gallon: The True Cost of Our Addiction to Oil*: www.terrytamminen.com
- Plug-in Hybrids: www.pluginpartners.org

parade because it contains hundreds of different chemicals, "dozens of which are recognized human toxicants, carcinogens, reproductive hazards or endocrine disruptors."[6]

Researchers found that a child riding inside a diesel school bus may be exposed to as much as four times the level of toxic diesel exhaust as someone riding in a car ahead of it. These exposures pose up to 46 times the cancer rate considered significant under US federal law.[7]

On Southern California's south coast, as many as 8,800 people die from exposure to diesel exhaust every year — four times more than are killed in auto accidents.[8] Overall, diesel exhaust from cars, buses, trucks, off-road equipment and cruise liners contributes to more than 125,000 cases of cancer a year,[9] almost 9% of all cancer cases in the US.

The problems begin at the wellhead, where a single drop of oil can change the taste of 14 gallons of water, and a single exploratory well dumps 25,000 pounds of toxic metals into the ocean.[10] Whenever there's a large-scale oil spill, the clean-up workers get very sick. In Ecuador, where oil is drilled for export to refineries in Los Angeles and San Francisco, the locals call it "the excrement of the devil."[11] The problems continue at refineries, where fugitive emissions poison the air of people living nearby, and cancer rates are elevated as far as 30 miles downwind from a facility.[12]

The solution is remarkably simple: stop using oil. By switching to plug-in electric hybrid vehicles powered by clean electricity from the sun, wind, tides, and deep rock's geothermal

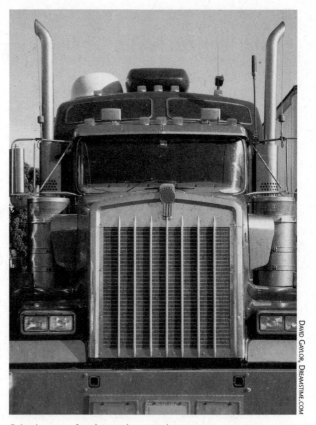

DAVID GAYLOR, DREAMSTIME.COM

Bringing you food, goods — and cancer.

energy, of which North America has an ample supply, and by rediscovering walking, cycling and the bus or train, we can leave this fossil-fuelled world and enter a world where oil no longer causes cancer, asthma, global warming and warfare.

The challenge is not technical: hybrid vehicles already exist, and plug-in hybrids are just one step away from mass production. (See Solution 82). The challenge is political, to shake people out of the cancer-causing comforts that oil has given us, realize that a world without oil will be far more healthy, peaceful, sustainable and civilized, and make it happen.

# The Way We Farm

Treat the Earth well. It was not given to you by your parents. It was loaned to you by your children.

— Kenyan proverb

Is modern industrial farming responsible for a share of the cancer epidemic? The evidence seems to say yes.

### Industrial Farming Deprives the Soil of Essential Minerals

The use of chemical fertilizers has increased yields but depleted the soil. Comparing the mineral content of food grown in the 1940s and 1950s with that grown today, researchers in Britain, Canada and the US have all reported that levels of iron, calcium, sodium, copper and magnesium in food have fallen by around 50%.[1] Meats and cheese have lost 50% of their iron; broccoli has lost 63% of its calcium; potatoes have lost 100% of their vitamin C.[2]

The soils have also lost selenium, an important antioxidant that is known to protect against cancer.[3] Selenium levels in soils vary, but its uptake by plants has been inhibited by modern fertilizers, as well as by mercury pollution and acid rain from burning fossil fuels. Since 1978 selenium levels in the British diet have fallen by almost 50%.[4]

### Industrial Farming Deprives Plants of Phytonutrients

Plants evolved over millions of years, so they know how to fight off disease. When they sense an attack coming, they generate phytonutrients to defend themselves. When we eat the plants, we acquire their disease-fighting compounds. When they have been sprayed with pesticides and fungicides, they are no longer attacked, and they don't generate the phytonutrients.

A particular nutrient in organic food may in fact help prevent cancer. In Britain two pharmaceutical researchers, Professors Gerry Potter and Danny Burke, discovered an enzyme that is highly over-expressed in cancer cells but not in normal tissue. Thinking (correctly) that its purpose might be to attack the cancer cells, they developed a drug to trigger it, which is going through clinical trials.

Potter then found a natural trigger in *resveratrol*, an antioxidant phytoestrogen found in grapes and red wine that is converted into the anticancer agent *piceatannol* when it interacts with the enzyme.[5] The piceatannol then attacks the cancer cell. When Potter's research team looked for similar compounds in other plants, however, they found no trace until they looked at food grown organically, where they found them everywhere — especially in globe artichokes, cabbage, broccoli, rosehips, peppers, red fruits and berries, apples, pears and various herbs. They named the compounds *salvestrols*.

The logic is simple. Plants that grow organically generate salvestrols as a natural defensive response against fungus and disease. When farmers use pesticides and fungicides, the plants don't need to bother, so the enzyme that evolved in our bodies over millions of years to kill cancer cells waits in vain, and the cancer cells are able to multiply without the body's natural defense. So while it is important to eat fruit and vegetables to protect yourself against cancer, they must be *organic* if you want to get their benefit.

Organic foods also contain higher levels of the cancer-fighting antioxidants that attack the

- Antioxidants in organic food:
  www.organic-center.org/reportfiles/Antioxidant_SSR.pdf
- Pesticides in produce: www.foodnews.org
- Salvestrol food supplements: www.salvestrols.ca
- Salvestrol cancer research: www.salvestrolscience.com

dangerous free radicals.[6] Organic corn contains 58% more antioxidants than corn grown with chemicals; strawberries 19% more. Organic produce also contains more ascorbic acid, which the body converts to vitamin C.[7] In contrast to the low mineral content of conventional food, organic crops maintain their minerals because the farmers build their soil with organic matter.[8]

## Cancer Among Farmers

Since 1975 studies have consistently shown that farmers develop and die of more cancers than the general population.[9] Although they are healthier than most people, and don't drink or smoke as much, the excess of cancers suggests that the causes must be among things they are exposed to, including engine exhaust, pesticides, solvents and sunlight. This growth in farming-linked cancers has occurred in all industrial countries, suggesting a common exposure to harm.[10]

## Industrial Farming Leaves Pesticide Residues

Modern farming also leaves cancer-causing residues on much produce. Apples, bell peppers, celery, cherries, imported grapes, nectarines, peaches, pears, potatoes, raspberries, spinach and strawberries are all consistently contaminated with pesticides.[11] Pesticides are showing up in the amniotic fluid of unborn babies[12], in mothers' breast milk[13] and in the bodies of farm workers. When pesticides also disrupt the endocrine system, they may contribute to the risk of cancer at a much lower level of contamination than has otherwise been assumed to be safe.[14]

If biotech corporations such as Monsanto succeed in their global goal of selling genetically modified seeds that have been engineered to resist pesticide use, the result will be an utter disaster for cancer prevention. We *must* return to organic agriculture.

Can organic farming feed a hungry world? The answer is a resounding yes. The results of 200 studies show that if the whole world were to go organic, there would be 75% more calories for everyone on the planet.[15] (See Solution 89)

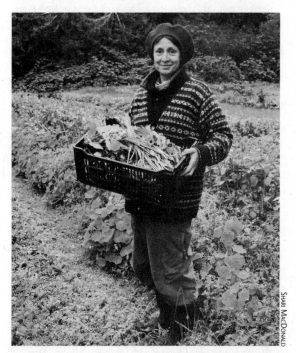

Nikki Spooner gathering organic salad greens at Varalaya organic farm, Mayne Island, BC. www.varalaya.ca

# The Food We Eat

Health is the birthright of every living organism.

— Sir Albert Howard

During the millions of years when our bodies evolved, the food we ate was fresh, raw, mostly plant-based and organic. Even cooking is a relatively recent invention.

It's our contention, backed by some very good evidence, that the best diet for a long and healthy life consists of foods that are fresh, organic, mainly vegetarian and mostly raw and unprocessed, with natural sugars and salts.

The typical American and Canadian diet, by contrast, seems almost designed to make us sick. It is heavy on meat, protein and fat; packed with refined sugar and added salt; processed with preservatives, color and artificial flavors; and neither fresh, raw nor organic. It also encourages obesity, which is a risk factor for several kinds of cancer.[1]

In 1982 cancer researchers noted an interesting phenomenon. When immigrants from a country with a low rate of cancer, such as Japan, moved to the United States, they "caught up" to the higher American cancer rates within two or three generations.[2] In the 1940s, when breast cancer in Japan was particularly rare, less than 10% of the calories in a typical Japanese diet came from fat. A typical American, by contrast, gets up to 40% of his or her calories from fat.[3]

*The China Study*, the first long-term study of diet, lifestyle and disease, was conducted by a large team under the direction of nutritional biochemist Colin Campbell of Cornell University.[4] Published in 1990, and reinforced with a follow-up study in 2001, it examined the health and diet of people in 24 provinces in rural and urban China and Taiwan who ate locally produced food, including many who were too poor to eat animal-based food. It produced 8,000 links between diet and disease and found that:

- Those who ate the most plant-based food were the healthiest.
- Those who ate the most animal-based food got the most chronic diseases.
- Provided there is variety, quality and quantity, a plant-based diet can be healthy and nutritionally complete without animal-based food.
- The greatest benefits came to those who ate the greatest variety of plant food, with the least heating, salting and processing.

In 1997 the World Cancer Research Fund and the American Institute for Cancer Research published a massive *Expert Report* that summarized the research into cancer and food and came to very similar conclusions.[5]

- *The China Study*: www.thechinastudy.com
- Health and Vegetarians: www.vegsoc.org/info/health3.html
- Meat Consumption and Cancer: www.cancerproject.org/survival/cancer_facts/pdfs/meat_and_cancer.pdf
- The Organic Center: www.organic-center.org
- Phytochemicals: www.vegetarian-nutrition.info/vn/phytochemicals.htm

Other studies have shown that:

- Greek women who eat plenty of fruit have a 35% lower risk of breast cancer; those who eat plenty of vegetables have a 47% lower risk.[6]
- German vegetarians have a 56% reduced incidence of colon cancer.[7]
- Japanese women who eat meat daily have an 8.5 times greater risk of breast cancer than those who rarely or never eat meat.[8]
- British women who ate more than 90 grams of saturated fat a day had 2 times the risk of breast cancer than those who ate 37 grams.[9]

As is so often the case, however, there is conflicting evidence. In 2004 a study by the Harvard School of Public Health found that fruit and vegetables gave no protective effect for breast cancer.[10] In 2005 a large European study came to the same conclusion,[11] and in 2006 an eight-year study of 49,000 women showed that a low-fat diet with more vegetables, fruits and grains reduced the incidence of breast cancer by only 9%, while increasing the risk of colorectal cancer by 9%.[12] The studies did not include food eaten during childhood, or by their mothers during pregnancy.

Unless such studies include a control group eating organic food however, the science may be invalid, since non-organic food is deficient in the very anti-oxidants and phytonutrients that are part of the body's defenses against cancer.[13] Many studies have documented the numerous health benefits of organic food compared to conventional food.[14]

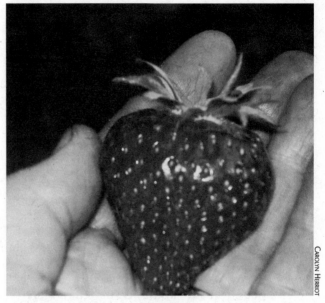

CAROLYN HERRIOT

A fresh, locally grown, organic Totem strawberry, moments before being eaten.

Non-organic food is often contaminated with pesticides, even perchlorate from rocket fuel and other contaminants.[15] Meat and fish are generally contaminated with chemicals that accumulate as they move up the food chain, concentrating in the body fat of each species that eats them. When they are eaten by humans, and then by breast-feeding infants, the contaminants are multiplied many thousands of times over.

Researchers in Seattle found that as soon as parents switched to organic produce and grains, the pesticide levels in their children's bodies dropped to zero within just a few days — but went back up again when they returned to a conventional diet.[16]

The overall weight of evidence is clear. If you switch to a diet that is mostly organic, low-fat and vegetarian, you will live a longer, healthier life.

# Awash in Pesticides

Future historians will be amazed by our distorted sense of proportion. How could intelligent beings seek to control a few unwanted species by a method that contaminated the entire environment and brought the threat of disease and death even to their own kind?

— Rachel Carson, *Silent Spring*, 1962

In the early 1950s, a serious outbreak of malaria in Borneo spurred the World Health Organization (WHO) to spray huge quantities of dichlorodiphenyl-trichloroethane (DDT) to kill mosquitoes carrying the disease. The mosquitoes died and malaria declined, but then came a surprising domino effect. The thatched roofs of local houses caved in because the DDT also wiped out a parasitic wasp that controlled thatch-eating caterpillars. Then DDT-poisoned insects were eaten by lizards, which were in turn consumed by cats. When the cats died, rats flourished, and humans were soon threatened by typhus and plague. To cope with the rats, WHO parachuted 14,000 live cats into Borneo.[1]

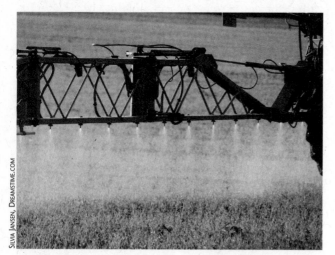

Much of the concern about pesticides focuses on residues left on foods, but another major concern is the higher rate of some cancers experienced by farmers and farm workers using chemical sprays.

SILVIA JANSEN, DREAMSTIME.COM

The story of Operation Cat Drop vividly illustrates how *not* taking into account the remarkable interconnectedness of nature can trigger dire outcomes.

During the early decades of the 20th century, tens of millions of humans died from malaria, yellow fever and typhus, including many soldiers. When the Swiss chemist Paul Müller discovered in 1939 that DDT could cheaply and effectively kill insects carrying infectious diseases, it was celebrated around the world as "miraculous." Many other synthetic pesticides created in the 1940s were the by-products of research to develop deadly chemical weapons.

After World War II, the use of DDT and other new pesticides multiplied exponentially, including a whole range of household and agricultural products. Practically everything was sprayed: forests, wetlands, lawns, parks, campgrounds, schools, hospitals, ships, aircraft, entire cities and crops of all kinds. "DDT is good for me-e-e" was a popular jingle in the late 1940s and early 50s.

Then came the domino effect, not as fast and furious as in Borneo, but serious indeed. In 1962 Rachel Carson documented the devastation to wildlife in her bestseller *Silent Spring*, and scientists since have gradually pieced together the full range of problems associated with pesticide use:

- The development of pesticide-resistant insects that survive the most poisonous assaults and pass on their genes to future generations.

- The persistence of many pesticides in the environment and long-distance transport to remote locations, such as the Arctic.

- The accumulation of pesticide traces in human, animal and plant tissue.
- The increased vulnerability of fetuses, infants, young adults and people who are genetically susceptible.
- The detection of many routes of exposure including food, water, air and soil.[2]
- The ability of many pesticides to mimic hormones in wildlife and humans, causing health effects at minute doses.

In 2004 the Ontario College of Family Physicians released a landmark pesticide literature review, after scrutinizing more than 12,500 studies conducted from 1990 to 2003. The review concluded that there is "consistent evidence of the health risks to patients with exposure to pesticides," naming brain cancer, prostate cancer, kidney cancer, pancreatic cancer and leukemia among a broad range of negative health effects. [3]

The physicians' study also found consistent links between parents' occupational exposure to several agricultural pesticides and effects on the growing fetus, ranging from damage to death.[4]

The International Agency for Research on Cancer (IARC) has identified over 45 pesticides as potential or known carcinogens. Almost half of these are still registered and in common use in the US and Canada, including the herbicide atrazine; the insecticides dichlorvos, dicofol and lindane; and the fungicides captan, pentachlorophenol and creosote.[5]

Despite the continuing obsession with dandelion-free lawns, and agriculture's ongoing addiction to petrochemical pesticides and fertilizers, there are several encouraging signs:

- Increased public awareness about the links between toxic substances and cancer.
- A growing movement to prohibit the cosmetic use of pesticides, including Quebec's 2006 province-wide ban.
- The exploding consumer demand for organic food.

**Pesticide use increases:** In 2004 a surge in the worldwide pesticide market led to record sales of $32 billion. This reflected a rise of 4.6% after inflation, the largest single-year growth for 10 years.[6] The main beneficiaries were the six multinational corporations that control approximately 80% of the agrochemical market — Bayer, Syngenta, BASF, Dow, Monsanto and DuPont.[7]

- *How Pesticides Work:* www.epa.nsw.gov.au/envirom/pesthwwrk.htm
- *Lawn and Garden Pesticides: Reducing Harm* (10 min. video): www.cape.ca
- Ontario College of Family Physicians *Pesticides Literature Review:* www.ocfp.on.ca search for "Environment & Health"
- *Our Children's Toxic Legacy: How Science and Law Fail to Protect Us from Pesticides,* by John Wargo, Yale University Press, 1998
- *Pesticides and Human Health:* www.panna.org/campaigns/docsDrift/PSR_PcidesHumanHlth.pdf

# For Everyone's Sake, Stop Smoking

**Quitting smoking is easy. I've done it a thousand times.**

— Mark Twain

Globally, smoking kills five million people every year, the equivalent of 30 Boeing 747 jets crashing every day. "One hundred million people died from smoking in the 20th century," stated Gérard Dubois, president of the French Alliance Against Tobacco. "If nothing changes, one billion people will die in the 21st century."[1]

Until 2002 scientists assumed nicotine dependence did not occur until adolescents smoked at least ten cigarettes per day. That was before a landmark study carried out at the University of Massachusetts Medical School concluded that 40% of all youth who had *ever* smoked reported symptoms of dependence after just a single puff. Teenage girls took an average of just three weeks to become addicted once they began smoking occasionally, while half of the boys were hooked within six months.[2]

Once addicted to nicotine, smokers resort to any number of shaky reasons not to stop, which speaks volumes about the remorseless grip of nicotine addiction. Many of their excuses are catalogued at the website www.WhyQuit.com — which shatters them all. Many smoking addicts liken cigarettes to a "friend" of sorts. The WhyQuit site responds:

> **What kind of 'friend' would deprive you of oxygen, take away your ability to smell, burn your clothes, destroy your teeth, harden your arteries, elevate your blood pressure, daily feed you 4,000+ chemical compounds, together with over 50 known cancer-causing agents,[3] before finally killing you with cancer, a stroke, a heart attack or emphysema?[4]**

Most smokers would indeed like to butt out for good, but of the more than 15 million Canadians and Americans who try quitting every year, only 2 million succeed. This sounds discouraging, but over time, about half of all smokers are able to quit permanently.[5] The idea is to try and try again. One Canadian study concluded that it takes men 3.5 attempts and women 2.5 attempts to quit for good.[6]

As a result of widespread public health campaigns, the public accepts that smoking causes lung cancer — accounting for 80% to 85% of lung cancers. Most of the remaining 15% to 20% are linked to second-hand smoke, air pollutants such as diesel soot, radon gas and workplace exposures including asbestos, arsenic and chromium. Smoking is also linked to cancer of the pharynx, larynx, oral cavity, nasal cavity and sinuses, esophagus, stomach, pancreas, cervix, kidney, ureter, bladder, colon[7] and breast.[8]

About 200,000 Canadians and Americans will be diagnosed with lung cancer this year.

- DeFacto, the website Canadian tobacco companies tried to shut down (en français): www.defacto.ca
- Physicians for a Smoke-Free Canada (includes the *Heather Crowe Campaign*): www.smoke-free.ca
- Second Hand Smoke: www.cancer.gov/cancertopics/factsheet/Tobacco/ETS
- What's in a Cigarette?: www.quitsmokingsupport.com/whatsinit.htm
- World Health Organization Tobacco Free Initiative: www.who.int/tobacco/en

With a five-year survival rate of less than 20%, over 180,000 will die.[9] Lung malignancies are among the most lethal of cancers.[10] When we include the other tobacco-related cancers, smoking accounts for 30% of all new cancer diagnoses — nearly half a million people a year.

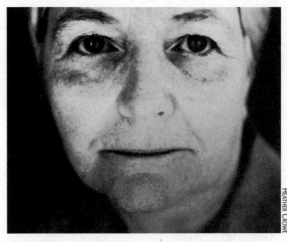

Heather Crowe died at age 58 from lung cancer caused by second-hand smoke.

## Innocent Bystander: The Power of One

"There is no risk-free level of exposure to second-hand smoke," the US Surgeon General made crystal clear in June 2006.[12] Breathing second-hand smoke is estimated to cause 3,300 lung cancer deaths a year among adult non-smokers in the US[13] and Canada.[14] Where bans are not yet in place, many hospitality industry workers are at risk. Second-hand smoke became the focus of Heather Crowe's final mission in life. "My goal is to be the last person to die from second-hand smoke," the Ottawa non-smoker told Canadians in 2003. She was 58 years old and had recently been diagnosed with lung cancer caused by constant exposure to second-hand smoke at the restaurants where she had worked as a waitress for 40 years. She knew her cancer was terminal, and she dedicated her remaining life to a better future for other workers exposed to second-hand smoke. In May 2006 when Heather Crowe died of lung cancer, 80% of Canadians lived in communities that were protected from second-hand smoke in bars and restaurants; 25% of Americans lived in states that were similarly protected.[15]

## More Reasons to Quit!

Other than tobacco, there are more than 4,000 'ingredients' in a cigarette, says the website QuitSmokingSupport.com. Here are some of them:

- Ammonia: Household cleaner
- Arsenic: Used in rat poisons
- Benzene: Used in making dyes, synthetic rubber
- Butane gas: Used in lighter fluid
- Carbon monoxide: Poisonous gas
- Cadmium: Used in batteries

- Cyanide: Deadly poison
- Ethyl Furoate: Causes liver damage in animals
- Lead: Poisonous in high doses
- Formaldehyde: Used to preserve dead specimens
- Methoprene: Insecticide

- Napthalene: Ingredient in mothballs
- Methyl isocyanate: Its accidental release killed 2000 people in Bhopal, India in 1984
- Polonium: Cancer-causing radioactive element.

# Electromagnetic Radiation: We're the Experiment

They told us DDT was safe. They told us above-ground nuclear testing was safe. They told us cigarettes were safe. Now they tell us blanketing us in electromagnetic radiation is safe.

— Juanita Cox and Jerry E. Smith

Electricity makes humans tick. Our physical bodies "work" because electrical impulses and currents stimulate and choreograph all the remarkable systems — muscles, heart and lung tissue, brains, eyesight, hearing — that make us vital and alive. The world we live in also abounds with natural electric and magnetic energies, and our bodies are finely tuned to operate within these age-old forces.

But we are now being swamped with man-made electromagnetic energy[1] — some call it electrical smog — and since 1979, alarm bells have been sounding over its health risks.

Can man-made electricity make us sick? The evidence is becoming clearer that the answer is yes.

EMR — electromagnetic radiation — is energy in wave form. An electric field is created around any power cord or electronic gizmo when it is plugged in — even in the "off" mode — and a magnetic field is produced when it's turned on, causing a current to move through the cord. The strength of the electric field (voltage) is the same at any setting and drops off with distance; the strength of the magnetic field depends how much current flows into the device and how close we are to it. In the case of home appliances, magnetic fields can vary enormously, then drop off to zero within a few feet or even inches.[2] The fields are gauged in tesla (T) or gauss (G) — named after the early electricity pioneers — and can be measured with a gaussmeter.

Over the past 120 years, "wired" electricity has spread into nearly every corner of our lives. "Wireless" followed, with radio, television and cellphone signals being beamed from antennae and satellites in the radio-wave segment of the electromagnetic spectrum.

Until 1979, evidence about health problems linked to electromagnetic energy was not widely publicized. That year, however, American scientists Nancy Wertheimer and Ed Leeper released a study showing an association between children living near power lines and a two- to threefold increase in deaths from cancer, notably leukemia.[3] Since then hundreds of researchers around the world have studied the health effects of man-made energy, with varying and contradictory results and often colored by politics and vested interests. Evidence has emerged linking EMR with cancers of the brain, breast and lymphoma, in addition to leukemia.[4]

In June 2001 an expert panel of the World Health Organization classified extremely low-frequency magnetic fields — including the energy from residential power lines — as a possible human carcinogen. They concluded that children regularly exposed to magnetic fields above 4mG have a two-fold increase in risk for leukemia.[5]

- *Cell Phones: Invisible Hazards in the Wireless Age*, by Dr. George Carlo and Martin Schram, Carroll & Graf, 2001
- Council on Wireless Technology Impacts: www.energyfields.org
- *MicroWave News*, a Report on Non-Ionizing Radiation: www.microwavenews.com

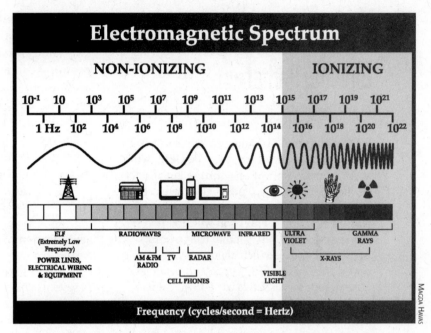

# Electromagnetic Spectrum

**NON-IONIZING** **IONIZING**

$10^{-1}$  $10$  $10^3$  $10^5$  $10^7$  $10^9$  $10^{11}$  $10^{13}$  $10^{15}$  $10^{17}$  $10^{19}$  $10^{21}$

$1\,Hz$  $10^2$  $10^4$  $10^6$  $10^8$  $10^{10}$  $10^{12}$  $10^{14}$  $10^{16}$  $10^{18}$  $10^{20}$  $10^{22}$

ELF (Extremely Low Frequency)    RADIOWAVES    MICROWAVE    INFRARED    ULTRA VIOLET    GAMMA RAYS

POWER LINES, ELECTRICAL WIRING & EQUIPMENT    AM & FM RADIO    TV    RADAR    X-RAYS

CELL PHONES    VISIBLE LIGHT

**Frequency (cycles/second = Hertz)**

MAGDA HAVAS

Over the past 120 years, wired electricity has spread into nearly every corner of our lives. With wireless technology, the Earth is being blanketed with EMR, exposing users and non-users alike.

Since 1985 engineers have curtailed EMR levels in many wired electrical appliances to reduce the health risks, says Louis Slesin, editor of *Microwave News*. For color TVs, lead was added to the glass of the cathode ray tube, absorbing any troublesome x-rays. For video display terminals (VDTs), the risk of miscarriage was eliminated when a Swedish union forced the electronics industry to reduce stray emissions to a very low level. For microwave ovens, radiation became "a non-problem" when the US FDA set tough leakage standards.[6]

"In these three cases, the EMR was an unwanted by-product of the electric device. For cellphones, however, it is the radiation itself that conveys the message."[7]

In the past decade, wireless has gone wild. In 1995 there were 10 million mobile-phone subscribers worldwide. In June 2006 the world's two-billionth cellphone customer was connected, doubling the mark passed in 2004. Nokia, the world's largest handset manufacturer, has predicted that by 2015 four billion people will be using a mobile.[8]

This is a massive human experiment. More than two billion people — including young children — are putting transmitters against their heads, allowing radiation to oscillate at 800 to 1600 million times per second. Seventy to 80% of the energy from a mobile phone penetrates the user's skull. Many studies suggest there are no problems associated with cellphones, but a University of Washington analysis of more than 250 research papers on the health effects of cellphone frequencies showed that nearly 60% reported some form of biological effect, including DNA damage. "Radiation is not as safe as the cellphone industry asserts," concluded Dr. Henry Lai.[9]

With wireless fidelity (Wi-Fi) making the Internet so widely accessible, and with tens of thousands of cellphone masts and broadcast towers scattered throughout North America, EMR pollution has become very widespread. Even if we don't use wireless technologies, we are constantly exposed. There is simply no place to hide.

# Cancer Hazards of Ionizing Radiation

C ancer is mind-boggling in its complexity. One cause, however, is crystal clear — the intense energy known as "ionizing radiation."

If you look at the right side of the electromagnetic spectrum (p. 49), above visible light and ultraviolet (UV) rays you will find two types of ionizing radiation: gamma, which occurs naturally, and x-rays, which are man-made. Along with naturally occurring alpha and beta particles, all four are classified as "known human carcinogens".

Ionizing radiation is one of very few substances classified as a "complete carcinogen," earning this designation because of its ability to do three things: initiate, promote *and* accelerate cancer. "Virtually every human tissue has been associated with radiation-induced cancer, but some appear to be more sensitive than others, including the breast, thyroid, lung, colon, stomach, liver and skin," explained Dr. Rosalie Bertell, a long-time nuclear industry critic.[1]

Here are three more facts about ionizing radiation's lethal character:

- There is no safe dose.
- Fetuses, infants and children are more vulnerable than adults.
- The individual doses we receive accumulate throughout life, lingering in our bones, organs and teeth.

**Natural "background" radiation** accounts for just over 80% of all human exposures, according to the US National Academy of Sciences. Individual doses can vary widely

**A primary goal of the Breast Cancer Fund is to help break our reliance on the status quo and reverse this profound, yet insupportable commitment to the medieval age of mammography. It is of the highest importance that we free up the resources and thinking necessary to develop affordable screening technology that can find breast cancer earlier than mammography and without invasive radiation.**

**— Andrea Ravinett Martin (1946-2003), founder of the Breast Cancer Fund**

depending on where you live (higher altitudes = greater exposure) and where you work (miners and jet pilots are more exposed, for example). Despite its "natural" designation, background radiation is hazardous, and it contributes to our burden of cancer — about 1%. But it's also a fact of life: we're all bombarded with this natural radioactivity from many sources, including the sun and outer space, Earth's own crust and simply from eating and breathing.

Radon gas, another natural form of ionizing radiation, seeps out of rocky soils containing uranium and can travel through both earth and water into our basements and water supplies. Vapors can accumulate to hazardous levels, and radon gas and its "daughters" are estimated to cause up to 22,000 premature lung cancer deaths every year in the United States,[2] with smokers at higher risk. Fortunately, most cases of excess radon can be reduced to safer levels. (See Solution 9.)

**Man-made ionizing radiation** made its debut in 1895 when Wilhelm Conrad Roentgen first detected its presence and named his discovery the "x-ray." Soon after, Marie and Pierre Curie purified radium from uranium ore — a painstaking, dangerous task that induced the leukemia that killed Madame Curie in 1934.

The early use of x-rays was free and easy, as doctors thought radium was completely safe, with "absolutely no toxic effects." Trial and a lot of deadly errors later, however, the new technology was reined in to (somewhat) safer exposure levels. Meanwhile, many other "hot" products, such as radium water ("liquid sunshine"), and radioactive hair tonics and toothpastes all went to town, capitalizing on slick marketing and radiation's imagined health-giving properties. Many of today's applications are interesting (if less fanciful): porcelain dentures, the mantles of camping lanterns, smoke alarms and optical lenses all contain radioactive elements.[3] These are minor sources of radioactivity, and reasonably harmless, but the earliest versions of glow-in-the-dark watches weren't so innocent. They caused lethal bone cancers in many of the female "dial painters" of the 1920s.[4]

During World War II, the Manhattan Project gave birth to the world's first atomic bombs, with their lethal, long-lasting side effects. Radioactive fallout from the Hiroshima and Nagasaki bombs, nuclear weapons testing in the 1950s and 60s, and the recent widespread use of depleted uranium to harden tips of armor-piercing missiles and bullets all contribute to the worldwide burden of radioactivity — and cancer.

**Medical applications** account for more than 90% of all non-background ionizing radiation. Now, here's a shocker: Catherine Caulfield, in her excellent book, *Multiple Exposures: Chronicles of the Radiation Age*, concludes that half of all medical radiation is unnecessary. Most people think these applications are safe, but we need to

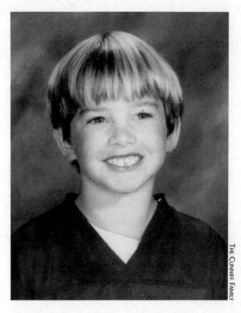

THE CUNNIFF FAMILY

"Exuberant, mischievous, loving" Danny Cunniff died at age 7 from acute myeloid leukemia (AML). He was hit by a car at age 2 and subsequently had five or six CT scans to his head and body, in effect exposing him to ionizing radiation at very high rates. CT scans must be calibrated for a child's height and weight.

be far less casual about them. The use of whole-body computed tomography (CT) or CAT scans, for example, has skyrocketed over the past 15 years, with worrisome consequences. "We do x-rays on children when the expected health benefit is greater than the tiny increased risk of eventual cancer," comments pediatrician Alan Greene. "A typical x-ray delivers 0.01 REM. CT scans give us much more information, but they also deliver as much radiation as getting 300 regular x-rays — or 600 if the CT scanner has not been adjusted for children."

To prevent cancer, reducing exposure to ionizing radiation must be a major part of the equation.

# Radiation and Nuclear Power

I'd put my money on the sun and solar energy. What a source of power! I hope we don't have to wait 'til oil and coal run out before we tackle that.
— Thomas Edison (1847-1931)

After years in the doldrums, nuclear power's boosters are back, promoting it as a way to produce energy without fuelling global warming. We could not disagree more.

Nuclear power is a cancer machine. All nuclear radiation is cumulative in our bodies and carries a risk for harm, including cancer, and every step in the nuclear chain increases the risk of cancer to those who are exposed, even at low doses. The risks of dying from cancer due to exposure to radiation are 37.5% higher for women than men, and 300% to 400% higher among babies than among adults.[1] There is no safe threshold for exposure to radiation: the greater the exposure, the greater the risk.[2]

The concern has always been about *external* radiation, as received by victims of the atomic bombings of Hiroshima and Nagasaki. In 2004, however, the British Committee Examining Radiation Risks of Internal Emitters (CERRIE) stated: "Tougher action is needed to allow for new information about the risks from *internal* radiation. Uncertainties about the risks mean that in some cases we might be exposed to ten times the risk previously thought."[3]

Among children under ten who lived near New York and New Jersey nuclear plants, the incidence of cancer increased 4 to 5 years after the level of strontium-90 in their teeth from radiation increased, declining again 4 to 5 years after it dropped. Similar results have been found in the UK, Canada, France, Germany and the former Soviet Union.[4]

In the US a study by the Radiation and Public Health Project found that the breast cancer in communities within 50 miles of a reactor increased by 14% to 40% while it was operating, compared to 1% a year in areas without a reactor.[5] And in North Wales, a study by the Low Level Radiation Campaign found that women under 50 who live in villages near the Trawsfynydd nuclear power station have 15 times more breast cancer than the national average.[6]

In the early days of nuclear power, scientists believed that as long as people received a "safe" dose of radiation, everything would be fine. The more they learned, however, the more they

- Campaign for Nuclear Phase-Out: www.cnp.ca
- CERRIE: www.cerrie.org
- Committee for Nuclear Responsibility: www.ratical.org/radiation/CNR
- *The Enemy Within: The High Cost of Living Near Nuclear Reactors*, by Jay M Gould, et al., Four Walls Eight Windows, 1996
- Greenpeace: www.greenpeace.org/international/campaigns/nuclear
- Institute for Energy and Environmental Research: www.ieer.org
- Life's Delicate Balance, by Janette Sherman: www.janettesherman.com
- Low-Level Radiation: www.ratical.org/radiation
- Low-Level Radiation Campaign: www.llrc.org
- Nuclear Policy Research Institute: www.nuclearpolicy.org
- Radiation and Public Health Project: www.radiation.org
- WISE Uranium Project: www.wise-uranium.org

lowered the allowable dose. Yet even these lower levels pose a risk that is several hundred times higher than that which is allowed for other kinds of pollution. A 15-country IARC study concluded that nuclear industry workers have a 1% to 2% increase in deaths from cancer.[7]

The uranium that must be mined as the fuel for nuclear power is also the deadliest metal on Earth. Uranium miners have a 2- to 5 times higher risk of lung cancer,[8] which continues among Navajo miners in Arizona, New Mexico and Utah and Dene First Nation miners at Port Radium in northern Canada.[9] Why should they suffer for our convenience?

Then there is the frightening possibility of a nuclear accident. Since the 1986 Chernobyl disaster in Ukraine there has been a 90-fold increase in thyroid cancer in the most contaminated areas of Ukraine, Belarus and Russia.[10] While the UN predicts that the disaster will ultimately cause 4,000 to 9,000 deaths from cancer, Greenpeace quoted studies that suggest as many as 93,000 deaths.[11] Who can be so confident as to promise that such an accident will never happen again?

Nuclear reactors also produce large quantities of radioactive waste that must be kept safe from earthquakes, sea-level rise and groundwater penetration for up to a million years.[12] No-one has found an acceptable solution to this yet, but nuclear proponents are willing to impose the problem on the next 40,000 generations.

Finally, there are concerns that nuclear power plants and their above-ground stored wastes might become a target for terrorists and that nuclear materials can be used to make a

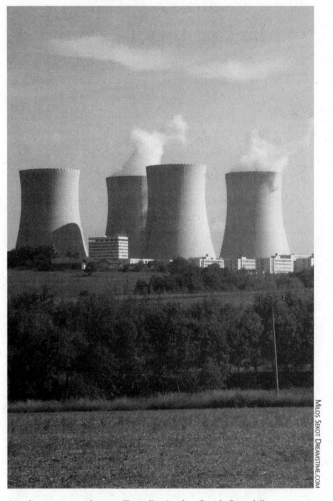

Nuclear power plant at Temelin, in the Czech Republic.

bomb. By 2003 there was enough plutonium in the world from nuclear power plants to make more than 300,000 nuclear bombs.[13]

If the taxpayers' money that governments propose spending on nuclear power is spent on measures to increase energy efficiency instead, it will yield as much as ten times more energy. It makes no sense at all — especially when there are so many other safe, sustainable, affordable ways to generate the energy we need.[14]

# The Cancerous Corporation

In Washington, the chemical
industry sets the agenda and has
overpowered the nation's system
of safeguarding the public health.[1]
— Russell Mokhiber,
Multinational Monitor

We can't stop cancer without ending the corruption of democracy by some of the world's largest corporations, and entering a new world of corporate social responsibility.

We could share many stories of companies whose directors knew that their practices were

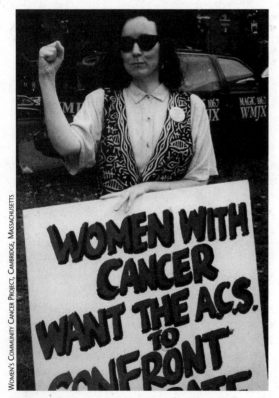

JeanMarie (Jeannie) Marshall was a writer and vocal member of the Women's Community Cancer Project in Boston. She died in 1995 from a rare cancer of the spinal cord, at age 37.

causing cancer, but who allowed things to continue while lying to the regulators, their workers and the communities that support them.

In *Trespass Against Us: Dow Chemical and The Toxic Century*, Jack Doyle chronicles Dow Chemical's "invent first and ask questions later" approach to selling chemicals; its persistent defense of the toxic herbicide 2,4-D and other hazardous chemicals; its promotion of silicon breast implants, vinyl chloride and perchloroethylene; and its "we can do no harm" culture.[2]

The tobacco industry does not do itself any favors. In an effort to distance itself from its reputation as the world's worst tobacco company, Philip Morris changed its name to Altria, perhaps hoping that people might associate it with "altruistic." In Britain Friends of the Earth declared British Allied Tobacco to be "one of the least responsible companies in the world."[3]

Then there's Grace, the global company that made vermiculite at its Libby, Montana, plant for use in attic insulation, fireproofing and fertilizers. The US government charges that during the late 1970s, after Grace learnt their vermiculite was contaminated with a form of asbestos, they failed to turn over the information and continued to distribute contaminated vermiculite in the Libby community.[4] Twelve hundred residents suffer from asbestos-related health problems, and more than 200 have died.

There have always been some "bad apples." The problem is much larger, however. Writing about the corporate corruption of science in a special 2005 issue of the *International Journal of Occupational and Environmental Health*, the

- Campaign for Corporate Responsibility: www.foe.co.uk/campaigns/corporates
- Center for Responsive Politics: www.opensecrets.org
- Holding Corporations Accountable: www.corpwatch.org
- Multinational Monitor: www.multinationalmonitor.com

editors stated: "There are simply too many bad apples to blame the problem on individual products, scientists or even corporations. The problem is with the barrel."[5]

What is it about our society that allows North American pesticide companies who sell 45,000 tons of pesticides a year in Central America to use free trade negotiations to undermine national legislation? There are an estimated 400,000 pesticide poisoning incidents in Central American countries every year, so their governments worked hard to control the most toxic pesticides. The pesticide industry, however, worked with committees of the Central American Free Trade Agreement to insert clauses that effectively circumvent any national legislation that might prove troublesome.[6] All in the name of free trade.

In 1970 the economist Milton Friedman, darling of the "free enterprise, minimum regulation" school of thought, wrote that "the social responsibility of business is to increase its profits … so long as it stays within the rules of the game, which is to say, engages in open and free competition without deception or fraud." He derided any talk about businesses needing to have a "social conscience" as "pure and unadulterated socialism."[7]

This assumes that governments will protect our health and the environment. This might work in the theoretical world that economists love, but in the real world there is always a power play going on, and corporations go to a lot of trouble to be players.

Step One is campaign donations, to buy a place at the politicians' table or golf club. The way to end this is to do as Canada has done and ban individual donations over $1,000 and all corporate and union campaign donations.

Step Two is to hire paid lobbyists in Washington (where they outnumber Members of Congress by 20 to 1[8]) who will lean on "their" politicians to weaken, delay or halt unfriendly legislation.

Step Three is to insert your people deep inside the regulatory system, creating "captive agencies" that serve corporate rather than public interests.

Step Four is to influence the public debate by setting up institutions whose staff use terms like "junk science" to attack anything that is not corporate-friendly, and "sound science" to describe corporate-friendly science.

Step Five is to seek to control the science that determines (e.g.) if a product is toxic or not (see Solution 26).

Step Six is to override national regulations under the rubric of "free trade"; and Step Seven is to move to a developing country with weaker regulations that is more easily controlled.

Let us be clear. There are many socially responsible corporations that contribute enormously to the public good, whose directors are ashamed at these crude and aggressive power plays by their colleagues that act like a cancer in the public body.

To counter this trend towards corporate power, we must step into the game and become players ourselves, defending the public body against these cancerous intrusions and steering instead towards a healthy, green, sustainable world.

# The Limits — and Corruption — of Science

W e put enormous faith in science, and we expect that the best research will be marshaled to protect our health and wellbeing. Such faith is often misplaced, however. Why?

- Most science — especially disciplines such as epidemiology — is inherently uncertain. Despite our wish for clear answers about the causes of cancer, science can rarely make absolute claims.
- Industry uses scientific uncertainty to keep hazardous substances in use.

PR agencies and industry front groups manufacture doubt and assail legitimate science to stall or paralyze the regulation of carcinogens and other toxic substances.

### Science is Inherently Uncertain
What could be more obvious than the connection between smoking and lung cancer? Yet, as Devra Davis explained in her book *When Smoke Ran Like Water: Tales of Environmental Deception and the Battle Against Pollution*, "It took fifty years of finding unmistakably higher levels of sickness and early death in smokers for us to reach the conclusion that cigarettes really are bad for you."[2] The US Surgeon General declared that smoking caused lung cancer in 1964, but indisputable proof of the link didn't come until 32 years later in 1996.

One of the "gospels" of human health research, cited in virtually all epidemiology textbooks, is Sir Austin Bradford Hill's *The Environment and Disease: Association or Causation?* Over the

All scientific work is incomplete — whether it be observational or experimental. All scientific work is liable to be upset or modified by advancing knowledge. That does not confer on us a freedom to ignore the knowledge we already have, or to postpone the action that it appears to demand at a given time.[1]

— Sir Austin Bradford Hill

years, Hill's insights have generally been reduced to a checklist of nine "criteria" — a word he never used — for establishing cause and effect and stripped of their larger meaning and context.[3] Rather than insisting on the rules that made him famous, Bradford Hill eventually came to this conclusion: *"Uncertainty about whether there is a causal relationship (or even an association) is not sufficient to suggest that action should not be taken."* Despite the topsy-turvy sentence structure, this is the precautionary principle through and through.

### Uncertainty Undermines Regulation
Uncertainty is often the excuse for stonewalling the banning or restriction of toxic substances. For over 20 years, the solvent trichloroethylene (TCE) was hung up in controversy at the US National Toxicology Program over its classification as a "known human carcinogen." With corporate scientists leading the charge, TCE's producers demanded virtually flawless human studies as proof of its danger. No cell cultures or rodent experiments were allowed into discussions. In 2001, to the veiled but obvious satisfaction of the chemical industry, the proposal to upgrade TCE as a "known human carcinogen" was turned down.[4] It's a common ruse: Scientific standards that are supposed to protect public health are used to sidestep stricter regulations and phase-outs.

- "Doubt Is Their Product," *Scientific American*, June 2005
- *The Republican War on Science*, by Chris Mooney: www.waronscience.com
- The Weekly Spin: www.prwatch.org

## Subverting Science, Manufacturing Doubt

In 2005 the *International Journal of Occupational & Environmental Health* published a special issue, *Corporate Corruption of Science*, full of evidence on the "substantial tradition of manipulation of evidence, data and analysis, ultimately designed to maintain favorable conditions for industry." One of the red flags is the explosion of corporate funding of university research, which grew from $264 million in 1980 to $2 billion in 2001.[5]

In their book *Trust Us, We're Experts: How Industry Manipulates Science and Gambles with Your Future*, Sheldon Rampton and John Stauber offered a whole slate of examples that demonstrate how corporations — behind the cover of public relations — "manufacture" and then promote fictitious evidence to cover their assets.

Another corporate trick is to characterize minute amounts of a hazard as trivial, with analogies like this: "It's the equivalent of one drop of gin in 660 tank cars full of tonic." This *does* sound trivial, but don't be fooled: the gin and tonic analogy accurately describes the seemingly infinitesimal fraction, one part per trillion, at which some hormones and hormone disruptors can play havoc in our bodies.

The corporate undermining of legitimate science also includes influence over governments. In September 2005 *Scientific American* reported:

> **Large swaths of the government in Washington are now in the hands of people who don't know what science is. More ominously, some of those in power may grasp how research works but nonetheless are willing to subvert science's knowledge and expert opinion for short-term political and economic gains.**[6]

Science in the public interest has taken major blows in Canada as well. In his book *Corrupt to the Core*, the former government microbiologist Dr. Shiv Chopra describes Canada's Health Protection Branch's failure to protect public health, and his firing in 2004 for blowing the whistle on conflicts of interests in the government's drug approval process.[7]

We need to staunchly protect and support science in the public interest — and the scientists who are deeply devoted to it.

**"Junk science" — a term coined by corporations to describe research they don't like.**

— Diana Zuckerman

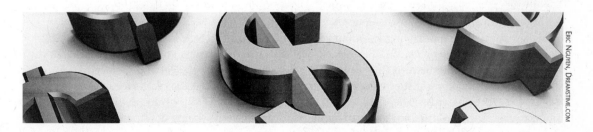

Eric Nguyen, Dreamstime.com

# Big Pharma and the War on Cancer

Well-established oncologists practicing in large urban areas can gross well in excess of a million dollars a year.

— Guy Faguet

When the US National Cancer Act was passed in December 1971, effectively firing the first shot in the War on Cancer declared by President Richard Nixon, leading scientists promised Congress a cure in time for the American Bicentennial in 1976.[1] Despite a $100 million boost to the National Cancer Institute's research budget, 1976 came and went with little progress. So did 1986. And 1996.

In 2006 Dr. Guy B. Faguet, a long-time cancer researcher for the National Institutes of Health, wrote a blistering critique called *The War on Cancer: An Anatomy of a Failure, A Blueprint for the Future*. He echoed what critics have been saying for a long time: the "war's" victories have been relatively minor, the costs for laboratory research huge[2] and the continued suffering from cancer enormous.[3]

But there *are* some undisputed winners: the drug companies and suppliers of radiation treatment and mammography screening equipment, for example. In 2006 cancer drugs were expected to be the fastest-growing class of pharmaceuticals in the world, exceeding $37 billion in sales.[4] The aging baby boomers will help this lucrative market explode over the next three decades. (See p. 6)

Chemotherapies are one part of a much larger issue — we're a society besotted by prescription medications and over-the-counter remedies. But there is a price to pay for our pill-popping habits. In *Prescription for Disaster*, Thomas J. Moore recommended that we put drugs much higher on our list of concerns about day-to-day cancer hazards: "There might be trace amounts of a suspected carcinogen on an apple, possibly a little more on the burnt material on a barbecued steak. That exposure is tiny compared to swallowing several pills a day for months or years on end."[5]

Of the top 50 pharmaceuticals on the market at the time of Moore's exposé, human evidence of cancer was reported for 4 drugs, animal evidence implicated 12, 2 caused cell mutations and 19 weren't tested for cancer risk. Giving the untested ones the benefit of the doubt, Moore said, "Eighteen of the top 50 drugs have measurable cancer risks."[6]

We need to get this legal drug trade under control.

It is clearly evident from Guy Faguet's book and others[7] that public health will be better served when pharmaceutical companies are compelled to:

- Stop funding clinical trials.
- Stop paying for and providing medical education.
- In the US, close the "chemotherapy concession."
- Stop direct-to-consumer advertising.

## Stop Direct Funding of Clinical Trials

Traditionally in Canada and the US, clinical cancer trials have been sponsored and funded by each country's National Cancer Institute, but this is rarely the case now. The "promise" of the human genome project and its potential for profits compelled the pharmaceutical industry to sponsor and fund trials for most anticancer drugs currently being developed.[8]

### Stop Providing Medical "Education"

Physician and former editor-in-chief of the *New England Journal of Medicine*, Marcia Angell pulls no punches: "We need to end the fiction that big pharma provides medical education. Drug companies are in business to sell drugs."[9] They need to stop pouring money into medical schools and teaching hospitals, she added, stop supporting continuing education and medical meetings, and stop funding professional associations. "Doctors not only receive biased information, but learn a very drug-intensive style of medicine."

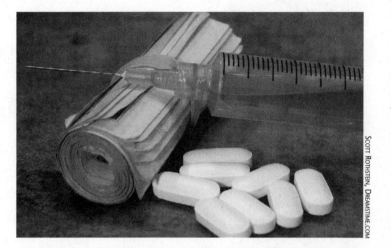

### Close the "Chemotherapy Concession"

In the US, medical oncologists who offer drug services at their offices can profit directly from prescribing certain pharmaceuticals, purchasing chemotherapy drugs in bulk and selling them to patients at retail prices, with markups "ranging between 10% or 20% to as high as 200%."[10] "Well-established oncologists practicing in large urban areas can gross well in excess of a million dollars a year," Guy Faguet reported.[11]

### Stop Direct-to-Consumer Advertising

Spending on the direct-to-consumer advertising of prescription drugs skyrocketed in the US from under $100 million in 1990 to $4.1 billion in 2004.[12] "The purpose and the effect of these commercials is to increase pressure on doctors to prescribe the latest, most expensive me-too drugs," wrote Marcia Angell.[13] Although the practice is illegal in Canada, Health Canada opened the door in 1996 by allowing "help-seeking" ads ("Ask your doctor about this condition"), and "reminder ads" (using a brand name only) in 2000. Still, Big Pharma forges on. The prescription drug Diane-35 was advertised to a target audience of young women for mild acne and birth control, with neither use approved by Health Canada. One ingredient of the drug, cyproterone, is associated with liver toxicity and causes changes to liver cell DNA. "A potential link to liver cancer remains an open question," wrote the Canadian Women's Health Network in a letter to the Canadian government demanding that the advertising stop.[14]

If pharmaceutical companies want to help win the war on cancer, they should donate 10% of their profits from the sale of cancer drugs to cancer prevention. Not screening, not "preventative drugs," but genuine prevention.

# Who Is Protecting Us?

The US regulatory system for chemical products is tailor-made for fraud.

— Peter Montague

Life is precious, and most people do not want to lose it. So we elect governments and pay them taxes to protect us. There are penalties for drunk driving, and even corrupt businessmen sometimes go to jail.

But when it comes to the multitude of hazardous substances we are so widely exposed to, almost nothing happens. Only a very small handful have been banned. The rest remain at large. The same applies to electromagnetic radiation from a host of electronic devices and power sources, where there are no legislated standards in Canada or the US to protect us from harm, and to our food, where nothing prevents producers from selling junk food that is known to be harmful.

Despite the Bush administration's fierce assault on environmental protection,[1] the situation is not all bad. Some local and state laws ban smoking in public places, and Canada (but not the US) bans tobacco advertising. The nuclear industry is highly regulated but not enough to protect those who live nearby. (See p. 52)

There are some ineffective federal regulations to limit air pollution from traffic, oil refineries, chemical plants and incinerators; there are some controls on the use of pesticides; and there are some city bylaws in Canada and a provincial law in Quebec banning the cosmetic use of pesticides.

There are federal bans, strengthened by global treaties, on only a small number of the most toxic chemicals. The US and Canada finally required companies to report their annual chemical emissions, after much industry resistance; and there are a few brave local efforts such as San Francisco's ban on the use of harmful chemicals in plastic baby bottles, pacifiers and toys, after the California legislature failed to act.

When it comes to the vast mass of chemicals, however, no one is protecting us. Only in California do citizens have the right to know if there are carcinogens in

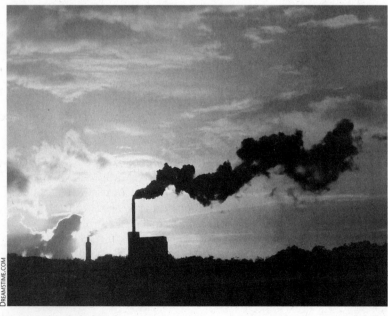

DREAMSTIME.COM

Pretty – but lethal

their products. Canada requires labeling for the ingredients in cosmetics but not to say which are harmful.

How did things get to be this bad? When the chemical industry grew rapidly after World War II, its products were allowed to be marketed without proof of safety.[2] We became the living experiment. Only when there was obvious evidence of harm did people start demanding changes.

When the US Congress passed the Toxic Substances Control Act in 1976, following the public outcry after Rachel Carson's book *Silent Spring*, 60,000 chemicals were "grandfathered" so that industry could continue producing them without health and safety data. The difficulties that the EPA has faced in trying to regulate chemicals are such that even in the case of asbestos, a known carcinogen that has caused at least 200,000 deaths in the US, industry was able to get the EPA's case overturned in the courts after ten years of EPA effort.[3]

For new chemicals, industry's only obligation is to report any ill effects to the EPA — not the public — using its own studies (or hiding them, as is often the case).[4] Canada finally brought in requirements for testing new chemicals under the Canadian Environmental Protection Act in 1988.[5]

Whenever the public demanded stricter controls, the chemical industry manipulated the science, dominated the regulatory process, used aggressive litigation and defended its right to go on polluting. It bullied the scientists, the regulators, the media, publishers and even their advertisers. A Wild West attitude prevailed, supported by industry-funded lobbyists and campaign donations to politicians. "I doubt you could find a single federal scientist who actually believes in his or her heart that the chemical regulatory system is presently protecting the public adequately from unwanted assault by industrial poisons," said Peter Montague.[6]

In response to the problems, Canada has prepared a new list of chemicals that must be tested, and the European Union has introduced comprehensive legislation known as REACH (see Solution 69). There are still two fundamental problems, however. The first is that all future testing must be done for very low as well as for high doses, to test for the risk of harm from endocrine disruption (see p. 32); and all previous testing must be repeated for low doses.

The second is that since we are being exposed to so many chemicals in combination, they must be tested in combination. When Peter Montague calculated how much time would be required to evaluate 1,000 chemicals in 11-chemical combinations at 15,000 tests a year, as *The Wall Street Journal* reported they hoped to, the answer was millions of times longer than the universe has existed. Montague then looked at just 3-chemical combinations. That would need 166 million tests and take 11,000 years.[7]

The numbers prove the nonsense. The entire regulatory structure must be rebuilt on the foundation of the precautionary principle. Instead of asking "How much harm can we get away with?" we must ask "How much harm can we avoid?"[8]

# What Are Cancer Charities and Hospitals Doing to __Prevent__ Cancer?

Priorities [of the Amercian Cancer Society] remain fixated on damage control — screening, diagnosis and treatment — with indifference or even hostility to cancer prevention.
— Dr. Samuel Epstein[1]

The cancer lottery's promotional brochure proudly declares the Ferrari F430 to be one of the most famous and sought-after automobiles in the history of motoring: "Every inch of this sleek, 490 hp beauty was inspired by Ferrari's celebrated F1 Racing Division."[2]

In 2005 this top-of-the-line speedster was one of three grand prizes in Alberta's Cash & Cars for Cancer lottery, luring millions of dollars to the province's coffers for cancer research.

To keep up with the crushing burden of cancer, North American cancer charities and hospitals need to move at warp speed, much faster than the Ferrari F430.

Meanwhile we wonder if this irony has occurred to cancer fundraisers: cars, and all gas-dependent vehicles, cause cancer. Among others, benzene, formaldehyde and polycyclic aromatic hydrocarbons in vehicle exhaust are known carcinogens. No surprise, but next to none of the funds raised in lotteries like Cash & Cars go to cancer prevention.

- Canadian Strategy for Cancer Control Best Practices Review: www.ohcow.on.ca/press_release/cancerpreventionreport.htm
- *Chasing the Cancer Answer*: www.cbc.ca/consumers/market/files/health/cancer
- Dr. Samuel Epstein's Cancer Prevention Coalition: www.preventcancer.com
- *The Cancer Industry* by Ralph Moss, Equinox Press, 1996

If you look carefully at the partnerships between cancer charities and corporate sponsors, you'll find many similar alliances with companies that broadcast carcinogens far and wide as part of their daily business. The Canadian Cancer Society (CCS) is in league with General Motors of Canada, Pratt & Whitney (aircraft turbines), PetroCanada and Alcan (aluminum smelters), to name just four. Other partners profit handsomely from cancer treatments, including most of the major pharmaceutical companies, such as Novartis and Pfizer.

The drug company AstraZeneca is also a CCS partner. Before Astra merged with Zeneca in 1999, the latter was a North American subsidiary of Imperial Chemical Industries in Great Britain, one of the largest producers of pesticides in the world. Zeneca was also the primary maker of tamoxifen (Novaldex) — still produced under the AstraZeneca banner — the world's most popular drug for metastatic breast cancer. In the 1980s Zeneca created the annual October event in the US called National Breast Cancer Awareness Month. AstraZeneca currently runs a string of cancer centers in the US under the name Aptium Oncology.[3] As cancer activist Judy Brady of San Francisco pointed out: "They cause it, they treat it, they control cancer care centers and they have the pink ribbon to cover it all up. They didn't miss a trick."

Nearly five decades ago, Dr. Wilhelm Heuper of the US National Cancer Institute offered his reasons why primary prevention of cancer languished: "The goal of curing the victims of cancer is more exciting, more tangible, more glamorous and rewarding than prevention."[4] To put it a little more bluntly: there is no profit in prevention — which is as true today as it was in 1962.

There is a lengthy history of cancer agencies establishing alliances with corporations that have big profits at stake, as longtime American Cancer Society critic Dr. Samuel Epstein, now in his eighties, has repeatedly argued in his crusades for prevention. In his books *The Politics of Cancer* and *Cancer-Gate: How to Win the Losing Cancer War*, Epstein repeatedly assailed what he called "the world's largest non-religious charity" for failing to embrace prevention.

During a debate in 2005, Dr. Michael Thun of the American Cancer Society acknowledged the ACS connections to corporations: "That can be construed as an inherent conflict of interest, or it can be construed as a pragmatic way to get funding to support cancer control."[5]

"Cancer control," to the ACS, means almost total focus on "lifestyle" factors for primary prevention — smoking, diet, alcohol consumption, physical exercise and exposure to the sun's UV rays. These are sometimes called the "low hanging fruit" of prevention — they're easiest to pick off because they focus on personal habits, rather than the far more complex and confrontational task of stopping the poisoning of our air, water, soil and food.

Are cancer agencies and charities willing to take on this bigger challenge if it means colliding head-on with their corporate partners? Many doubt it, but there are some promising signs. Under its then CEO Julie White, in 2002 the Canadian Cancer Society called for a ban on

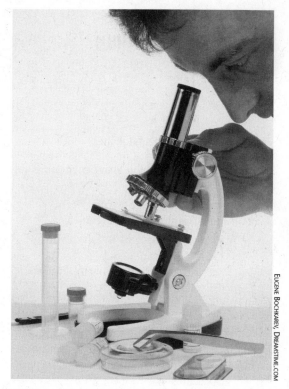

Searching for ways to cure cancer.

lawn and garden pesticides containing carcinogens. It also adopted the precautionary principle (although still struggled with a decision to ban asbestos) and endorsed the Canadian Strategy for Cancer Control's 2005 *Best Practices Review and Recommendations* for preventing occupational and environmental cancers.

The Canadian TV special *Chasing the Cancer Answer* threw down the gauntlet in Spring 2006, questioning why the CCS knowingly tolerates carcinogens such as formaldehyde in everyday consumer products, and asking them to act more boldly for prevention. It is surely inevitable that cancer agencies and societies around the world will soon awake to the challenge of cancer prevention — not just screening and early detection, but real prevention.

# Prevent Cancer Now

Cancer prevention deserves to be put on a resource footing equal to that of the search for the cure ... for every dollar spent on the search, a dollar must be spent on preventive action.[1]
— Dr. Ross Hume Hall

The overall goals of this book are:

- To inform you about the many environmental causes of cancer.
- To show you that there are practical solutions to almost all these causes.
- To inspire you to become involved with others so that we can work together to implement the solutions, and stop cancer before it starts.

The changes needed are huge — and it's not just cancer. By working together to eliminate the hazardous substances that are causing cancer, and by restoring nutritional quality to our food, we will also address the root causes of many other ailments and diseases.

To achieve these changes, we need to build a movement in which so many people stand up and say *"Enough — Prevent Cancer Now!"* that governments, health agencies and businesses are forced to pay attention and change their priorities.

We need to build a movement that involves everyone — you and your neighbors, teachers and

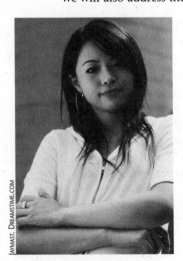

Are we going to remove the threat of cancer from her generation?

nurses, workers and business owners, grandparents and teenagers, musicians and artists, city councilors and government staff, scientists and technicians, farmers and gardeners, and volunteers and staff from citizens' organizations and cancer societies the world over.

The old approach has failed. We need to adopt a new approach based on the precautionary principle and a clear commitment to prevent cancer *now*, before it begins.

### Sweden's Environmental Objectives

To build this movement, we need clear goals that we can unite behind, with target dates for their achievement. In 1999 the Swedish Government determined "to pass on to the next generation a society in which all the major environmental problems have been solved."[2] They established 16 environmental quality objectives to be achieved by 2020, including:

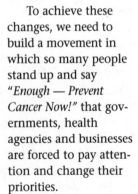

- Clean Air: so as not to represent a risk to human health or to animals, plants or cultural assets.
- A Non-Toxic Environment: free from manmade or extracted compounds and metals that represent a threat to human health or biological diversity.
- A Protective Ozone Layer: to provide long-term protection against harmful UV radiation.
- A Safe Radiation Environment: to protect against the harmful effects of radiation.
- Good Quality Groundwater: to provide a safe and sustainable supply of drinking water.

"For this to be feasible," the government writes, "every sector of society must assume its share of responsibility. Public agencies, organizations, enterprises and individuals must devote more attention to environmental issues and sustainable development."

**Ten Goals**

Here are some objectives we need to organize around:

1. That the public has a right to know about product ingredients and workplace exposures.

2. That all health-related decision-making be based on the precautionary principle, using toxics use reduction, alternatives assessment and substitution.

3. That half of all cancer funding should be directed to the primary prevention of cancer.

4. That corporate law require directors to minimize harm to local communities, public health and the environment, while pursuing private profit.

5. That all junk food be eliminated from schools, hospitals and television advertising.

6. That all hazardous chemicals and air pollution be eliminated by 2025.

7. That all harmful man-made radiation be reduced to safe levels by 2025.

8. That there are no more teenagers smoking by 2025.

9. That there has been a **nationwide transition** to organic farming by 2025.

- Breast Cancer Action (US): www.bcaction.org
- Cancer Prevention Coalition (US): www.preventcancer.com
- Cancer Prevention and Education Society (UK): www.cancerpreventionsociety.org
- Collaborative for Health and the Environment (Global): www.healthandenvironment.org
- Health and Environment Alliance (Europe): www.env-health.org
- Prevent Cancer Now (Canada): www.preventcancernow.ca
- Prevention Is the Cure (New York): www.preventionisthecure.org

10. That there is an accelerated elimination of ozone-depleting substances so that the ozone layer is healed by 2025.

For the USA, two further goals are needed:

1. That democracy is reclaimed from corrupted electoral processes.

2. That corporate influence is eliminated from campaign financing, as Canada did in 2005/2006.[3]

The way to succeed is to organize and link together. We urge you to join organizations that are working towards these goals, and to bring your personal talents and commitment into play.

If we continue on our present course, we are heading towards an increasing incidence of cancer, not towards a reduction. It is not enough to seek to *control* cancer. We need to *prevent* cancer.

If we achieve these goals, we will put a major dent in future cancer rates, while helping our ecologically challenged civilization to steer down a wiser path towards a more sustainable, green, peaceful future.

It is a simple but compelling vision. If you **have children** or grandchildren, what do they think? We doubt that they'll hesitate.

# Part II

## 101 Solutions

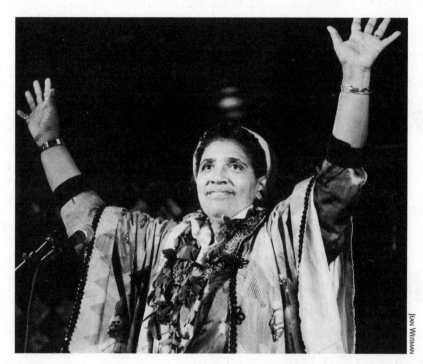

Audre Lorde 1934-1992

"When I dare to be powerful, to use my strength in the service of my vision, then it becomes less important whether or not I am unafraid."

# 1

## Open Your Eyes

We are unwilling victims in a huge radiation, chemical and genetic engineering experiment, without our informed consent.

— Lynn Howard Ehrle,
Organic Consumers Association

You're probably surprised to see that our first solution for individuals isn't about tobacco. We'll get there in Solution 3, but first we'd like you to consider the larger picture and what you can do about it.

Nearly half of all North American males and more than one third of females will be diagnosed with a malignant tumor at some point in their lives, not including non-melanoma skin cancers.

Dying prematurely from cancer robs more years from our average life expectancy than any other disease, what insurance specialists call "potential years of life lost," or PYLL. Cancer is far and away the leader in PYLL in Canada and the US, miles ahead of respiratory illness, car accidents, suicides and strokes, and it accounts for more than twice the number of early deaths from heart disease. In 2001 Canadian females lost 498,000 years of potential life to cancer, while males lost 469,000 years. This is a tragedy of epic — and epidemic — proportions.

Cancers frequently strike the most vulnerable among us — poor people at the margins, young children and elderly citizens with fragile immune systems. They also strike people who are healthy and robust.

Good personal habits will certainly reduce your cancer risk. But the bigger picture must also include environmental hazards we can't stop at the front doorstep, despite the healthiest lifestyle choices.

Human body burden tests provide dramatic evidence that hundreds of novel chemicals such as dioxins, fire retardants and PCBs, as well as radioactive materials, are trespassing into our bodies. They enter as invisible hitchhikers on the food we eat, the air we breathe and the water we drink. Many pass easily through our skin. Infants are exposed *in utero*, even before conception in some instances. Human semen and ova are often surrounded by a profusion of toxic substances.

The striking thing is that this is not news at all. Over 40 years ago, in *Silent Spring*, biologist Rachel Carson wrote, "For the first time in the history of the world, every human being is now subjected to contact with dangerous chemicals, from the moment of conception until death." Our governments have never acted boldly on what Carson called the "golden opportunity" to stop cancer — by applying primary prevention.

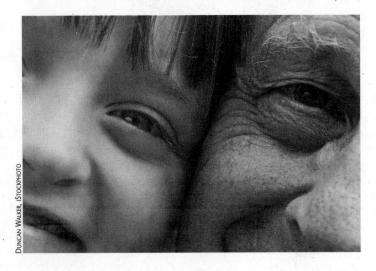

DUNCAN WALKER, ISTOCKPHOTO

## Smoking and Lung Cancer: The Bigger Picture

Our cancer agencies have done a good job educating us about tobacco. Almost everyone is aware that smoking causes lung cancer. But did you know that:

- One in five women diagnosed with lung cancer has never smoked?

- More than 20 substances other than tobacco — including coal tar and beryllium — also initiate lung cancer?

These links to cancer came to light in the workplace, when people exposed to these substances were found to experience higher rates of lung cancer. They were "dying for a living," as one Canadian labor union put it.

- Chemical Body Burden: www.chemicalbodyburden.org
- Chemical Trespass: Pesticides in Our Bodies: www.panna.org
- Toxic Nation Report Card (Canada): www.toxicnation.ca
- Scorecard, the Pollution Information Site (US): www.scorecard.org, then click on Health Effects
- State of the Evidence: What Is the Connection Between the Environment and Breast Cancer? www.breastcancerfund.org/evidence
- Your Body Burden: www.ewg.org

Between the good personal habits we choose and the environmental hazards we can't easily avoid because they're invisible trespassers, there are many cancer-causing substances that we *can* eliminate. Many we rarely connect to cancer because they're so much a part of daily life. Consider:

- The cars we drive, which run on carcinogenic petroleum products.
- The clothes we wear — not-so-natural cottons and synthetics, perma-pressed and dry-cleaned with chemicals that include perchloroethylene and formaldehyde.
- Personal and household products, even cleaners, that contain known carcinogens.
- The food we eat, processed, packaged, scarce on "value," and laced with toxic additives and traces of pesticides.
- The toxic indoor air in our homes, schools and workplaces.
- The perfect lawn and flawless bed of roses that depend on chemicals to keep them blooming.
- Numerous prescription drugs that cause hormone havoc *and* cancer.
- Many job-related carcinogens.

It would be easy to throw up our hands and say *everything* causes cancer — but it doesn't. As individuals, we can significantly reduce our exposure to man-made and natural carcinogens, just as we can change our personal habits. In this section of the book, we will take a very complex subject and transform it into what we hope are simple, practical, workable solutions that will help reduce the heavy burden of cancer in our lives.

# 2

# Adopt Healthy Habits

**Bicycling is a big part of the future. It has to be. There's something wrong with a society that drives a car to work out in a gym.**

— **Bill Nye, the Science Guy**

Do healthy habits play a positive role in cancer prevention? Read on!

## Get Physically Active

Surprisingly, the jury is still out on some familiar "steps to health," such as getting sufficient physical exercise.

"Medical researchers agree that, at the very least, regular exercise can make people feel better, and feel better about themselves," wrote Gina Kolata of the *New York Times* in late 2005, [but] there is less agreement on whether it can prevent cancer." For two common cancers, however, breast and colon, the evidence is "promising," Kolata explains, with at least 50 studies showing positive results as a preventive for colon cancer.[1]

There is evidence that exercise may also reduce the risk for prostate cancer.[2] Exercise also helps us trim extra body fat, which is a known risk for cancer. We say that's good enough for us, so let's get active! For adults to get and stay fit, the American Cancer Society (ACS) recommends engaging in moderate activity — such as brisk walking, dancing, canoeing, yoga — for at least 30 minutes, five or more days a week.

## Drive Less: Cycle, Walk, Jog and Bus More

This is not just a matter of fitness. Driving your car, especially in heavy traffic, exposes you to a host of carcinogens, including benzene, formaldehyde and diesel particulates.[3] Recent California research found that 90% of the cancer-causing air pollution in the state's south coast region came from vehicle emissions, mostly

from diesel exhaust.[4] Driving behind diesel buses or mid-size trucks with low tailpipes is especially unhealthy because it subjects drivers to much higher levels of carcinogenic soot from diesel exhaust. Whenever possible don't exercise in heavily polluted air. Opt for your local park, hiking and biking trails or the beach.

## Drink Alcohol Moderately

Alcohol is an established cause of cancers of the mouth, pharynx (throat), larynx (voice box), esophagus, liver and breast; it may also increase the incidence of colon cancer. "People who drink alcohol should limit their intake to no more than two drinks a day for men and one drink a day for women (who are physically smaller and metabolize alcohol more slowly)," advises the ACS. A drink is defined as 12 ounces of beer, 5 ounces of wine or 1.5 ounces of 80-proof distilled spirits.[5]

On the brighter side, the anti-oxidant benefits of resveratrol in red wine may help prevent prostate and other cancers. Still, moderation is "a good thing."

## Practice Safe Sex

Sexually transmitted viruses and bacteria can increase the risks for cervical cancer (human papillomavirus from genital herpes and chlamydia), liver cancer (hepatitis B and C) and Kaposi's (herpes simplex virus 8), as well as for the human immuno-deficiency virus (HIV) that is a risk factor for Kaposi's sarcoma and non-Hodgkin's lymphoma.[6] Until a sexual relationship is long-term and monogamous, gays and heterosexual couples

- *The Complete Cancer Cleanse: A Proven Program to Detoxify and Renew Body, Mind and Spirit*, by Cherie Calbom, John Calbom and Michael Mahaffey. Nelson, 2003.

should always use a condom and spermicide. Lesbian sexual activity is not risk free, as is often assumed; until the partnership is long-term and monogamous, it's wise to use a female condom.

### Practice Sun Sense, But Get Your Vitamin D

Sunscreens have long been promoted as one of the best ways to avoid the harmful UV radiation that causes skin cancers, along with wearing protective clothing and shunning the midday sun. But sunscreens can create a false sense of security, leaving you vulnerable to the most harmful UV-A rays that can trigger melanoma, the deadliest type of skin cancer.[7] So keep covering up while ducking the sun's strongest rays between 11am and 3pm, especially if you're fair-haired and light-skinned.

However, it is critically important to get enough Vitamin D — the sunshine vitamin — because it reduces the incidence of breast, prostate and colon cancer.[8] Food — especially organic — can be a good source: organ meats, eggs and especially fish oils contain this important vitamin. It's especially crucial during the dark winter months to get sufficient D, so top up with vitamin supplements, in consultation with a knowledgeable health professional.

### Detoxify

Body burden testing tells us that virtually all humans in industrialized countries are contaminated with scores of man-made toxic substances. Our livers, kidneys and lungs are especially overtaxed in their attempt to detoxify all these "foreigners," including many carcinogens.

Regular detoxing under the supervision of a qualified professional can help restore well-being.

### Make Life Worth Living

Connect often with the astonishing wonders of the natural world. Nature herself lays the foundation for our good health, and the more contact we have with her, the happier and healthier we are.

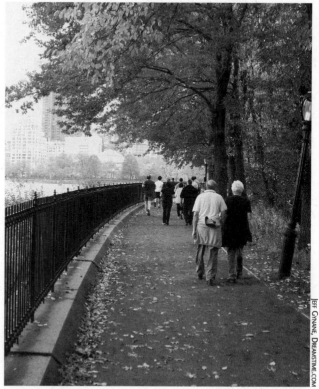

JEFF GYNANE, DREAMSTIME.COM

# 3

# Avoid All Tobacco Smoke

A cigarette for the beginner is a symbolic act. "I am no longer my mother's child, I'm tough, I'm an adventurer ...." As the force from the psychological symbolism subsides, the pharmacological effect takes over to sustain the habit.
— Philip Morris report, *Why One Smokes*, 1969[1]

Smoking cigarettes isn't just a "habit," as Philip Morris finally but silently admitted on its website in 1999.[2] It's an extremely stubborn, dogged addiction that is often lethal.

I (Liz) was hooked on cigarettes for more than 20 years, from my early teens to my mid-30s. For me, smoking was less a symbolic act than a case of "monkey see, monkey do." My parents and one older sister smoked, and so did many other adults I respected, including the medical doctor who lived next door. At 16, I was not only immortal — weren't we all then? — but convinced I could give up cigarettes any time I chose. This boast later proved to be hugely mistaken. (Only a seriously addicted person would venture out in a howling Canadian snowstorm to buy cigarettes. I did this several times over the span of my smoking "career." Never, ever did I set off in similar weather for fruits and veggies.) It took ten years and several failed attempts for me to finally put down those aptly named "coffin nails" for good.

One thing I'm certain about, having fallen into the trap several times when I tried unsuccessfully to quit: I am still addicted to cigarettes. A single puff would probably put me right back

en route to a pack a day. Smoking is not just a physical addiction; it's psychological too.

If you don't smoke, please be wise and never start. If you're one of the 70% of adult smokers who at any given time truly want to stop smoking,[4] our deepest wish is for you to find the strength to quit for good. And, if at first you don't succeed, join the club! Research shows that the more times a smoker earnestly tries to stop, the better the chance of ultimately succeeding. This was certainly true in my case — I knew deep down I really wanted to be a non-smoker, and finally just got tired of all that quitting.

Some approaches that helped me and other quitters:

- Hypnosis and meditation
- Vitamin therapy and juicing
- Acupuncture
- Quitting with a buddy or smoking cessation group
- Working closely with a family doctor and naturopath
- Using the nicotine patch and gum.

If you can't quit for yourself, then do it for your spouse, your kids or your favorite waiter at the local pub (if smoking is still allowed there). Everybody wins. You'll be free of a dangerous addiction, and those around you will stop being exposed to your second-hand smoke, which kills over 40,000 Canadians and Americans every year, and is a known cause of lung cancer, heart disease, chronic lung ailments such as bronchitis and asthma, and low birth weights in newborns.[5]

**Fact:** Nearly 200,000 Americans and Canadians will die from lung cancer this year, and 87% of these deaths will be directly related to smoking. Another 300,000 will die from smoking-related diseases such as emphysema, stroke and heart disease. The lifetime risk of developing lung cancer is 1% for non-smokers and about 30% for heavy smokers.[3]

Despite the tobacco industry's longstanding deceit, nearly all of us know about the connection between lung cancer and smoking. But it's not just lung cancer. Tobacco use is also a major cause of these cancers: larynx, oral cavity, esophagus and bladder cancer.

Smoking "substantially elevates" death rates for these cancers: kidney, pancreas and cervical[7] cancer. And it's "associated" with these cancers: stomach, liver, prostate, colon, rectum[8] and breast.[9]

"Former smokers tend to have a healthier lifestyle, with less alcohol consumption, a better diet and a higher level of physical activity than current smokers," reports McGill University in Montreal. "Former smokers are also more likely to practice preventive health measures."[10]

All true in my case. And the best bottom line: I *love* my life and myself far more as a non-smoker!

**Fact:** Cigarette smoke contains more than 4,800 different compounds, 69 of which are known and probable carcinogens.[6] These include benzene, formaldehyde, arsenic, numerous polycyclic aromatic hydrocarbons (PAHs) and vinyl chloride.

**Fact:** The more years and the higher number of tobacco products you smoke daily — this includes pipes and cigars, as well as cigarettes — the greater your risk of lung cancer. The good news is that if you stop smoking, the risk of lung cancer decreases each year as normal cells replace abnormal cells. After ten years, the risk drops to a level that is one-third to one-half the risk for people who continue to smoke,[11] and the danger of lung cancer continues to fall, the longer you're tobacco-free.

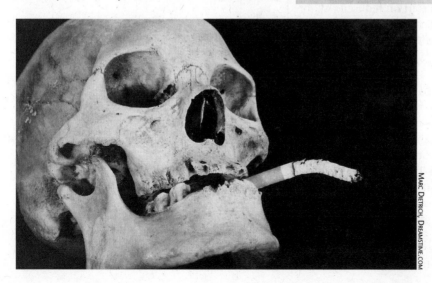

MARC DIETRICH, DREAMSTIME.COM

When we think about diseases caused by smoking, we automatically think of lung cancer, but more than a dozen other cancers are linked to tobacco use as well, as are heart disease, stroke and emphysema.

# 4

# Eat a Healthy Diet

> Populations around the world that practice a very low-fat vegetarian diet, in general, have the lowest rates of cancer.
>
> — Hans Diehl, *Diet for a New Century*

Here are four healthy diet principles to reduce your cancer risk:

- Eat plenty of fresh, ripe, locally grown, organic fruits and vegetables, whenever possible. Raw or lightly steamed veggies are more nutritious than cooked; fresh is better than frozen; frozen is better than from cans, which may have hormone disruptors in their plastic lining.

- Drink generous quantities of healthy liquids, including pure water cleansed of chlorine residues and other contaminants, various teas, such as green, Chai, white and rooibos,[1] and freshly juiced fruits and vegetables.

- Start your cancer prevention diet in the womb. No kidding. If your mother ate nutritious food while you were *in utero* and breastfed you for at least six months, you really did get a head start on reduced risk for cancer later in life. The good news: *From a cancer prevention standpoint, it's never too late to improve your diet.*

- Take good quality food supplements, including vitamins, minerals and other elements that build immunity, such as salvestrols and precursors to glutathione, a known anti-cancer agent. We *should* be able to get everything a healthy body needs from our meal plates, but too much North American food is sadly lacking in nutrients because of the harmful effects of modern farming and food processing practices (see p. 40).

Are you skeptical about organic food? Think it's too expensive, hard to get, or no more nutritious or safe than non-organic food? Then consider these points:

- Cost: *Mothers and Others for a Livable Planet* demonstrated in a shopping basket comparison that, with modest adjustments in buying habits, the cost of organic food was about equal to the cost of food treated with pesticides and grown with chemical fertilizers. The two key changes? Buying in bulk and substituting vegetable proteins for most meats.

- Food value: Many studies have shown the nutritional superiority of organic over non-organic crops. A 2001 literature survey by Virginia Worthington found that organic crops contained "significantly more vitamin C, iron, magnesium and phosphorus, and significantly less nitrates than conventional crops."[2, 3]

- Pesticide residues: Do they cause cancer? Dr. Charles Benbrook, Chief Scientist at The Organic Center, says one third of the population is vulnerable.[4] In a 2001 study of 96 children in the Seattle area, only one child showed no measurable concentration of any of the organophosphorus metabolites from pesticides. This child's parents bought exclusively organic produce and did not use any pesticides at home.[5]

- Supplements: The American Medical Association used to believe it was unnecessary for North Americans to take vitamins. But in 2002, this mainstream doctors' group concluded: "Pending strong evidence of effectiveness from randomized trials, it

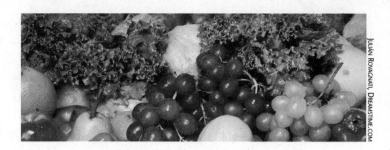

Fruits and vegetables contain thousands of phytochemicals, and many are powerful anti-cancer agents. Organic produce is best.

appears prudent for all adults to take vitamin supplements."[6]

## Ten Foods and Drinks to Limit or Eliminate

- All charred foods, which create *heterocyclic aromatic amines*, known carcinogens. Even dark toast is suspect.
- Well-done red meat.[7] Medium or rare is better, little or no red meat is best.
- Sugar, both white and brown (which is simply white sugar with molasses added).[8]
- Heavily salted, smoked and pickled foods, which lead to higher rates of stomach cancer.
- Sodas/soft drinks, which pose health risks, both for what they contain — sugar and various additives — and for what they replace in the diet — beverages and foods that provide vitamins, minerals, and other nutrients.[9]
- French fries, chips and snack foods that contain trans fats.[10]
- Some food and drink additives, including aspartame.
- Excess alcohol. (See Solution 2)
- Baked goods, for the *acrylamide*.
- Farmed fish, which contains higher levels of toxins such as PCBs.

## Ten Foods and Drinks for Cancer Protection

- Cruciferous vegetables: broccoli, cauliflower, cabbage, Brussels sprouts, bok choy and kale. These score high for containing many anti-cancer substances, such as the *isothiocyanates*.

- Globe artichoke for very high levels of *salvestrols*.[11]
- Dark greens, such as spinach and romaine lettuce, for their *fiber*, *folate* and a wide range of cancer-fighting *carotenoids*. Other dark-colored veggies, too, such as beets and red cabbage.
- Grapes and red wine, especially for the *resveratrol*.[12]
- Legumes — beans, peas and lentils, for the *saponins*, *protease inhibitors* and more.
- Berries, particularly blueberries, for the *ellagic acid* and *anthocyanosides*.
- Flaxseed, especially if you grind it yourself and consume when fresh, for the essential fatty acid *alpha-linolenic acid*, *lignans* and other "good fats."[13]
- Garlic, onions, scallions, leeks and chives, for many anti-cancer substances including *allicin*.
- Green tea, for its anti-cancer *catechins*, a potent anti-oxidant.
- Tomatoes, for the famous flavenoid *lycopene*.

- Fats and Cholesterol: www.hsph.harvard.edu/nutritionsource/fats.html
- *The Food Revolution: How Your Diet Can Help Save Your Life and the World*, John Robbins. Conari, 2001: www.foodrevolution.org
- *Foods That Fight Cancer: Preventing Cancer Through Diet*, Richard Béliveau and Denis Gingras, McClelland & Stewart, 2006
- Guide to Food Additives: www.cspinet.org/reports/chemcuisine.htm

# 5

# Switch to Safe Personal Products

**M**any products that we use daily and never think twice about can be hazardous to our health. American and Canadian consumers are poorly protected by the health and safety agencies that are supposed to be watching out for us.

**Personal Care Products (for men too)**
Count 'em up! Men use about 10 personal care products each day, and women closer to 20, including 6 cosmetics. North Americans spend an astounding US$35 billion a year on toothpaste, cosmetics, hand creams, soaps, shampoos, deodorants, hair dyes, fragrances and so on. They *should* be safe, and we trust that they are.

Our advice? Trust less and investigate more, because there are very few regulations governing the use of ingredients in personal care products. Words such as "herbal" and "all-natural" are essentially meaningless in a marketplace with limited standards. Still, some excellent products are available on store shelves and online.

• The Environmental Working Group's *Skin Deep* is an online, brand-by-brand guide to nearly 15,000 personal care products, ranking them according to their toxicity. "Our investigation of product safety shows cause for concern, not alarm. Much more study is needed to understand the contribution of exposures from personal care products to current human health trends."[2] It adds, however, that over

• *Skin Deep*: www.ewg.org/reports/skindeep
• *The Green Guide*: www.thegreenguide.com

If Canadians don't know about the potential short-term effects of beauty products, neither are they informed about the huge gaps in knowledge surrounding cosmetic safety. New research shows cosmetics and toiletries sometimes contain a potentially dangerous cocktail of carcinogens, mutagens and reproductive toxins that can alter the function of hormones, and in rare circumstances, lead to infertility.
— *Ottawa Citizen*, March 5, 2006[1]

30% of the products in the survey contained one or more ingredients classified as a possible human carcinogen, and 1 in every 120 contained known or probable carcinogens.

• *The Green Guide* offers a critique of personal care products, including many brand names. Aubrey Organics, Aveda, Burt's Bees and Dr. Hauschka are among the best. *The Guide* also publishes a small, downloadable *Dirty Dozen Shopper's Card: 12 Ingredients to Avoid in Personal Care Products*, including several carcinogens and endocrine disruptors, such as formaldehyde (disguised as Quaternium 15), fragrances with phthalates, the preservative parabens and phenylenediamine (PPD), used in many hair dyes.

**Pharmaceutical Drugs**
Always be cautious about taking prescription medications. With the help of a knowledgeable health professional, try the most natural, non-prescription remedies first. Many pharmaceuticals do have benefits that outweigh the risks, but cancer has sometimes been an unexpected side effect. Be especially cautious of hormone-based drugs. An excellent resource for women is the book *Hormone Balance* by Dr. Carolyn Dean.[3]

Ask your physician to photocopy the details of *any* prescription drug suggested for you from the "bible" of drug information, the *Compendium of Pharmaceuticals and Specialties*. Read Thomas

Thanks to the US Campaign for Safe Cosmetics, by Spring 2006, more than 300 cosmetics and body care products companies had promised to replace ingredients linked to cancer, birth defects, hormone disruption and other negative health effects with safer alternatives.

Moore's *Prescription for Disaster*. The subtitle is instructive: *How to Get the Greatest Benefits from Prescription Drugs, Over-the-counter Medications and Natural Compounds at the Lowest Risk.*[4]

**'Use Daily' shouldn't be dangerous advice.**

150 cosmetics companies agree: Beauty products don't need to be toxic. Every day, we use as many as 25 personal care products on our bodies. Some of the chemicals in these products are linked to cancer, infertility and birth defects—and most have never been evaluated for their health effects.

More than 150 cosmetics companies are leading the way in cleaning up their industry. These companies have signed a pledge—the Compact for Safe Cosmetics—to remove hazardous ingredients. Now, all cosmetics companies should sign the Compact and prove that their concern for their customers is more than just skin deep.

**The Campaign for Safe Cosmetics**
www.SafeCosmetics.org

Has your favorite brand pledged to make safe products?

CAMPAIGN FOR SAFE COSMETICS

**Breast Implants**

We don't recommend this kind of surgery — and especially not for young adults — for cosmetic reasons alone. Women who have had mastectomies and are seeking reconstructive breast surgery with implants need to be skeptical of studies paid for by breast implant manufacturers and organizations representing plastic surgeons that often obscure possible dangers. Pay attention to two studies by the National Cancer Institute: one found that women with implants are more likely to die from brain tumors, lung cancer, other respiratory diseases and suicide, compared to other plastic surgery patients. The other found a 21% increased risk of cancer for women with implants, compared to women of the same age in the general population.[5, 6]

**Clothing**

Here's to 100% *organic* cotton, linen, wool and hemp. Abstain from garments made from petroleum-based synthetics, especially polyvinyl chloride (PVC) raincoats, patent vinyl pants, laminated aprons and so on. Shun regular cotton, which is doused with pesticides, herbicides and defoliants, bleached with chlorine, dyed with heavy metals and aromatic amines and made wrinkle-free with formaldehyde.

And then there are shoes. There are too many carcinogens to list here, including chromium, formaldehyde and coal-tar derivatives, which are created in the manufacture of most footwear. Check out www.treehugger.com for PVC- and animal-free options — even Stella McCartney vegan boots!

**Bras**

In their 1995 book, *Dressed to Kill: The Link Between Breast Cancer and Bras*, authors Singer and Grismaijer report that the longer women wore bras each day, the higher their breast cancer risk.[7] Their hypothesis? Bras bind and constrict lymphatic circulation, preventing the flushing of cancer-causing toxins from breast tissue. The authors' methodology was criticized by many scientists, but there have been other hints of such a link. A study in the May 1999 *Lancet* concluded that pre-menopausal women with fibrocystic breast disease have an almost six-fold higher risk of breast cancer.[8] Since there are case studies of women relieved of fibrocystic breast disease when they went bra-free, this surely ought to rouse the cancer agencies to undertake more investigation.[9]

# 6

## Live in a Healthy Home

> Whatever we do to our home, we do to ourselves.
>
> — Athena Thompson, author of
> *Homes That Heal and Those That Don't*

For the most part, we're blissfully unaware that the environment *inside* our homes is far more toxic than the air outdoors, even in cities where trucks and factories belch noxious pollution.[1]

Entire books have been written about how to make our homes truly healthy places to live, and we enthusiastically recommend these two, which are loaded with useful information and resources:

- *Home Safe Home: Creating a Healthy Home Environment by Reducing Exposure to Toxic Household Products* by Debra Lynn Dadd, Jeremy P. Tarcher/Penguin, 2005.

- *Homes That Heal and Those That Don't: How Your Home Could Be Harming Your Family's Health* by Athena Thompson, New Society Publishers, 2004.

Toxic homes can trigger health consequences other than cancer, such as allergies, multiple chemical sensitivity, chronic fatigue syndrome and asthma, so the whole picture needs addressing. But let's focus on three cancer concerns:

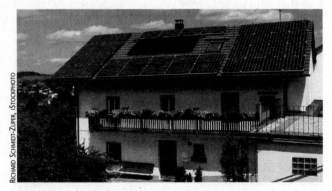

Building 'green' is becoming mainstream.

- Construction materials and finishes
- Air and water systems
- Home furnishings.

In Solutions 7 and 9, we'll take a closer look at household products — such as cleaners, paints and art supplies — and radon gas and electromagnetic radiation (EMR).

In *Cancer Where You Live* (p. 36), we saw that our homes are built with many toxic products. Particleboard and plywood contain formaldehyde; toxic adhesives, sealants and caulks, and solvent-based paints release volatile organic compounds (VOCs), such as toluene and benzene; wall coverings and blinds are often made with PVC. And that just skims the surface of our building challenges.

If you have the resources to remodel your home or build one from scratch, a whole new era has dawned in healthy building materials over the past few years. Non-toxic products include insulation made of 100% recycled denim or cellulose, emission-free wheat straw fiberboard; reclaimed wood, ultra-low VOC paints and finishes, and healthy roofing and driveway materials.

### Make Sure Your Indoor Air Is Fresh

- Reduce or eliminate the toxic products and furnishing that pollute your indoor air. Open the windows daily and let the sun shine in.
- Equip your house with an energy recovery ventilator to provide fresh and filtered air at close to room temperature.
- House plants such as aloe vera, English ivy, ficus benjamina (fig) and the peace lily will

RICHARD SCHMIDT-ZUPER, ISTOCKPHOTO

remove at least some carcinogens, including formaldehyde and benzene.

- Install air filters and change them regularly.

## Make Sure Your Water Is Pure

Alas, it may be contaminated with pollutants such as chlorine and its by-products, cadmium, lead, flouride, VOCs, solvents and pesticides. As Athena Thompson says, "Ultimately, we must restore the purity of our water by dealing directly with the sources of toxins in our global environment. In the meantime, we must take the matter into our own hands by installing whole house and point-of-use water filtration systems."

## Home Furnishings

We recommend the use of:

- Healthy flooring options such as natural cork, linoleum with jute backing, engineered hardwood with ultra-low VOC finishes, natural stone tiles, pigmented concrete and area rugs made from natural fibers and non-toxic dyes, instead of carpets.
- Certified organic fabrics for bedding, towels and upholstered furniture; cotton or hemp shower curtains; certified organic window covering or naturally finished wood shutters, louvers or metallic venetian blinds.
- Natural wall finishes such as plaster and water-based zero- or low-VOC paints.
- Mattresses made from natural materials such as certified organic cotton or pure-grown wool; bed frames and kitchen cupboards made of wood that is free from toxic glues, particleboard and chemical stains.

- *Building for Health*, healthy and environmentally sound building materials and home comforts: www.buildingforhealth.com
- Building Green: www.buildinggreen.com
- Environmental Home Center: www.environmentalhomecenter.com
- *Guide to Less Toxic Products*: www.lesstoxicguide.ca
- *How to Grow Fresh Air: 50 Houseplants That Purify Your Home or Office* by Dr Bill Wolverton, Penguin, 1997.
- Kitchen water filters: www.consumersearch.com
- Toxic carpeting: www.holisticmed.com/carpet
- Treehugger: www.treehugger.com

## Is there a Bau•biologist in the house?

The primary focus of the relatively new science called Bau-Biologie — originally developed in Germany — is how buildings affect the health of their inhabitants and how to improve the health of both. Bau-biologists perform full-spectrum evaluations, based on measurable standards:

- Exposures to chemicals, both as shorter-term gases in the air (VOCs) and as longer-term molecules that attach to house dust.
- Building and finishing materials made of natural, renewable, biodegradable resources, which are considered more compatible with the human body.
- Exposures to micro-organisms, including mold and bacteria, and other micro air pollutants such as dust and dander.
- Thermal and moisture conditions.
- Electromagnetic fields, both man-made and natural
- Radiation from various sources, natural and man-made.

Bau-Biologie is a field with many facets and interpretations, says Debra Lynn Dadd, "but at its heart, it's about practical ways to support life, whether that be our own bodies or the larger ecosystems that sustain us."[2] (See bau-biologieusa.com)

# 7

# Clean Your Home Safely

*The easiest first step to creating a non-toxic home is to replace all the heavy-duty chemicals you use ... with simple, inexpensive and natural materials you probably already have in your kitchen.*
— Debra Lynn Dadd, *Home Safe Home*

There are two ways to keep your home as non-toxic and carcinogen-free as possible.

- Reduce traces of cancer-causing substances that hitchhike invisibly into your house via the air, water and food and aboard your feet.
- Stop buying products that contain carcinogens or that create carcinogens when you use them.

It will be impossible to prevent hazardous man-made substances from getting indoors until manufacturers go green. Until then, toxins will continue to travel far and wide and into our living spaces, but at least we can lessen the load:

- Leave your shoes at the door, because dirt tracked in on footwear nearly always carries toxic intruders such as pesticides, solvents and heavy metals.
- Dust is a major magnet for toxins, so mopping floors and cleaning carpets twice a week with a HEPA (high-efficiency particulate-absorbing) filter-equipped vacuum and dusting regularly with a clean, damp cloth are strongly advised.
- Buy carcinogen-free products. Given poor government regulation, this is easier said than done. We buy products in good faith believing them to be safe when used as directed, but this is a costly delusion. Many cleaners are laced with such "everyday" carcinogens as formaldehyde, nitrobenzene, methylene chloride, napthalene and perchlorethylene. Many household products also contain reproductive toxins or hormone

disruptors, while others cause liver, kidney and brain damage, allergies and asthma.

Please take this issue seriously — then take action. Entire books and websites have been devoted to healthy personal and home products for a good reason. Make *Home Safe Home* by Debra Lynn Dadd your bible of healthy, prudent home products.

You might expect cleaners, of all household products, at least to be *clean* — not carcinogenic. The *Guide to Less Toxic Products* will help you find out what's good, what's not so good and what should never be bought at all.

For the simplest approach, we recommend plain water, a spray bottle, a microfiber cloth and some elbow grease. This deceptively simple combination is good for dusting and shining just about everything in your house, especially hard surfaces. Your windows will be nearly as brilliant as the day they were glazed.

You can also make your own cleaners and polishes from scratch. It is a myth that the only cleaners that work must have a pungent chemical odor. You need just six ingredients:

- White distilled vinegar — disinfects and deodorizes.
- Lemon juice — cuts grease and polishes metal.
- Baking soda — has many cleaning and deodorizing uses.
- Washing soda — is a stronger alternative to baking soda.
- Borax — kills mold.
- Olive oil — mix with vinegar for furniture polish.

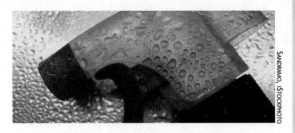
SANDRAMO, iSTOCKPHOTO

For specific cleaning tasks, see *Recipes for Safer Cleaners* at the Healthy Child, Healthy World website, where you'll find simple mixtures for cleaning kitchens, bathrooms, living rooms, floors, carpets and laundry, as well as metal polishes and air fresheners.

You can buy healthy cleaning products at a natural health store, or online from companies such as Seventh Generation (seventhgeneration.com), Nature Clean (natureclean.ca) or Ecover (ecover.com), one of the pioneers of healthy, eco-friendly cleaning products.

## Other Household Solutions

- Air fresheners: Often contain napthalene and formaldehyde. Try zeolite or natural fragrances from essential oils.
- Art supplies: Epoxy and rubber cement glues, acrylic paints and solvents, and permanent markers often contain carcinogens. See *The Healthy Artist's Guide to a Less Toxic Studio*: www.environmentaldefence.ca/toxicnation/artist/index.htm
- Automotive supplies: Most are toxic. Keep them safely away from the house and dispose safely at a hazardous waste disposal center.
- Candles: Avoid artificially scented paraffin candles that produce combustion by-products, including soot. Beeswax only, with cotton wicks.
- Carpet and upholstery shampoos: Use only wet-clean, natural ingredients.
- Dry-cleaning: Choose clothes that don't need perchlorethylene to clean them. Ask for

- CancerSmart Consumer Guide: www.leas.ca/CancerSmart-Consumer-Guide.htm
- Chemical Glossary: www.lifekind.com/catalog/chemical_glossary.php
- Debra Lynn Dadd's *Home Safe Home*: www.dld123.com
- Environmental Home Center: www.environmentalhomecenter.com
- *Guide to Less Toxic Products:* www.lesstoxicguide.ca
- Microfiber cleaning cloths: www.ecomall.com/greenshopping/micro.htm
- *Recipes for Safer Cleaners:* www.healthychild.org
- *Safe Substitutes at Home: Non-toxic Household Products:* http://es.epa.gov/techinfo/facts/safe-fs.html
- Simple, sustainable living: www.eartheasy.com
- US EPA: www.epa.gov: search "indoor air quality" and "volatile organic compounds"

the wet-cleaning option at your local cleaners, or seek dry-cleaners that use liquid CO2 or citrus juice cleaners.

- Flea, tick and lice control: Avoid lindane-based pesticides. Search online for "natural flea control."
- Paints and varnishes: Always choose low- or no-VOC finishes.
- Household pesticides: Go natural! See www.panna.org/resources/advisor.dv.html
- Microwaves: *Never* microwave or heat food in a plastic container.

Plastics: Avoid polyvinyl chloride (PVC) products and PVC plasticizers, DEHP, phthalates; polyethylene; Teflon-coated kitchenware (C-8, a suspected carcinogen), styrene products, and acrylic plastics from acrylonitrile.

- Safe plastics: www.care2.com/channels/solutions/guides/473
- Spot removers: www.care2.com/channels/solutions/home/559

For every toxic household problem, there *is* a solution.

# 8

## Treat Your Garden with TLC, not 2,4-D

> Show me your garden and I shall tell you what you are.
>
> — Alfred Austin

Remember, it's a *garden*, not a battlefield. Many North Americans spray-bomb their lawns, flowerbeds and vegetable patches with copious quantities of pesticides, as if dandelions were a mortal enemy. There are several other toxic booby traps in many backyards, too.

It's time to declare peace throughout your land.

### Say Adios to Lawn and Garden Pesticides

If you want to understand why it's so important to go pesticide-free, read *Pesticides and Human Health: A Resource for Health Care Professionals*, by Physicians for Social Responsibility and Californians for Pesticide Reform. Despite its title, the 60-page report is written in plain, understandable, convincing language at www.pesticidereform.org.

If it's your heart's desire, you *can* have a gorgeous, lush, healthy lawn — without a particle of poison. For starters, apply these 3 simple steps:

1. Mow high, using a mulch mower.
2. Water infrequently, but deeply.
3. Over-seed in springtime.

For more details, visit www.organiclawncaretips.com. If you don't want to spend the whole summer "doing the grass," go to *Organic Lawn Care for the Cheap and Lazy*: www.richsoil.com/lawn.

To gradually eliminate lawn weeds without poisons, try corn gluten, a non-toxic by-product of corn processing. It kills weed seedlings within days of application and adds nitrogen to the soil. One application before weeds emerge reduces their survival by about 60%, according to Iowa State University research. After several years of consistent application, corn gluten can provide up to 90% weed control.[1]

For your flowers and veggies, there are many non-toxic and less-toxic options to ward off the predators, but not beneficial bugs. Our favorite — mainly because of the name, we admit — is Holy Terra Products, with its all-natural Anti-Pest-O products that "repel rather than kill" insects: www.antipesto.biz (Keep checking, it's not available in Canada or western US yet).

### Step off the Gas

Every spring and summer weekend, 50 million Americans and (once the snow melts) several million Canadians mow their lawns using a whopping 800 million US gallons of gasoline a year.[2] Gas mowers are not just annoyingly noisy; they are far more polluting than cars per hour, and they also emit carcinogens such as benzene

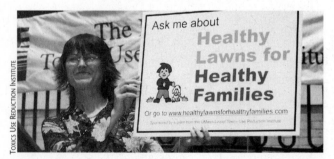

TOXICS USE REDUCTION INSTITUTE

Tessa David, Director of the North Central Regional Solid Waste Cooperative, holds up a poster about the Town of Westford, Massachusett's pesticide-free lawn care project, funded by the Toxics Use Reduction Institute (TURI).

- Carolyn Herriot, *A Year on the Garden Path: A 52-Week Guide to Organic Gardening*, New Society Publishers, 2006: www.earthfuture.com/gardenpath
- Backyard burning: www.epa.gov/msw/backyard
- Canadians Against Pesticides Green Alternatives: www.caps.20m.com/alternatives.htm
- CCA wood alternatives: www.toronto.ca/health/factsheet_ptw.htm
- Carole Rubin, *How to Get Your Lawn and Garden Off Drugs*, Harbour, 2003.
- Least Toxic and Non-Toxic Alternatives: www.pesticideinfo.org/Alternatives.html
- Ozone water treatment: www.mainstreamozone.com/ozonefaqs.shtml
- Ten Ways to Go Organic: www.bbc.co.uk/gardening/basics/techniques/organic_tenwaysorganic.shtml

and 1,3 butadiene. The same goes for gas-powered weed whackers and leaf blowers. The new generation of manual lawn mowers are lightweight and far easier to push than their ancient predecessors. They tackle two cancer-related problems at the same time: more exercise for the pusher, and no airborne pollutants for the neighborhood.

## Grow Organic Food

The healthiest food is ripe, freshly picked organic food, so why not grow it yourself? Even a window box can raise a crop of organic tomatoes. If you have never grown food before, try an easy book such as *A Year on the Garden Path* to get you started. You'll learn that it's all about building your soil with compost, manure and leaf mulch so that plants are strong and healthy and resist pests. It's also about encouraging the bugs and beetles so that they keep each other in balance. It's about working *with* Nature, instead of against her.

## Ban the Burn Barrel

A 2005 *New York Times* story reported that burn barrels are the largest source of dioxin emissions in the nation — and dioxins, in case you'd forgotten, are among the most toxic chemicals ever created.[3] At least 14 states, including Maine, New Mexico and California, have banned the backyard burning of domestic wastes.

## Avoid Pressure-treated Wood

Healthy Child, Healthy World suggests testing the soil around wood treated with chromated copper arsenate (CCA), covering deck play areas with blankets and making sure children wash their hands if they've had contact. Replace CCA-treated wood with safer alternatives such as naturally rot-resistant domestic woods, for example, cedar, redwood or black locust.

## Say No to Plastic Grass

Really, just say no. Plastic grass — a polyethylene-polypropylene blend — is fashioned from finite fossil fuels.[4] (And what on Earth is the dog supposed to do?)

## Choose Healthy Pools and Hot Tubs

Chlorinated water produces toxic by-products, including trihalomethanes (THMs) and chloroform. You can avoid these by using Earth- and body-friendly treatments for your pool and spa — ozone and salt water are two alternatives to explore. They may be more expensive at the outset, but healthier over the long term. Another option highly recommended by healthy-home guru Debra Lynn Dadd is a chlorine-free combination that uses a water conditioner and hydrogen peroxide.[5]

# 9

# Minimize Your Exposure to Radiation

Despite its immense usefulness, medical exposure [to ionizing radiation] is a cause for concern because of its magnitude, because its use is growing so rapidly and because so much of it is unnecessary.

— Catherine Caulfield[1]

All forms of radiation — especially ionizing radiation, which is cumulative throughout our lives — contribute to our burden of cancer. The larger the dose, the greater the risk.

We can't escape small, steady doses of "background" ionizing radiation that reach Earth from the sun and distant stars, or — down here on solid ground — are emitted from rocks, soil, water and even the most wholesome food. People who live or fly regularly at high altitudes are more exposed than others, but we're all awash in this natural radioactivity. And yes, it does cause a small percentage of our human cancers.

## Radon Gas

One naturally occurring source of ionizing radiation that we *can* escape, more or less, is radon gas, a naturally occurring carcinogen that can migrate from some types of rock into the lower levels of our homes in gaseous form, or through water supplies. Elevated levels of radon have been found in all 50 American states, so the US government recommends annual home testing. Canadians, who are generally less aware of this hazard, should also take note and check their homes and workplaces regularly. "Seal tight, ventilate right" is the byword.

## Man-made Radioactivity

We advise paying special attention to the medical uses of ionizing radiation, including mammograms for breast cancer screening, x-rays, commuted tomography (CT) scans and other applications of nuclear medicine, which account for more than 90% of our average lifetime exposure to man-made ionizing radiation.[2]

- Take seriously all medical x-rays, especially CT scans[3] for children,[4] and other forms of nuclear medicine. We tend to be very casual about this form of ionizing radiation and wrongly assume it's risk-free.

- Since ionizing radiation exposure is cumulative, we need a complete record kept from birth onwards to provide an up-to-date sum of our lifetime exposure to radiation. (Remember those wallet cards listing all your childhood vaccinations?) The US FDA offers a rudimentary X-Ray Record Card as a model (see box): Medical radiation information should be digitalized, with electronic storage and retrieval of images in a secure, central database so that repeat x-rays are not required.

- Ask to know the exposure information when you are asked for an x-ray, as a basic right, and ask about safety measures. Make sure that parts of the body not being x-rayed, especially the breasts and genitals, are carefully shielded.

- Women should demand non-ionizing radiation alternatives to screening mammography, such as thermography, MRIs and transillumination procedures, in combination with thorough, competent clinical breast exams and correct self-examination techniques. Until suitable, safer alternatives to mammography are available, women must demand that screening mammography not begin until age 50, since the evidence shows few benefits.[5]

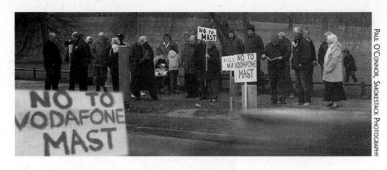

PAUL O'CONNOR, SMOKESTACK PHOTOGRAPHY

Demonstrators in Britain campaign against the installation of cellphone antennas.

## Electro-magnetic Radiation (EMR)

At the opposite end of the electromagnetic spectrum from powerful gamma, beta and x-rays is non-ionizing energy, which is mostly *man-made*. We're swimming in radio waves and microwaves, and with new electronic gizmos appearing with dizzying regularity, our exposure to non-ionizing EMR keeps rising.

There is no indisputable link between cancer and radio frequency or microwave energy, but there is sufficient evidence of a connection to childhood leukemia, breast and brain cancer to warrant "prudent avoidance."

The good news is that exposure to EMR can be reduced. With precaution as your watchword, and the aid of a good EMF detector (such as the Trifield), you or a trained technician can check the areas in your home or office where you spend the most time. In *Homes That Heal and Those that Don't*, Athena Thompson counseled that bedrooms, especially, should be as free of EMR as possible, with low electric and magnetic fields. It is also wise to check these electrical sources:

- Power lines into your home
- Electric razors, hair dryers, blenders, coffee grinders, microwaves and other kitchen appliances
- Televisions, and other home entertainment equipment
- Computers, printers, copiers, fax machines, scanners and CD/DVD burners
- Clock radios in the bedroom, electric blankets and waterbeds, in-floor or ceiling electric heating

## Cellphones and Power Lines

While research continues to determine the long-term safety of cellphones, these recommendations make sense:

- Where possible, use a corded (not portable) land-line telephone for day-to-day communications. Use cellphones only for emergencies.
- Avoid using digital cordless phones that radiate continuously even when not in use.[6]
- If you do use a cellphone, use an earpiece/headset on the speakerphone setting. Text messaging is also a good way to reduce exposure.
- Turn your cellphone off when not it's in use. Even in "standby mode" it periodically radiates energy.
- Avoid living near a cellphone transmitter tower; the evidence of harm is enough to warrant great caution.

- *Citizen's Guide to Protecting Yourself and Your Family From Radon*: www.epa.gov/radon/pubs/citguide.html
- Mammography Screening and New Technologies; www.bcaction.org/Pages/GetInformed/MammographyAndNewTech.html
- SARVALUES Facts and Figures on Cellular Phone Radiation: www.sarvalues.com
- Trifield EMF meter: www.trifield.com/EMF_meter.htm
- What Is Nuclear Medicine?: www.umm.edu/radiology/nucmed.htm
- X-Ray Record Card: www.fda.gov/cdrh/consumer/record_card.pdf

# 10

# Make a Difference

I have, despite all disillusionment, never,
ever, allowed myself to feel like giving up.
This is my message today: it is not worthy
of a human being to give up.

— Alva Myrdal, winner of the
1982 Nobel Peace Prize

A young girl is walking along a beach at low tide, picking up stranded starfish one at a time and tossing them into the water. An older man comes along and says, "Why are you wasting your time? Tomorrow the beach will be covered again with starfish. You won't make any difference." "Oh, no?" the little girl replies. She picks up a starfish and tosses it into the sea. "See? It made a difference to that one."

Here are ten steps you can take for cancer prevention:

## Step 1. Read the Best Books about Environmental Links to Health

- *Silent Spring* by Rachel Carson, published in 1962, is astonishingly prophetic 45 years later. The chapter "One in Every Four" discloses a fact about the early 1960s that was almost unthinkable at the time — that one in every four Americans was destined to contract cancer at some point in their lives. Today, more than a third of women and nearly half of all men in Canada and the US will be diagnosed with cancer at some point in their lives; one in four will die from the disease. In the 45 years since *Silent Spring*, we have tragically neglected to heed Carson's advice and seize the golden opportunity for cancer *prevention*.

- *Living Downstream: A Scientist's Personal Investigation of Cancer and the Environment* was written by the poet and biologist Sandra Steingraber, who is worthy in every sense to be called this generation's Rachel Carson. In her own words: "*Living Downstream* was written not only to scrutinize evidence with a scientist's disinterested objectivity, but also to remind us all — scientists and non-scientists alike — that behind every data point is a human life."

- *Our Stolen Future: Are We Threatening Our Fertility, Intelligence, and Survival?* is a scientific detective story by Theo Colborn, Dianne Dumanoski and John Peterson Myers (Dutton 1996). Colburn has been pioneering the research about hormone disruption and is one of the true heroes of our time. See www.ourstolenfuture.org.

## Step 2. Demand Non-toxic Alternatives

Make good use of toll-free telephone numbers on everyday products that have dangerous ingredients in them. Choose safer products for use in your home and share good info with your family and friends.

- *The Guide to Less Toxic Products*: www.lesstoxicguide.ca
- *Safe Substitutes at Home: Non-toxic Household Products*: http://es.epa.gov/techinfo/facts/safe-fs.html

## Step 3. Write Letters to the Newspapers and to Governments

Ask what cancer societies and health institutions in your community are doing to *prevent* cancer, and offer suggestions from this book. Send a copy of your correspondence to other levels of government. Let your elected representatives know that primary prevention is the single best way to reduce the epidemic rates of cancer we're experiencing.

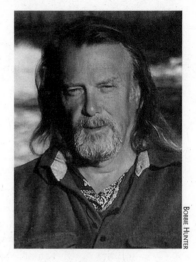

Bob Hunter was the intrepid co-founder of Greenpeace, a fearless and funny journalist, and a passionate environmentalist all his life. He died in 2005 at age 63 of prostate cancer.

BOBBIE HUNTER

### Step 4. Use Your Consumer Clout

Use your consumer clout and encourage your friends and neighbors to do the same. Buy local, fresh organic food. Join a Community Supported Agriculture or brown box group. If neighborhood stores aren't supplying organic produce, speak up — your voice and dollars will make a big difference. Alternatively, start a local buying club with friends and family to purchase healthy food at economical prices, and obtain the safest possible consumer products of all kinds that are not available locally.

- Community Supported Agriculture: www.nal.usda.gov/afsic/csa
- Buying Clubs USA: www.allspecies.org/neigh/foodbuyclub.htm
- Buying Clubs Canada: www.life.ca/nl/63/food.html

### Step 5. Join a Cancer Prevention Action Group

- Prevent Cancer Now (Canada): www.preventcancernow.ca
- Cancer Prevention Coalition: www.preventcancer.com
- The Breast Cancer Fund: www.breastcancerfund.org
- Breast Cancer Action: www.bcaction.org

### Step 6. Organize Your Own Cancer Prevention Action Group

You could start by obtaining one of the videos listed in Solution 25 and inviting your friends to watch it with you. Then discuss a plan of action.

### Step 7. Get Involved Politically

For starters, vote in every election: it *does* make a difference. Join a political party and work with others to write cancer prevention action resolutions for its policy platform. Tell your elected representatives about this book; better yet, give them a copy. Donate another copy to your local cancer agency.

### Step 8. Plan to Leave a Healthy Legacy

There's a lot of work to do, and it would be good to know that your intentions lived on after your death by making a generous bequest to a cancer prevention group.

### Step 9. Never Give Up on the Quest for Cancer Prevention

We need to "de-normalize" cancer, just as earlier generations de-normalized slavery, smallpox and — more recently — smoking in public places. If not us, who?

### Step 10. Have a Natural Funeral

Carcinogenic embalming fluid, with its use of cancer-causing formaldehyde, is a very *un*healthy legacy to leave.

- *You Can't Take It With You*: www.nrdc.org/onearth/04win/briefings.asp
- The Natural Death Centre: www.naturaldeath.org.uk

# 11
# Create a Healthy Pregnancy

If we want to have good health for the whole of our lives, and if we want to protect the health of our children, we can start early — before we conceive the next generation.[1]

— Sat Dharam Kaur, ND

A healthy pregnancy *and* cancer prevention both begin well before that remarkable moment when sperm meets egg.

It's apparent that later life cancers may originate from prenatal exposures (see p. 14), but the hazards do not always fall neatly into pre- and post-conception time slots. The harm to an infant's health can sometimes begin before conception, from damage to the mother's egg or father's sperm — or perhaps from chemical

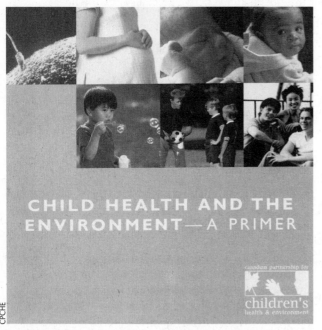

CPCHE

The cover of the excellent resource, *Child Health and the Environment — A Primer,* by the Canadian Partnership for Children's Health and Environment (www.healthyenvironmentforkids.ca)

exposures several generations prior, as the emerging science of epigenetics reveals.[2]

Would-be parents of both sexes need to protect themselves from workplace hazards,[3] eat healthy — preferably organic — food with a minimum of meat, drink plenty of pure water, and make their home a safe place to conceive and raise children. Some health professionals suggest detoxifying with saunas and juice fasts to improve the likelihood of successful conception and to reduce the burden of toxic chemicals that may later affect your baby-to-be.

Now let's suppose you're already pregnant. Our best advice is to swear personal, unswerving allegiance to the precautionary principle throughout your pregnancy, and (ideally) forever. The mistaken belief that a fetus is protected by the placenta was shattered by the tragedies of thalidomide and diethylstilbestrol (DES), drugs prescribed to pregnant women decades ago.[4] We now know that developing infants are exposed to virtually all the pollutants that circulate and are stored in the blood and tissues of their mothers: "The umbilical cord carries not only the building blocks of life, but also a steady stream of industrial chemicals, pollutants and pesticides that cross the placenta as readily as residues from cigarettes and alcohol"*(Body Burden: The Pollution in Newborns).*[5] (See p. 4.)

It is not possible to keep all man-made pollutants out of our bodies — that won't happen until they are banned forever from air, water, soil, food and consumer products. But there are many ways to reduce your exposure, and your developing infant's:

- The *First Steps Program* by biologist, mother and cancer survivor Sandra Steingraber, is based on advice in her superb book, *Having Faith: An Ecologist's Journey to Motherhood*.[6] It is sponsored by Healthy Child, Healthy World, which has many more outstanding resources for parents and babies at all stages of development: www.healthychild.org

- *10 Steps to Reduce Risks If You're Pregnant*: www.thegreenguide.com (Search "Pregnancy Risks")

Some other advice while you're pregnant:

- Reduce indoor air pollutants. Keep your house well ventilated and use simple, home-made cleaners (see Solution 7). *Home Safe Home*: www.dld123.com

- Don't smoke, and eliminate all exposure to second-hand smoke.

- Remove your carpets if possible, and replace with healthy flooring (see Solution 6).

- Avoid home improvement projects that require the use of hazardous materials.

- Eat organic, fresh, local food whenever possible. Pay attention to freshwater fish advisories for pregnant women, and restrict consumption. If you do eat meat, trim fat even from organically raised meat products.

- Don't use toxic pesticides on the lawn or in your home. There are many better choices.

- Avoid solvents in dry-cleaning fluids, gasoline, spot removers and carpet cleaners. Stay away from fresh paint.

- Find out about releases of industrial pollutants in your community.
  For the US: www.scorecard.org.
  For Canada: www.pollutionwatch.org

- "Recognize that that you have an intimate relationship with tap water whether you drink it or not. Breathing, not drinking, is our main route of volatile pollutants in tap water" (Sandra Steingraber).

- Avoid traffic exhaust, refueling your car (benzene) and diesel emissions.

- While you wait for your new arrival, join the Coming Clean campaign for organic personal care products: www.organicconsumers.org/bodycare.

---

- The *Health Before Pregnancy Environment Checklist* offers commonsense advice on air quality, food, everyday chemicals and renovations to avoid during the crucial preconception period: www.healthbeforepregnancy.ca

- For more information on preconception health care, see the Center for Occupational and Environmental Medicine: www.coem.com

- The June 15, 2002 edition of *American Family Physician* addresses a wide variety of maternal health issues, including environmental exposures: www.aafp.org

- Foresight — The Association for the Promotion of Preconceptual Care is packed full of useful information: www.foresight-preconception.org.uk

# 12

# Create a Healthy Home for Your Baby

The precautionary principle has been around a long time, probably as long as human mothers... It's the credo that prompts us to buckle seat belts, get out of the pool when lightning flashes, and throw away the mysterious leftovers discovered in the back of the refrigerator.

— Sandra Steingraber

Infants and children are not just small adults. They absorb more toxic substances because, pound for pound, they eat, drink and breathe more than grown-ups do. Children live closer to the ground where toxins often accumulate in higher concentrations than they do up in adult territory. Your baby's kidneys and liver — the body's main detoxing organs — and its immune system do not function fully at birth, so the less exposure to toxic products at this earliest stage of life, the better.

The last skill you might put on a list called "The Top Ten Most Useful Talents for Brand New Parents" would be Becoming a Household Detective. (Maybe later, when they're teens...) However, it is essential to scrutinize your home with great care well before your new baby arrives to make it as non-toxic as possible, so get out your magnifying glass.

You don't have to start from scratch, because Healthy Child, Healthy World, based in Los Angeles, has a terrific resource called *The Household Detective* that offers practical information on how to protect infants and children from toxins at home. It includes chapters on household cleaners, toys, art supplies, pest control, air quality, food and water, pets, "toxic trash" and a superb compilation of resources to help parents locate non-toxic alternatives. The fee for membership includes a copy of the handbook. *The Household Detective* also deals with issues related to asthma, allergies, autism, ADHD and other health problems that burden far too many of today's kids.

Or you can solve the major toxic "crimes" in the household yourself:

- Cribs, mattresses and bedding: Go for natural products, such as 100% wooden cribs with no chemical preservatives or finishes, or buy second-hand at yard sales and freshen up with a heavy metal-free, no-VOC (volatile organic compound) paint. Choose certified organic cotton and wools for the mattress, and formaldehyde-free crib blankets and sheets, not perma-pressed or treated with toxic flame-retardants.

- Carpets and flooring: Remove the carpets and replace them with wood floors finished with no-VOC products, natural linoleum, a green flooring product such as cork, as long as the veneers are not backed with vinyl or binders like formaldehyde, or area rugs made from natural materials (not petroleum) that

## CAUTION: Don't use "anti-bacterial" cleaners

There *are* some good, useful germs, so don't scrub down the nursery with cleaners containing "germicidals" and "anti-bacterials." The excellent book *Green Living* explains that infants need both good bacteria and bad to prime their immature immune systems. "Germ-killing soaps are unnecessary and even risky. Most anti-bacterials contain pesticides and, sometimes, even formaldehyde...A common ingredient, triclosan, actually mutates the genes of the bacteria, raising concerns about the creation of 'superbugs' and antibiotic resistance."[1] For "hot spots" — kitchen counters, baby's change table — that need to be disinfected, try a natural botanical product such as Benefect (www.benefect.com).

are easily washed with water (not dry-cleaned) and/or vacuumed regularly. Use a HEPA (high-efficiency particle arrester) vacuum cleaner to gobble up — and not redistribute — the toxic dust that is part of daily living.

- Paints, wallpapers and window coverings: Stay away from PVC plastics. Go for environmentally and baby-friendly paints.

- Electromagnetic fields: Best-case scenario is no electrical equipment close to your baby at all. Do your best to place the crib away from electrical currents. Check levels with a Gauss meter (see Solution 9).

- Toys: Avoid plastics, especially soft toys containing PVC or hormone-disrupting phthalates. Go for all-natural fiber and wooden products.

- Baby clothes: Aim for 100% certified organic fibers. Hand-me-downs washed in natural soaps are also a good choice.

- Diapers: If you can find a diaper service offering chlorine-free laundering and organic, all-cotton products, sign up! See www.diaperpin.com

- Personal care products for babies: At the time of writing, there were no regulations defining the word "organic" for personal care products for babies or adults. So be a healthy skeptic when it comes to words like "all-natural," "organic" and "healthy." Seek out trusted sources such as Debra Lynn Dadd's *Home Safe Home*: www.dld123.com.

- Canadian Partnership for Children's Health and Environment: www.healthyenvironmentforkids.ca
- *Children's Environmental Health Resource Sampler*: www.phpartners.org/cehir/sampler.html
- *The Green Guide: Better Basics for Your Baby's Room*, Issue 102, May-June 2004. Also offers information on furniture, clothing, paints, varnishes and cleaning products (Subscription fee): www.thegreenguide.com
- Green Home: www.chec.greenhome.com/products
- *Guide to Natural Baby Care: Non-toxic and Environmentally Friendly Ways to Take Care of Your New Child* by Mindy Pennybacker and Aisha Ikramuddin, John Wiley & Sons, 1999
- Healthy Child, Healthy World: www.healthychild.org
- *Out of Harm's Way: Preventing Toxic Threats to Child Development — Personal Guidelines for Parents and Future Parents*: www.psr.org
- *Ten Steps to Our Children's Toxic-Free Future*: www.safer-products.org

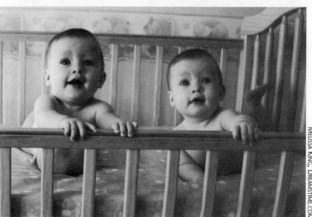

MELISSA KING, DREAMSTIME.COM

Among many 'healthy home' issues for babies is electro-magnetic radiation (EMR). Tip #1: Since magnetic fields penetrate through walls, a computer at the adjacent wall in the room next to the crib may expose your baby to magnetic fields. Tip #2: Avoid buying radio-powered toys for children; instead find ones with wires attached.

# 13

# Breastfeed Your Baby

Why is breast milk best? For starters, human babies are far less mature at birth than the offspring of most mammals, and their body systems — including digestion and immunity — develop best when fed milk from their own species.

There's much more: Human breast milk is alive and brimming with immune boosters and anti-infective agents. It contains living cells that actually "eat" germs and is one of the few

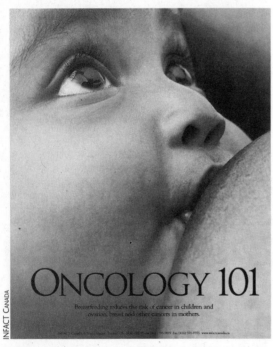

ONCOLOGY 101

Breastfeeding reduces the risk of cancer in children and ovarian, breast and other cancers in mothers.

"Breastfeeding reduces the risk of cancer in children and ovarian and other cancers in mothers."
INFACT Canada

The promoters of infant formula often proclaim that their latest blend is "closer than ever to breast milk." Dr. Jack Newman, a Toronto pediatrician and passionate advocate of breast-feeding, responds with some basic geography: "Yes," he says, "closer than ever. Just like Montreal is closer to Vancouver than Halifax is."

substances that can attack viruses. Further, breast milk is always free, constantly the right temperature and convenient, especially in the middle of the night. For a lyrical and scientific summary of the merits of human milk, we recommend *Having Faith: An Ecologist's Journey to Motherhood*, by Sandra Steingraber.

For new mothers who are unable to breast-feed their babies, another emerging option is donated human milk, collected and pasteurized at a regional "milk bank." Once a common practice, present-day milk banks at the Children's and Women's Health Care Centre in Vancouver, British Columbia, and the Mothers' Milk Bank in Austin, Texas, are at the forefront of a welcome revival.

On the whole, breast-fed infants grow up to be more intelligent and less obese than their formula-fed peers; they have fewer allergies, less asthma and a decreased incidence of heart disease and diabetes. And cancer? Breast-fed daughters have lower rates of breast cancer when they grow up, and mother's milk also protects against some childhood cancers, particularly leukemia.[1] Moms who have breast-fed their infants also benefit by incurring lower rates of breast and ovarian cancers.

Despite these remarkable advantages for both babies and their mothers, a depressing fact of life, especially in industrialized countries, is that the lipids (fats) in human breast milk are contaminated with trace pollutants that have hitchhiked up the food chain into all of our bodies and concentrate in fatty cells, including mother's milk.

- *Child Health and the Environment — A Primer*:
  www.healthyenvironmentforkids.ca
- *In Harm's Way: Toxic Threats to Child Development*:
  http://psr.igc.org/ihw-project.htm
- Infant Feeding Action Coalition of Canada:
  www.infactcanada.ca

Most persistent toxic substances are lipophilic — they cling to fat molecules and become more concentrated the higher they go. As Sandra Steingraber points out, human adults are not at the top of the food chain — a lactating mother's breast is. This means that breast milk has a higher concentration of toxic substances than any other food. Restoring the purity of breast milk is surely the best reason there is for applying the precautionary principle to prevent hazardous and potentially cancer-causing substances in the first place.

So, what's a new mother to do in the meantime? Answer: continue to breast-feed. The authors of the landmark Environmental Working Group study, *Mothers' Milk*, which found record levels of toxic fire retardants in the breast milk of 20 first-time American moms, are unequivocal: "The evidence is clear: Women should breast-feed their children and continue to do so for as long as possible...Breastfeeding may even reverse some of the damage caused by chemical exposures in the womb."[2]

When toxic substances are prohibited, their presence in breast milk soon declines. As the 2005 *Child Health and the Environment Primer* explains: "While DDT and PCBs are still found in breast milk, levels have declined steadily since these substances were discontinued and/or banned in the 1970s. Dioxin levels have also dropped in breast milk, alongside and following regulatory controls."[3]

In Sweden and other European countries, levels of toxic fire-retardants (PDBEs) in breast milk, which began to increase in the 1970s, are now falling in the wake of a ban in the late 1990s. In Canada and the United States (other than California), where controls are less stringent, trace amounts of these contaminants continue to increase in human milk. The message doesn't get much simpler: We must act quickly with much safer substitutes.

Although the lipids in most infant formulas are from sources lower on the food chain than human milk, there are other concerns about breast milk substitutes:

- Mixing formula powders with drinking water can expose babies to a variety of contaminants. As the Environmental Working Groups pointed out, "Infants under four months of age get more than seven times the dose of chemicals in tap water than an adult would get."[4] Chlorine by-products, pesticides, solvents, nitrates and arsenic are among chemicals of concern in many tap water supplies. Effective home water filters are a must.
- Polycarbonate plastic baby bottles can leach the hormone disruptor bisphenol-A (BPA) into formula when heated.[5] Opt for good old-fashioned glass baby bottles instead. (Google on "Evenflo Glass Baby Bottles")

When it comes to getting our babies off to the very best start in life, pure and untainted breast milk is their birthright — and our first responsibility.

# 14

# Feed Your Kids Organic Whole Foods

Here are the top three reasons why organic food is best for babies (and all of us):

1. It reduces exposure to chemical pesticides.
2. There is evidence that organic food can protect us against cancer (see p. 42).
3. It's wiser to err on the side of precaution — to be safe rather than sorry.

We add these two extra morsels of advice:

- Set a great example for your kids by eating well yourself.
- Develop a thick skin.

- Downloadable wallet card of foods with the most pesticide residues: www.foodnews.org
- Eating Organic for Less than Processed Food: www.mercola.com/2005/feb/16/organic_food.htm
- Environmental Working Group: www.ewg.org (search Food Safety)
- *Good Stuff — Baby Products*: www.worldwatch.org/node/1478
- *Guide to Food Additives*: www.cspinet.org/reports/chemcuisine.htm
- Healthy Snacks: www.enviroalternatives.com/foodsnacks.html
- No Splenda or Aspartame: www.generationgreen.org/2005-01_lead-story.htm
- *Organic: A Choice for Our Children*: www.drgreene.com/21_868.html
- Organic Food and Pesticide Residues: www.consumerreports.org

When you choose organic, you're not only protecting your family's health, you're helping to protect the environment, too. The environment is our groundwater ... it's our world. Organic is healthy for farmers, healthy for plants, healthy for animals, and healthy for kids. It's a legacy we can feel good about leaving to future generations.

— Dr Alan Greene

This last advice is obvious but often overlooked. "Do as I do, not just as I say" will pay big dividends for both you and your kids. And the thick skin? You'll need it to fend off the billions of dollars' worth of advertising aimed directly at your children to lure them into consuming sugary, low-nutrient fast food that's contaminated with pesticides.

"For every $1 spent by the World Health Organization on trying to improve the nutrition of the world's population, $500 is spent by the food industry on promoting processed food" (International Association of Consumer Food Organizations).[1] So be prepared to be relentlessly badgered for junk food "treats" when your toddler starts watching TV and sets off to kindergarten.

News Flash! *Healthy food for kids doesn't have to be boring!* It can be delicious, packed with good nutrition and fun to eat. Snacks such as berry blends, smoothies with fresh peaches and yogurt, fruit kabobs and seasoned nut and seed mixes can all leave kids smiling and satisfied.

Dr. Alan Greene, the Palo Alto, California-based pediatrician whose website, www.DrGreene.com, gets several million hits a month, is an organic food advocate. In *Organic: A Choice for Our Children*, he offers practical suggestions about feeding kids healthy foods and says "fun presentation" really helps: "Preschool children often love food that is shaped like something interesting — a face, a clown, a dinosaur, a favorite hero, etc." He adds, "When all else fails, sneak it in. Make zucchini bread, carrot muffins. Add shaved vegetables or pieces of fruit to virtually any baked good."[2]

One of the keys is to start children on the path to lifelong healthy food habits as soon as they're ready for their first pureed mouthful. Mothers and Others for a Livable Planet's *Guide to Natural Baby Care* recommends that parents go organic when making the transition to baby's first food. Commercial products such as Earth's Best and Gerber's Tender Harvest win their applause, as does homemade fare, which is not as labor-intensive as it may sound. (Got a blender? Go!)

Organic foods are becoming more and more widely available, and prices are coming down. Careful bulk shopping for fresh, whole food will actually lower your grocery bill if you've previously been buying mostly processed foods.[3]

One final piece of advice: Urge your local cancer society to recommend organic fruits, veggies and other whole foods. It's good for all of us, and the planet too.

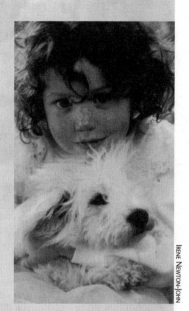

Nancy and Jim Chuda of California did everything possible to protect the health of their young daughter, Colette. They even fed her organic baby food produced by Nancy's own baby-food company, Baby's Choice. But at age four, Colette was diagnosed with a rare cancer known as Wilm's Tumor, and died in 1991 at five years of age. Genetic testing showed that Colette's cancer was not inherited. The Chudas suspected environmental contamination, a hunch that was given credence by a study associating Wilm's Tumor with pesticide exposure.[6] The Chudas transformed their grief into action by creating a coalition now called Healthy Child, Healthy World, dedicated to protecting children by eliminating environmental toxins including pesticides on food. See www.healthychild.org

Colette Chuda

IRENE NEWTON-JOHN

University of Washington researchers tracked a group of preschool children — 18 with organic diets and 21 with conventional diets — and analyzed their urine for evidence of exposure to five different kinds of toxic pesticides. They found that the average total was six- to almost nine times higher for children with conventional diets than for children with organic diets. Conclusion? Consuming organic fruits and vegetables can provide a relatively simple means for parents to reduce their children's pesticide exposure.[4]

# 15

## Take Action for Healthy Schools

**Studies show that one-half of our nation's schools have problems linked to indoor air quality. Students, teachers and staff are at greater risk because of the hours spent in school facilities and because children are especially susceptible to pollutants.**

**— Environmental Protection Agency (EPA).[1]**

Just how quickly kids get exposed to toxins in school became clear when the ABC Television show *Good Morning America* conducted an experiment in a classroom at P.S. 8 in New York City in October 2005.

> **First, we applied Glo-Germ, a non-toxic powder only visible under ultra-violet light, in areas where pesticides are most likely to be sprayed or settle, like baseboards, windowsills and desktops. Then we invited the kids to play. After only 20 minutes, we showed them the stunning results. Using UV light, we found traces of Glo-Germ all over their clothes, hands and faces.[2]**

### How to know if your school has environmental problems

❑ The building is new or newly renovated, and smells like paint, varnish or glue.
❑ The building is fully carpeted.
❑ Your child goes to school healthy, but comes home ill, cranky or exhausted.
❑ Your child comes home with odors clinging to his or her clothing.
❑ Building maintenance and repair costs are often cut at budget time.
❑ Fumes are seeping into the building.
❑ The building and grounds are routinely treated with pesticide sprays.
❑ Construction work is messy, and debris surrounds the school.

Cleaning up schools is critical to good health. More than 50 million students and 5 million teachers and support staff in the US are exposed daily to radon, asbestos, chemical fumes, pesticides, molds, lead and other toxins.[3] These are just a handful of many health-threatening problems found in and around our children's schools.

In addition to cancer, there are a host of environmentally linked health and learning woes facing today's students — asthma, attention deficit disorders, autism, allergies, and so on. The good news is that, when risks associated with cancer are addressed, the triggers for many other disorders are also reduced or eliminated.

Here are some of the cancer prevention actions that all schools should act on:

- Reduce diesel bus emissions, e.g., siting of drop-off areas, unnecessary idling.
- Eliminate toxic products used for cleaning and maintenance.
- Eliminate toxic art supplies.
- Stop all pesticide use, indoors and out.
- Protect against radon.
- Eliminate asbestos.
- Phase out the use of polyvinyl chloride (PVC).
- Improve indoor air quality. Eliminate chemical off-gassing from carpets, paints, flooring, cabinets, etc.
- Eliminate chromium copper arsenate from wooden playground equipment.
- Eliminate electromagnetic radiation from the siting of radio or cell towers at schools.
- Control dust (the purveyor of many toxic substances).

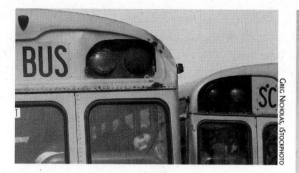

GREG NICHOLAS, ISTOCKPHOTO

- Avoid proximity to dirty industries, toxic waste sites and nuclear facilities.

This last concern is different. What can parents do when a school or playground has been sited near a major pollution source? The best strategy is to avoid such insanity in the first place; therefore, an active interest in school siting ought to be a top priority for parents and child advocates — see the report *School Location Matters: Preventing School Siting Disasters.*[4]

All parents should be concerned about the state of their children's school. The Healthy Schools Network recommends these steps to organize a Healthy School action group:

- Ask your school or parent group to learn more about making your school a healthier place for all children.
- If they are too busy, create your own group.
- Commit to investigate a few simple but important issues.
- Ask others to join you. Investigate together and share information regularly.
- Create fact sheets that your group supports.
- Test your facts: visit your school principal or superintendent together and ask questions; review the fact sheet after your visit and edit if necessary.
- Pick your issues to work on (our priority here is cancer, so we suggest the cancer prevention issues listed above).

- The ABCs of Healthy Schools: www.childproofing.org/ABC.pdf
- Active & Safe Routes to School and International Walk to School Week: www.goforgreen.ca/asrts
- Back to School Environmental Checklist: www.besafenet.com/checklist.pdf
- Beyond Pesticides School Publications and Reports: www.beyondpesticides.org/schools/publications
- Childproofing Our Communities: www.childproofing.org
- Citizens for a Safe Learning Environment (Canada): www.chebucto.ns.ca/Education/CASLE
- Clean School Bus USA: www.epa.gov/cleanschoolbus
- Community Organizing for Environmental Health: www.eco-act.org/programs.html
- The Edible Schoolyard: www.edibleschoolyard.org
- Electric and Magnetic Fields: www.cehn.org/cehn/resourceguide/emfs.html
- Generation Green's School & Playground: www.generationgreen.org
- Green Flag Program: www.greenflagschools.org
- The Green Schools Initiative: www.greenschools.net
- Healthy Schools Network: www.healthyschools.org
- Illinois Healthy Schools Campaign: www.healthyschoolscampaign.org
- Indoor Air Quality Design Tools for Schools: www.epa.gov/iaq/schooldesign/
- Site Selection, National Clearinghouse for Educational Facilities: www.edfacilities.org/rl/site_selection.cfm

- Communicate as a group: create your own name and letterhead to establish a higher profile.
- Write letters; keep copies; track responses; see change happen.
- Celebrate with your school when you succeed in making positives changes.

# 16

## Keep Your Eyes Wide Open

**Children become aware of brands at a very early age. They are brand impressionable from as early as the age of one.**
— *International Journal of Advertising & Marketing to Children*[1]

Y ou're young and you've got almost your whole life ahead of you. So why should you worry about cancer? It mainly strikes older people, doesn't it?

Try looking at it from Tanya Thomas's point of view. She would say pay attention to cancer because it kills more children and youth than any other disease. She would urge you to be careful about what you eat and to know where your food comes from. She would tell you to look closely at the world, then ask critical questions and act with passion.

Tanya can't say this herself because she's one of many thousands of North American teens who have died from cancer this past decade. After two years of grueling treatments for a similar type of cancer that killed Canada's one-legged marathon hero, Terry Fox, Tanya passed away at age 17 in June 1999.

As a young girl, Tanya was curious about a lot of things, including some pretty strange human practices that most people don't think twice about. At age seven, for example, she asked her mother questions like this one: "Why do they test mascara on rabbits when rabbits don't wear mascara?"

After her cancer diagnosis at age 15, Tanya's questions got even more intense:

- Why is bovine growth hormone allowed in milk?
- Why are people only looking for a cancer cure and not the cause?
- Why do the cancer agencies accept donations from polluters?

We have a gut feeling that Tanya would know immediately that advertising and marketing are often hazardous to kids' health. She would get right away that hundreds of billions are being spent every year to persuade kids to do stupid, unhealthy things that are a recipe for cancer and other diseases later in life — or maybe sooner.

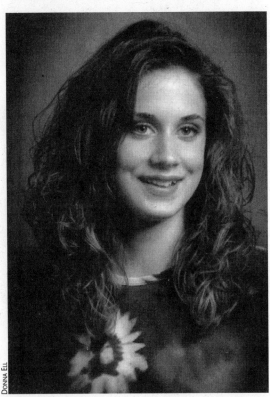

Tanya Thomas, 1982-1999.

- Center for a New American Dream:
  www.newdream.org/buy/buydifferent.php
- Don't Buy It — Get Media Smart!
  www.pbskids.org/dontbuyit

Tanya would get it. Do you?

Right now you have more money to spend than any other generation of kids in history — $170 *billion* every year, compared to $99 billion in 1994.[2] This makes you a very valuable target market. All sorts of companies want your money and your lifelong brand loyalty to the products they sell — food, clothing, computers, video games, athletic shoes, cellphones, cosmetics, candy, cigarettes, cars — and much more. They'll do a great deal to get your attention, and they're counting on you to pester your parents to spend money on stuff that's likely bad for your health.

You probably know that tobacco companies care more about their profits than they do about you (see Solution 17), but the same goes for many other corporations selling products to kids.

You've probably heard adults say things like "Children are our most precious asset" or "Kids are our future." But at the same time:

- Huge corporations are hooking you on fast food loaded with way too much sugar, risky chemical additives and dangerous trans fats.

- Your school grounds and parks are being sprayed with toxic pesticides. How much do they care about you if killing dandelions comes first?

- You're being exposed to scores of cancer-causing substances, and this exposure started even before you were born. Don't blame your mom for this. Toxic substances are everywhere in our "modern" environment, which is why they ended up in her body, and then became part of *your* "body burden" too.

- Your computers and other electronic gadgets are contaminated with heavy metals and toxic solvents.

You get the picture.

Meanwhile, the cancer society in your community urges you to eat lots of fruits and veggies, exercise regularly to keep your body weight healthy, never to smoke (or chew tobacco!) as well as staying away from tanning beds while practicing "sun-sense." And to limit consumption of alcohol — but hey, you're not supposed to be drinking at all at your age!

That's all good advice. But then why did Tanya Thomas get cancer? Her personal lifestyle was the best — she never smoked, she exercised regularly, always ate healthy food and even had friends join her boycott of fast-food restaurants. She was very conscientious about all of these things. So what caused her cancer?

If you're like Tanya, you'll see there's a lot more to cancer and cancer prevention than most adults usually talk about. Your "lifestyle" also includes things like cellphones, cosmetics, personal products such as nail polish, toothpaste and hair dyes — even the types of clothes and shoes you wear, plus the bus you ride to school, with its harmful diesel fumes. And then there are all the pollutants in the air you breathe and the water you drink...

Seeing and acting on this bigger picture is crucial to preventing cancer.

# 17

# Don't Be a Sucker to Big Tobacco. Kick Butts!

> **Are you kidding? We reserve that right for the poor, the young, the black and the stupid.**
>
> — Tobacco executive, on why he doesn't smoke

You already know that smoking is bad news for your health, so we won't even go there. If you do need some grisly evidence to stop you or your best friend from starting to smoke, take a look at the Tobacco Industry's Poster Child at www.tobaccofacts.org/poster. Not a pretty sight.

Instead, here's a question for you: Which age group is Big Tobacco's most important target market, by far? And here's a big hint (as if you need it ...):

To keep making their huge profits, tobacco companies in Canada and the US need 3,000 new suckers — oops, customers — to start smoking *every day* in order to replace the 1,400 people who die from tobacco-related diseases, plus all the smokers who finally (whew!) succeed in quitting.

- Asian American Youth Against Tobacco: www.aayat.org
- Children Opposed to Smoking Tobacco: www.costkids.org (see *True Ads*)
- Leave the Pack Behind (for college-age students): www.leavethepackbehind.org
- National African American Tobacco Prevention Network: www.naatpn.org
- Smoking Isn't Kool: www.sik.ca
- SWAT, Students Working Against Tobacco: www.gen-swat.com
- The Truth: www.thetruth.com
- You Are the Target: www.you-are-the-target.com
- Youth Anti-Tobacco Collaborative: www.notbuyinit.org
- WHUDAFXUP: www.whudafxup.com

One age group accounts for at least 90% of all these new smokers, and — another hint — it's *not* the 50-plus baby boomers or kids in kindergarten.

Answer: Well, you don't have to be a genius to figure out that the big tobacco corporations desperately need *teenagers* in order to stay in business, and they spend zillions on the youth market. Publicly, they say things like: "Minors should *not* smoke. Period." But behind closed doors they say things like: "They got lips? We want them."[1] That's what one tobacco company marketer said when he was asked if the young people they were targeting were junior high-school age or even younger.

So, if you're between 12 and 20, you'd better watch your back because *You Are the Target*, which also happens to be the name of a great book and website that exposes the obscene nature of Big Tobacco.

## Good News, Bad News

The good news is that teen smoking has declined in both Canada and the United States from the late 1990s to 2005.[2, 3] Knowing this, Big Tobacco has gone berserk promoting their products in the developing world, where smoking is growing in leaps and bounds among unsuspecting teens. As one tobacco executive bluntly said in 1998: "You know what we want. We want Asia."

The bad news? The evil tobacco companies are now targeting "young adults," since they've had less success lately with junior high and high-school youth because of tougher marketing restrictions — and smarter teens! So they're going after college and university students,[4] and particularly young women, black youth and other minority groups.

**Example 1:** In 2004 Brown & Williamson Tobacco (now RJR) released flavored cigarettes called Smooth Fusions. "With their ornate package designs and vivid, girly colors, these flavored cigarettes are clearly aimed at young women."[5]

**Example 2:** Khoa Ma, who was born in Vietnam, helped establish the Cincinnati, Ohio chapter of AAYAT, Asian American Youth Against Tobacco. "In many parts of the USA, minority communities are not very connected, they tend to be poor and have a hard time with the English language." The tobacco industry knows this. "When they show up to sponsor events like the Lunar New Year and pass out free tobacco products, these communities take the offer without any questions."[6]

**Example 3:** In 2004 Brown & Williamson Tobacco launched its Kool MIXX promotion, billed as a "celebration" of hip-hop music and culture. It featured cash prizes and a bunch of other enticements, including a Kool MIXX CD-ROM with mixing software, music files and, of course, special edition Kool cigarette packs that featured hip-hop designs and MIXX Stick radios.[7]

Good news, in this last case: Challenged by lawsuits in three states, R.J. Reynolds Tobacco, which had bought Brown & Williamson, agreed to "substantial limitations" on all future Kool MIXX promotions and agreed to pay $1.46 million to be used for youth smoking-prevention purposes.[8]

You get the idea. These tobacco guys *never quit*. So, take some advice from a bunch of youth anti-smoking activists: Don't be a sucker to Big Tobacco. Kick butts!

Dave Goerlitz, the main advertising man for Winston cigarettes back in the 1980s — and now a non-stop critic of Big Tobacco — was at an outdoor photo shoot one day with several RJ Reynolds tobacco executives. There were a lot of Winston cigarette cartons lying around, and Dave asked if he could take one. "Take them all," said one of the execs. Dave was surprised and asked, "Don't any of you smoke?" The executive shook his head and replied, "Are you kidding? We reserve that right for the poor, the young, the black and the stupid."[9]

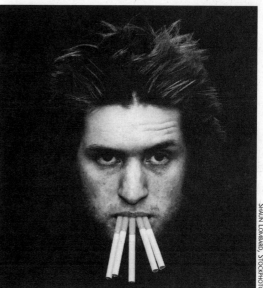

SHAUN LOMBARD, ISTOCKPHOTO

Addicted!

# 18

# Be Careful of Everyday Products

If you think you are too small to make an impact, try sleeping in a room with a mosquito.

— African proverb

Some risks we choose — like downhill skiing or skydiving — because they give us a big adrenaline rush.

Some risks we don't choose — or even know about. These include everyday things like drinking from plastic bottles, slapping on sunscreen, using make-up, and even talking on cell phones. *These are risky?* You're probably thinking, Get a life!

But not so fast. While we don't want to spoil anyone's fun, you'd be smart to get educated about virtually all the consumer products you buy and use. The old 1960s slogan, Question authority, question *everything*, is still good advice.

**Why do the cancer agencies accept donations from polluters? Why are people only looking for the cure, and not the cause?**
**— Tanya Thomas, 1982-1999**

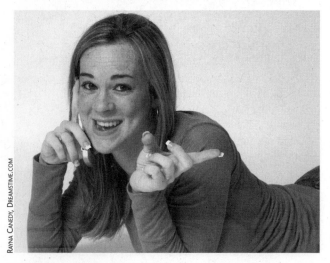

RAYNA CANEDY, DREAMSTIME.COM

It may be cool, but is it wise??

**Water Bottles**

Hikers, campers and high-school students love those clear and colorful plastic water bottles made from a polycarbonate plastic. They're tough, lightweight, absorb no flavors and don't give liquids inside a bad taste. But, wait a minute, they may leach a chemical called bisphenol-A (BPA). This is a problem because unimaginably small amounts of BPA can promote the growth of prostate tumors, affect breast tissue development and sperm counts and possibly create and enlarge fat cells.[1]

What to do? Avoid plastics with the recycling symbol #7, and go for the less risky types — HDPE (#2), LDPE (#4), polypropylene (#5) and PET (#1)[2]. And the very best choice? Skip plastics altogether and use glass bottles or containers made of stainless steel, both inside and out.

**Sunscreens**

We might not even be talking about sunscreens if big sections of the ozone layer that protect us from the sun's harmful rays hadn't been destroyed by man-made chemicals. Now we're paying the price with skyrocketing skin cancer rates, including a deadly type called *malignant melanoma*.

But don't bet your life on sunscreen. "Sunscreen ranks a distant second to sun *avoidance* — which means covering up and getting into the shade, especially during peak sunlight hours," advises *The Green Guide*'s product report on sunscreens.[3] When you compare the popular brands, some sunscreens contain downright hazardous chemicals, including some linked to cancer. "Sunscreens are imperfect … Picking a sunscreen that is right for you requires balancing the potential health risks of sunscreen ingredients with the known health risks of sun damage."[4] Zinc oxide is a sun *block* — it physically reflects the sun's rays, while sunscreens absorb them — but its bright white color turns some people off.

So, is it best to stay out of the sun totally? Here's where it gets even more confusing. While there's no question that overexposure to sunlight causes skin cancers, the latest research shows that Vitamin D from sunlight protects against several kinds of *internal* cancers. Some experts are advising people to get modest daily doses of unscreened sunshine all year round, including summer, when the sun's rays are strongest. But — and this is crucial — never, ever stay exposed to the point of sunburning or blistering.[5] How do you know when to get out of the sun? A short period of daily sunshine before mid-morning or later in the afternoon is a good idea, but be on your guard whenever the sun's heat feels "prickly." Do like people in the Mediterranean countries: spend the hottest hours inside or under a shady tree and wear loose, protective clothing and hats when you are in the sun.

## Tanning Beds and Sunlamps

These are not a good idea for anyone, at any age. It's a myth that getting a head start on an outdoor tan at an indoor tanning salon is a good idea. People who use these devices have higher risks of skin cancer.[6]

- Affluenza: www.pbs.org/kcts/affluenza
- Be Different. Live Different. Buy Different: www.ibuydifferent.org
- Campaign for Safe Cosmetics: www.safecosmetics.org
- The Case Against Indoor Tanning: www.skincancer.org/content/view/36/11
- Conscious Consumer: www.newdream.org/consumer
- Coop America: www.coopamerica.org
- Poisoned Cosmetics: www.nottoopretty.org
- Virtual House: www.healthychild.org. Search "Virtual House"

## Cosmetics and Personal Products

You want to look good, but you'll be shocked to find out how many ingredients are just plain bad for you. Sisters in Action for Reproductive Empowerment, a group of Asian-American teens in Marin County, California, closely looked at the chemical ingredients in cosmetics and personal products like lip gloss, hair dyes, mascara and scented skin cream. Like other investigators, they found many chemicals that can cause a long list of problems, including cancer.

## Cellphones and Cordless Phones

The makers of Mickey Mouse and Barbie want even the youngest preteens to go wireless. But if you're under 18, you're still growing, and that includes your brain, skull and nervous system. When you use a cellphone or cordless phone, an invisible stream of RF (radio frequency) energy is constantly penetrating your head. The long-term effects of RF are unknown, but there is enough evidence to be concerned, including the risk of cancer.[7, 8] We strongly advise that you use a cellphone or cordless phone for emergencies only.

# 19

# Make Your School Healthy

Walking to school can be really fun
Walk to school 'cause you're not dumb.
Walk to school and you'll feel great
Walk to school and you'll stay in shape!
— Rajbeer, Mr.Hoft's grade 5 class, Morton Way
Public School, Brampton, Ontario

Note to all students. Think about this: Without you, there wouldn't be any schools, which makes you Very Important People.

All too often, though, your schools are toxic places, especially in the downtown areas of big cities. But not just downtown. All schools everywhere have environmental problems, which in turn cause kids to have health problems. Think of all your friends with asthma, and allergies. Some things in schools can also cause cancer.

It's *your* school, and it shouldn't make you sick!

There's power in teaming up with custodians, teachers and even your parents to fix environmental problems at your school, such as bad air quality, toxic pesticide spraying or diesel bus fumes. (See Solution 15). But there's also a lot you can do with kids your own age.

### Start a Good Food Fight!

School food is often junk food — high-fat, sugar-drenched, nutrient-empty fillers — that may taste good, but it sure sets you up for getting fat and getting sick, both now and later. If you've seen the movie *Super-Size Me*, or have read *Fast Food Nation*, and you'd rather fuel your body with real food for a change, how about persuading your school to follow the example of The Edible School Yard at Martin Luther King Junior Middle School in Berkeley, California. There students grow, harvest and prepare healthy organic produce from a school garden (www.edibleschoolyard.org).

### Start a Revolution with Your $$$

Here's where you can make a really big difference. Companies know you and other kids your age have a lot of money to spend, and they want as much of it as they can get! Your consumer power can be huge, especially if a whole bunch of you get together to use it.

- Start by buying *less*. This is hard when companies hit you with hundreds of "buy me now" commercials 24/7 and "buzz" marketing, which makes it cool to have all the latest things. But the huge amounts of stuff we buy — there's just no nicer way of saying this — makes us the pigs of the world, and a lot of it is toxic.

- Spend your money on non-toxic school products. Here are some suggestions:

  - Lunch containers and thermoses: Go for stainless steel over plastic.

  - Clothing: Organic cotton and hemp keep toxic pesticides out of the water.

  - Shoes: Many athletic shoe companies are eliminating PVC from their products and

- The Green Flag Program: www.greenflagschools.org
- The Green Guide: www.thegreenguide.com
- Green Schools Checklist: www.epa.state.il.us/green-illinois/green-schools/green-schools-checklist.pdf
- The Green Squad, Kids Taking Action for Greener Healthier Schools: www.nrdc.org/greensquad
- Kids for Saving Earth (free environmental curriculum materials): www.kidsforsavingearth.org

The Prescott Valley (Arizona) Charter School 2006-2007 Green Flag Team. The Green Flag Program is a project of the national Child Proofing Our Communities Campaign, coordinated by the Center for Health Environment and Justice: www.chej.org.

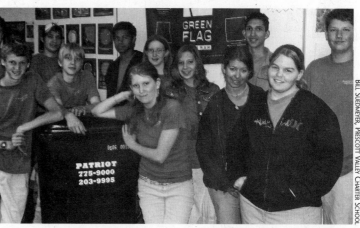

reducing VOCs (volatile organic chemicals). Get moving!

- Bags and Backpacks: Choose PVC-free. Check out hemp, recycled rubber or canvas products.
- Art supplies: check out the Twin Cities Green Guide: www.thegreenguide.org/article/arts/supplies
- Paper: Choose recycled, chlorine-free paper products.
- Computers: Go for products with the least solvents and the best recycling options.
- Ink and Toner Cartridges: Ask for remanufactured and recycled products.

## Tell *Channel One* to Butt Out for Good!

*Channel One* is not really a TV channel at all, but a commercial-crammed daily program beamed to more than 30% of all middle-school and high-school students in the US. In return for loans of television sets and other electronics, schools sign up for 12 minutes of programming for most schooldays, including 2 minutes of advertising. Sixty percent of the movie ads show actors smoking, with some predictable results. "Adolescents who see plenty of smoking on screen are nearly three times more likely to start smoking than those who see the least."[1] So, start the movement to butt out *Channel One* forever. And keep marketing and advertising off school buses, too — that's the latest way companies are trying to get into your head (and your wallet).[2]

## Students Environmental Bill of Rights

Ask your school board to sign the Students' Environmental Bill of Rights developed by the Labour Environmental Alliance Society and students, teachers and school support staff. This gives you and your family the right to know about toxic chemicals at school and invites school boards to make a commitment to finding healthy alternatives, for example, to floor strippers and solvent-based cleaners made with harmful ingredients. Go to www.leas.ca/Toxins-Free-Schools.htm.

## Skip the School Bus

Walk or bike to school — what a concept! In 2005 more than three million kids, parents and community leaders took part in International Walk to School (www.iwalktoschool.org), which happens each October in Canada, the US and 35 other countries. Why not join them to reduce your use of fossil fuels and all the resulting pollutants?

## Convert Your Schoolyard

*Learning Grounds* (www.evergreen.ca/en/lg/lg.html) brings students, teachers and neighbors together to transform asphalt and grass schoolgrounds into natural outdoor classrooms.

# 20

# Become an Activist

When I was 12, I co-founded Georgia Kids Against Pollution. The first thing we did was make posters. Then we went to Savannah and did a little protest and held a press conference. It was nerve-wracking!
— Illai Kenney

Clinton, Illai, Jean-Dominic and Elizabeth all stood up as young people and spoke out because they cared deeply about the world around them and were determined to make things better.

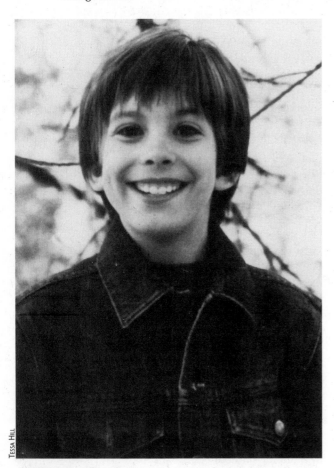

TESSA HILL

Clinton Hill, 1978-1989.

Rocking the boat early in life can make a lot of long-lasting ripples — and it can make the world a better, healthier place.

**Clinton Hill**, from Minneapolis, died from a brain tumor in 1989 at age 11, so he never really saw the amazing result of what he started. In the 1980s, Clint was a kid who looked around and saw that many humans were treating the world badly — poisoning skies and rivers, abusing plants and animals, and so on. He thought about it and even despaired about it, but Clint didn't stop there. He started a club called Kids for Saving Earth dedicated to "peaceful, Earth-saving actions."

By 2005 over 7,000 schools and concerned kids around the world had taken up Clint's passionate cause and his challenge. The two people he most inspired were his own parents, William and Tessa, who enthusiastically kept Kids for Saving Earth moving right along after Clint died. Although William also died from cancer in 1994, Tessa continues the work, inspiring a whole new generation to take action for a healthy Earth in memory of her wonderful, caring son.

In 2003, at just 14 years of age, **Illai Kenney** was already a veteran of several activist campaigns when she was honored with the David Brower Youth Award for her outstanding contribution to environmental causes. Illai, who lives near Atlanta, Georgia, co-founded Georgia Kids Against Pollution in response to the explosion of childhood asthma in that area and her desire to see urban youth connect with the world of nature outside Atlanta's city limits. Illai says, "We think young people would care if they knew about the problems, and if they have a chance to see natural areas where people have not taken over."[1] She continues to speak and act on behalf of many important issues, including clean air, clean water and energy efficiency to reduce global warming.

**Jean-Dominic Lévesque-René**, now in his early twenties, has been "watchdogging" pesticide issues since he was a 10-year-old on the cancer ward at Ste. Justine Hospital in Quebec, not far from his home in Île Bizard. While fighting his battle with non-Hodgkin's lymphoma, a cancer of the immune system, he began his environmental crusade to ban the use of pesticides, which he believed was at the root of his disease. In Île Bizard, golf courses make up about half the town's area, and Jean-Dominic learned that to keep them weed-free, heavy doses of toxic pesticides were the weapons of choice. Working with many other activists in the province of Quebec and elsewhere in Canada, Jean-Dominic and his friends have achieved remarkable success in their campaign against "cosmetic" (non-agricultural) pesticides. As a result of this work, the entire province of Quebec and nearly 200 municipalities in Canada now have bylaws and regulations severely restricting — and in some cases, totally banning — pesticides on public and private property.

**Elizabeth May** is now "old" by teenage standards, but at 18, after moving with her parents to Nova Scotia from the United States in 1972, she almost immediately got involved with Cape Breton Landowners Against the Spray, which was fighting to stop the spraying of forests with toxic pesticides such as 2,4,5-T (a close cousin to the notorious Agent Orange). Why did they choose someone so young and so new to Nova Scotia? Easy: Elizabeth already had a lot of experience as an activist. "I grew up in Connecticut, and at an early age, some of our sheep died for no apparent reason...We took the animals to the vet, and he couldn't figure out what happened. Some time later, I read Rachel Carson's *Silent Spring*, and I recognized the symptoms." At 12, Elizabeth wrote and asked if the town had been spraying the roadsides when the sheep died. "They had, in fact, sprayed organic phosphate insecticides and chlorinated hydrocarbons," Elizabeth says. "So the connection between our animals and pesticides at an early age certainly made me very concerned about what we were doing to the environment."[2]

Elizabeth, a hugely successful activist for many years, is now leader of the Green Party of Canada and generously shares her experience and very wise advice with kids of all ages.

- *How to Save the World in Your Spare Time* by Elizabeth May, Key Porter, 2006
- Illai Kenney: www.sierraclub.org/sierra/200505/step.asp
- Jean-Dominic Lévesque-René: www.sankey.ws/jeandominic.html
- Kids Against Pollution: www.kidsagainstpollution.org
- Kids for Saving Earth: www.kidsforsavingearth.org.
- YES! Helping Outstanding Young Leaders Build A Better World: www.yesworld.org

# 21

# Join the Activists

When I dare to be powerful — to use my strength in the service of my vision, then it becomes less and less important whether I am afraid.

— Audre Lorde

So, you have cleansed your cupboards of toxic products, switched to healthy organic food, changed your cosmetics, stopped smoking and started exercising regularly. That's great for you and your family and will definitely help to prevent your body burden of contaminants from increasing. It is not enough, however.

It's like using an umbrella when someone is spraying the air with a dangerous poison. After a while, you begin to ask, "Who the heck is spraying me, and how can I stop them? Why are these dangers there in the first place?" These are the questions that will turn you from a citizen into an activist.

The world is full of ordinary people who have become activists. They have one thing in common: they are fed up with complaining, and they want to DO something. Once started, they are persistent and unstoppable.

**Rachel Carson** (1907-1964) was a marine biologist who grew up in rural Springdale, Pennsylvania, where she developed a deep love of nature. As she became increasingly disturbed about the growing effects of pesticides on wildlife, she decided to write *Silent Spring*. It caused a huge storm, inspired millions to think more deeply about our behavior and launched the modern environmental movement. Two years after it was published, she died of breast cancer in 1964, age 57.

**Lois Gibbs** was a housewife living in Niagara Falls, New York, when she read a report about Love Canal, a toxic stew of 20,000 tons of chemicals that lay buried under her neighborhood. After her son was hospitalized with pneumonia, she went door-to-door with a clipboard, asking her neighbors to help. They stood up to the chemical company that dumped the wastes, and opposition from every level of government, but eventually won. As a result, 900 families were rehoused, and President Jimmy Carter launched the program that became known as Superfund to clean up hazardous sites nationwide. Lois went on to found the Center for Health, Environment and Justice where she works today, helping communities that face similar challenges.

There is no secret to becoming an activist. Simply make a pact with yourself: *I will do whatever it takes to help this world become healthy again.*

The Resources box lists websites for the personal stories of some of our planet's heroes who have devoted their lives to preventing cancer at its source. Thousands of others are equally persistent but less well-known.

We need many more people to become activists. Just think what we could achieve if everyone who shares our concern about cancer

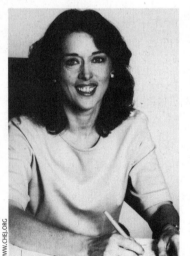

WWW.CHEJ.ORG

Lois Gibbs, founder of the Center for Health, Environment and Justice

> Unless someone like you cares a whole lot, nothing is going to get better. It's not.
>
> — Dr. Seuss, *The Lorax*

was to read this book, pick up their telephone, and start calling their friends saying "Let's DO something!"

Elizabeth May (See p. 107), one of Canada's most accomplished activists, has these words of advice:

**There is no formal school for activists. All of us learn from experience.**

**Refuse to be intimidated.** If you are told that a subject is too technical or scientific for you to understand, don't believe it. You may not be an expert. But you can read and understand what experts have to say.

**Be creative!** Every campaign and issue has its own dynamic. Let your creative juices flow. Maybe satire will work for you. Maybe song. Even conventional campaigns can attract people if you have an optimistic, innovative approach.

**Don't take no for an answer.** If you want to meet an elected official, call every day. Drop by the office and get to know the staff. Be persistent. Ask lots of questions. Do your homework.

**Be unfailingly polite.** Being persistent is not the same thing as being rude. You may be in this for the long haul, so don't burn any bridges.

**Leave no stone unturned.** Think about who knows who. How can you expand your network? Your allies may come from unexpected places, so do not make assumptions. Ask people for help.

- Anil Agarwal: www.cseindia.org/aboutus/anilji/anilji.htm
- Audre Lorde: www.indiana.edu/~glbtlib/reviews/r00801.html
- Bella Abzug: www.jwa.org/exhibits/wov/abzug
- Denny Larson: www.commongroundmag.com Search "Denny Larson"
- Diane Wilson: www.chelseagreen.com/authors/277
- Lois Gibbs: www.goldmanprize.org
- Margie Richard: www.goldmanprize.org Search "Margie Richard"
- Michael Lerner: www.commonweal.org
- Rachel Carson: www.rachelcarson.org
- Rosalie Bertell: www.cspi.org/womenspress/books/b/bertell.htm
- Rose Kushner: www.rkbcac.org/rose.html
- Sandra Steingraber: www.steingraber.com
- Sam Epstein: www.rightlivelihood.org/recip/epstein.htm
- Sharon Batt: www.canadiangeographic.ca/cea2005/en/winners.asp#health
- Susan Love: www.susanlovemd.com
- Terri Swearingen: www.sdearthtimes.com/et0897/et0897s17.html
- Von Hernandez: www.goldmanprize.org Search "Von Hernandez"
- Wilma Subra: www.commonweal.org/programs/fg_fenceline/subra.html

**When someone in government does something good for the environment,** be sure to give public credit and thanks. You can accomplish anything if you don't care who gets the credit.

**Remember that politics is also personal.** Watch out for burnout. You'll need the support of friends and family. Build love into your campaigns.

See *How To Be an Activist*: www.sierraclub.ca/activist-publication.

# 22
# Form a Local Group

You do not need to act alone. It is much easier and more fun working with others who think and feel the same way. You could join an existing environmental, women's, or health group or a church, labor, service or social justice group and persuade them to start a Prevent Cancer campaign.

If you want to form a new group, we suggest that you invite people to your home to discuss the idea. Make a flyer and post it on notice boards in community halls, cafés, shops, health clinics, colleges, libraries and women's centers. Send an e-mail to everyone you know. Many

- Activist Toolbox: www.ran.org/action/toolbox
- Activist Toolkit: www.onenw.org/bin/page.cfm/secid/5
- Activists Tools: www.environmentalleague.org/activist.html
- Breast Cancer Fund: www.breastcancerfund.org
- *Calling All Activists*, by Meghan Taylor: www.beyondpesticides.org/lawn/activist
- Community Campaign ideas: www.come-clean.org/stepscom.htm
- Fun with Fundraising: www.bcaction.org/Pages/Membership/FunWithFundraising.html
- *Preparing for a Campaign*, by Mary O'Brien: www.stopcancer.org/organize
- Starting a Nonprofit Society: www.snpo.org/resources/startup.php
- Toolkit for Boards: www.managementhelp.org/boards/boards.htm
- Virtual Activist: www.netaction.org/training

We climb to demonstrate our commitment, to ourselves and to others, that we stand for a world in which cancer is a thing of the past. We apply our courage and faith that anything is possible, if taken one step at a time. And we do it all as part of a team, climbers and supporters, knowing that there is more that we can achieve together than apart.
— Andrea Ravinett Martin

successful groups were started by just one or two people, such as the Women's Community Cancer Project (Boston), Breast Cancer Action Montreal and the Breast Cancer Research and Education Fund (St. Catharines, Ontario).

## The Breast Cancer Fund
Based in San Francisco, the Breast Cancer Fund (BCF) was founded by Andrea Ravinett Martin in her living room in 1992. At the age of 45, she had been treated for breast cancer, and both breasts had been surgically removed. Andrea wanted to transform the breast cancer epidemic from a private secret to a public health priority and persuaded anyone who would join to help her.

One of the group's first successes was to write and secure the passage of California legislation for a two-cent cigarette tax to fund breast cancer research and detection services for uninsured women. Then in 1995, Andrea and 16 other survivors climbed Mt. Aconcagua in Argentina and raised $1 million, saying that climbing mountains was like facing breast cancer. In subsequent years, survivors and supporters have climbed Mt. McKinley, Mt. Fuji and Mt. Shasta, winning worldwide attention and more donations.

In 1997 they funded and hosted the premiere screening of *Rachel's Daughters: Searching for the Causes of Breast Cancer*, reaching 3.2 million people through HBO in the first month. In 1999 they worked with legislators to increase the budget for the Centers for Disease Control's Environmental Health Laboratory from $7 to $21 million, to identify the environmental causes of breast cancer.

In 2000 the BCF ran a public awareness ad in Bay Area bus shelters called Obsessed with Breasts, which showed models with mastectomy scars (taken from Andrea's own scars), asking, "Society is obsessed with breasts, but what are we doing about breast cancer?" In 2001 they adopted the mission of identifying and advocating for the elimination of the environmental and other preventable causes of breast cancer.

They established a LifeLines program in 2002 to provide meals, transport, emergency funds and in-home care to low-income and uninsured women with breast cancer. They also organized International Hearings on Breast Cancer and the Environment for the California legislature, initiated the first International Summit on Breast Cancer and the Environment, and published the report *State of the Evidence: What Is the Connection Between Chemicals and Breast Cancer?*

In 2003 they worked with others to persuade San Francisco to adopt the precautionary principle (the first city in the US to do so), launched a Spanish language outreach program and initiated the Strong Voices Leadership Development Program to help people build leadership confidence and create a nationwide network of survivors who are willing to share their stories and inspire others to take action against breast cancer. That same year, Andrea died, two years after being diagnosed with a malignant brain tumor. Before she died, she had traveled to New

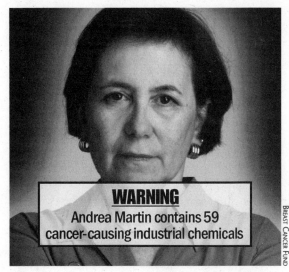

**WARNING**
Andrea Martin contains 59 cancer-causing industrial chemicals

Andrea Ravinett Martin's ad in the *New York Times*. She passed away in August 2003 following a two-year struggle with brain cancer.

York and Washington DC and was featured in a *New York Times* ad that said, "Warning — Andrea Martin contains 59 cancer-causing chemicals." Under Andrea's leadership, the Fund has grown to 70,000 supporters who continue to pursue her dream of a world without breast cancer.

We can all be leaders if we have the courage to take it one step at a time. There are many sources of advice that you can draw on to form a thriving group. Two that we recommend are *Calling All Activists*, by Meghan Taylor, and *Preparing for a Campaign*, by Mary O'Brien.

> **Over the years, her vision, her light, illuminates our lives. Sunlight for our cloud-filled days, moonlight and starlight, a nightlight to sooth our midnight fears.**
>
> **— Wanna Wright**

# 23

# Choose Your Priorities

O ne of the challenges of running a group is choosing what to do. What will bring the best results, while motivating your members to remain inspired and do more?

The following list contains activities that groups engage in to rid the world of the environmental causes of cancer and other diseases. Think of it as a giant undertaking that has yet to reach maturity. That moment will be reached when the groups recognize each other's existence and start working as one, using their combined pressure to change the direction of our civilization.

**There is no formal school for activists. No university degree qualifies the graduate to practice grassroots organizing. Environmental activists, like many other practitioners of social change, come in all shapes and sizes, from all walks of life, and even from all political parties. And all of us learn from experience.**

**— Elizabeth May**

To help you evaluate different ideas, score each question 0 (No) 1 (Maybe), or 2 (Yes).

A. Does this grab your attention?

B. Does it have an achievable short-term goal?

C. Does it contribute towards long-term success?

D. Add the total score for each idea.

| Ideas for Action Groups | A | B | C | D |
|---|---|---|---|---|
| 1. Become organized, with a website, nonprofit status and memberships | | | | |
| 2. Start a newsletter to keep in touch with your members | | | | |
| 3. Organize a fundraising run, walk, auction or mountain-climb | | | | |
| 4. Organize monthly meetings with a speaker, to build your membership | | | | |
| 5. Hold a monthly vegetarian potluck evening, with a speaker | | | | |
| 6. Write letters to the editor and submit articles to local papers | | | | |
| 7. Start a study circle to educate yourselves about the issues | | | | |
| 8. Run a booth at local community fairs and festivals | | | | |
| 9. Organize a petition that people can sign to express their concerns | | | | |
| 10. Use the arts and music to bring colour to a campaign | | | | |
| 11. Form partnerships with local organizations that share your concerns | | | | |
| 12. Organize a support group for people who have cancer | | | | |
| 13. Organize help for low-income families where someone has cancer | | | | |
| 14. Organize meetings with low-income and minority members of your community to learn about their health concerns | | | | |
| 15. Organize meetings with local health experts to discuss cancer prevention | | | | |
| 16. Organize a safe pregnancy study circle to learn how to avoid toxic dangers | | | | |
| 17. Organize a conference on the environmental causes of cancer | | | | |
| 18. Organize a local breast cancer mapping project | | | | |

|  | A | B | C | D |
|---|---|---|---|---|
| 19. Organize a film festival on cancer, toxics and the struggle for justice |  |  |  |  |
| 20. Invite people to run toxic-free movie nights in their homes to learn about indoor air pollution and safe, healthy products, followed by letter writing |  |  |  |  |
| 21. Go into local schools to talk to teenagers about the environmental links to cancer |  |  |  |  |
| 22. Persuade schools to offer healthy food and use non-toxic cleaning products |  |  |  |  |
| 23. Organize an organic food fair or banquet to promote safe, healthy food |  |  |  |  |
| 24. Organize local organic gardening and pesticide-free lawn workshops |  |  |  |  |
| 25. Organize a campaign to stop vehicle idling |  |  |  |  |
| 26. Campaign for a ban on smoking in all public places |  |  |  |  |
| 27. Campaign for a ban on the cosmetic use of pesticides |  |  |  |  |
| 28. Campaign for safe pest control in public housing, rental apartments and condos |  |  |  |  |
| 29. Build a partnership to develop a citywide plan to prevent cancer, like in Toronto |  |  |  |  |
| 30. Persuade your city to adopt the precautionary principle, like in San Francisco |  |  |  |  |
| 31. Campaign for more sustainable transport, walking, cycling and transit |  |  |  |  |
| 32. Meet with local labor unions to discuss their needs for a cancer-safe workplace |  |  |  |  |
| 33. Visit local dry cleaners and hairdressers and tell them about safe alternatives |  |  |  |  |
| 34. Start a campaign to persuade builders to adopt non-toxic building practices |  |  |  |  |
| 35. Start a campaign to shut down a local incinerator, to eliminate dioxin emissions |  |  |  |  |
| 36. Organize a toxic industry tour or a sustainable living tour, renting a local bus |  |  |  |  |
| 37. Create an awards night to honour those who are contributing to cancer prevention |  |  |  |  |
| 38. Research the toxic hazards in your community and organize meetings to publicize the results. (See www.scorecard.org or www.pollutionwatch.org) |  |  |  |  |
| 39. Form a Bucket Brigade to test for local air pollution (see Solution 26) |  |  |  |  |
| 40. Organize a toxic-free neighbourhoods campaign |  |  |  |  |
| 41. Help neighbours to campaign against cellphone towers and EMF pollution |  |  |  |  |
| 42. Start a campaign to persuade a local polluter to adopt clean production methods |  |  |  |  |
| 43. Buy shares in a local polluting company and organize a shareholder action |  |  |  |  |
| 44. Join national groups that are working for cancer prevention and toxics reduction |  |  |  |  |
| 45. Start a campaign to introduce Toxics Use Reduction legislation (see Solution 72) |  |  |  |  |
| 46. Start a campaign for Right to Know legislation about local pesticides, chemicals in consumer products and the use of chemicals by local industry |  |  |  |  |
| 47. Join the Campaign for Safe Cosmetics, and play an active part |  |  |  |  |
| 48. Campaign for corporate law reform to require corporate directors to consider the social and environmental aspects of their activities, as well as financial |  |  |  |  |
| 49. Create questionnaires for candidates in elections, and publicize the results |  |  |  |  |
| 50. Meet with local politicians to put the case for cancer prevention legislation |  |  |  |  |
| 51. Your idea: |  |  |  |  |
| 52. Your idea: |  |  |  |  |

To download this as a form, see www.preventcancernow.ca

# 24

# Tackle a Local Challenge

Never doubt that a small group of thoughtful, committed citizens can change the world. Indeed, it is the only thing that ever has.
— Margaret Mead, anthropologist

If you are a member of a local group, it is important to choose a challenge that can engage your community and give you a sense of achievement.

In San Francisco, Breast Cancer Action was founded in 1990 by Elenore Pred and other women with breast cancer. One of their campaigns, Stop Cancer Where It Starts, educates the public and local governments about the environmental links to cancer and pushes them to adopt legislation that will reduce people's exposure to known and suspected toxins. It also highlights their frustration with runs, walks and pink ribbons that do nothing to prevent cancer.

As a result of the campaign, on October 10, 2000, the City of Berkeley declared October as Stop Cancer Where It Starts Month and passed a motion committing the City to a wide range of measures (see box). Following their success, similar motions were passed in San Francisco, Oakland and Marin County (www.bcaction.org).

In Missoula, Montana, Women's Voices for the Earth (WVE) was formed in 1995 by women who felt that local environmental campaigns did not address the issues that mattered to them. Their mission is to empower women, who historically have had little power in affecting environmental policy, to create an ecologically sustainable and socially just society. As a result:

- Four of the state's five medical waste incinerators (burning plastic produces dioxin), were replaced with cleaner, waste disposal methods, as were the last municipal waste incinerator, in Livingston, and the Rocky Mountain Laboratories incinerator in Hamilton.

- Their outdoor environmental leadership program, Girls Using Their Strengths (GUTS!), registered over 7,500 new women voters in partnership with other women's organizations.

- Five conferences explored the environmental links to breast cancer.

- Chlorine bleaching was eliminated at Missoula's main pulp mill.

## Berkeley Stops Cancer Where It Starts

- Encourage local industries to work towards a goal of zero toxic emissions.
- Eliminate the use of PVC in new construction and renovations.
- Develop a healthy building ordinance/bylaw.
- Develop fact sheets on the links between cancer and carcinogenic chemicals and their alternatives to distribute to clinics, hospitals, nurseries and stores.
- Eliminate the use of pesticides in city parks and buildings.
- Replace City vehicles that run on diesel with cleaner fuel.
- Purchase totally chlorine-free paper products when they are available.
- Develop an ordinance/bylaw to substitute safer alternatives for PVC medical products as a condition of hospital operations.
- Work with other public facilities and institutions in Berkeley to promote pesticide bans and use safer alternative products and methods.

- With a Seattle group, they studied the role of flame-retardants in the breast milk of women in the Pacific Northwest.
- With the Campaign for Safe Cosmetics, they convinced several major cosmetics companies, including L'Oreal, Revlon and Unilever, to eliminate toxic chemicals from their products.

**Think Positive**

When you are campaigning, remember to focus on solutions. Negative campaigns are a wearying effort and turn people off. Build positive relationships and generate a hopeful vision of a healthy, sustainable future. Don't get trapped in anger and blame. Take a strong, determined attitude. We have a right to live in a world without the sicknesses and health assaults that result from pollution.

In Britain, the 100 groups in the Women's Environmental Network organize socials, conduct toxic tours, build local breast cancer maps, form organic food growing groups, organize environmental play workshops and run booths at fairs and festivals. The Network's national activities include Real Nappy Week (cloth diapers instead of disposables, www.realnappycampaign.com) and Stop Breast Cancer Before It Starts: www.wen.org.uk

**Think Big**

When you are planning your activities, remember to *think big*. Local campaigns are important, but we also need to link up with other groups to work on larger issues (see Solution 28). In Bangor, Maine, one of the Environmental Health

> ## Local Campaign Tools
> - *Dying from Dioxin*, by Lois Marie Gibbs. An organizing manual for local groups.
> - Investigate local polluters: www.scorecard.org, www.pollutionwatch.org
> - Pesticides Community Organizing: www.beyondpesticides.org
> - Refinery Reform Campaign: www.refineryreform.org
> - Right to Know Network: www.rtknet.org
> - Stop Cancer Where It Starts Campaign Guide: www.bcaction.org/PDF/SCWISGuide.pdf

Strategy Center's goals is to phase out all persistent toxic chemicals statewide within one generation. They also organize Toxic-Free Movie Nights, when members invite friends and neighbors into their homes to watch a video about removing toxic chemicals from the home and workplace, and write letters to the state governor urging him to phase out toxic chemicals from consumer products.

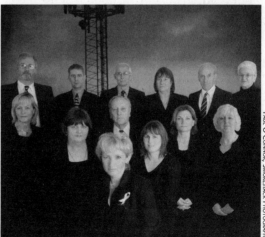

The Directors of SCRAM in front of a cellphone mast in the English village of Wishaw, one of many masts they are opposing. www.scram.uk.com

# 25

# Become a Research Wiz

Research is to see what everyone else has seen, and to think what no-one else has thought.

— Hungarian biochemist Albert Szent-Gyorgi, 1937 Nobel Prize for Medicine

Every action group needs someone who will read the reports and dig into the data. Two essential strengths for campaigning and advocacy work are the accuracy of your information and the solidness of your data. When you have these, people will respect you.

With this in mind, we are using this Solution to share some resources that will help you.

## Environmental Health News
Sign up for Above the Fold for a daily summary of stories from the world's papers: www.environmentalhealthnews.org.

Go to Google, click on "News," then "Edit this Personalized Page". If you enter "toxic" or "breast cancer," Google will send you up-to-date stories from all around the world that use these terms.

## What Do the Cancer Statistics Say?
Canada: www.cancer.ca, click on Canada-wide > Publications > Canadian Cancer Statistics
US: www.cancer.org/docroot/STT/STT_0.asp, www.seer.cancer.gov and www.seer.cancer.gov/csr/1975_2001
Global: www-dep.iarc.fr
World Cancer Report: www.iarc.fr/WCR

## What Is Carcinogenic?
IARC's full list of carcinogens: monographs.iarc.fr/ENG/Classification/index.php
National Toxicology Program: http://ntp.niehs.nih.gov, click on *Report on Carcinogens*

National Institute for Occupational Safety and Health: www.cdc.gov/niosh/npotocca.html
California's list: www.oehha.ca.gov/prop65/prop65_list/Newlist.html

## Cancer and the Environment
For solid science and great discussions, join the Collaborative on Health and the Environment: www.healthandenvironment.org
*Environmental and Occupational Causes of Cancer: A Review of Recent Scientific Evidence*: www.healthandenvironment.org/wg_cancer_news/216
*Key Scientific Reviews and Studies on the Relationship Between Cancer and the Environment*: www.cancerpreventionsociety.org/importantStudies.htm
*Fetal Origins of Cancer*: www.healthandenvironment.org/wg_cancer_news/365
*Toxicant and Disease Database*, links between chemical contaminants and 183 diseases: database.healthandenvironment.org
*Breast Cancer and Environmental Risk Factors*: envirocancer.cornell.edu
*State of the Evidence 2006*, draws on 350 studies linking breast cancer to chemicals and radiation exposure: www.breastcancerfund.org
*Toxic Beginnings: A Lifetime of Chemical Exposure in the First Year*: www.net.org/health/toxic_beginnings.pdf
*Environmental Health Perspectives*, read in over 190 countries: www.ehponline.org
*International Journal of Occupational and Environmental Health*: www.ijoeh.com

Eggs from a herring gull colony in Lake Ontario, showing eggshell thinning due to DDT, and dead chicks due to dioxin-like chemicals.

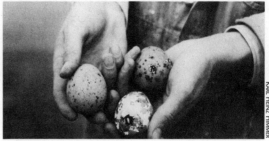

### Are There Hazardous Chemicals in My Neighborhood, Home or at Work?
Canada: www.pollutionwatch.org
Priority List of Hazardous Substances:
www.atsdr.cdc.gov/cercla
Material Safety Data Sheets: www.msds.com
Household Products Database:
www.householdproducts.nlm.nih.gov
ToxTown: www.toxtown.nlm.nih.gov
TOXMAP: www.toxmap.nlm.nih.gov
TOXNET: www.toxnet.nlm.nih.gov
ToxSeek: www.toxseek.nlm.nih.gov
US Envirofacts by zipcode: www.epa.gov/enviro
US pollution by zipcode: www.scorecard.org

### Environmental Health Resources
Environmental Research Foundation:
www.rachel.org
University of Pittsburgh Center for Environmental Oncology: www.environmentaloncology.com

### Great Videos
*Blue Vinyl*: www.bluevinyl.org
*A Civil Action* (local video stores)
*Chasing the Cancer Answer* (CBC, Wendy Mesley):
www.cbc.ca/consumers/market/files/
health/cancer
*Erin Brokovich* (local video stores)
*Exposure: Environmental Links to Breast Cancer*:
www.whenvironments.ca/video1.html
*A Healthy Baby Girl*: www.wmm.com/
catalog/pages/c139.htm
*If You Love Our Children: Children's Health and the Environment*: www.whenvironments.ca/
video2.html

*The Insider* (local video stores)
*Rachel's Daughters*:
www.wmm.com/catalog/pages/c401.htm
*River of Broken Promises*:
www.environmentalhealth.org/pubs-for-sale.html
*Toxic Trespass: Children's Health and Environment* (NFB, 2007)
*Trade Secrets, A Bill Moyers Report*:
www.pbs.org/tradesecrets

### Great Books
*Cancer Wars: How Politics Shapes What We Know and Don't Know About Cancer*, by Robert Proctor
*Cancer-Gate: How to Win the Losing Cancer War*, by Sam Epstein
*Diamond: A Struggle for Environmental Justice in Louisiana's Chemical Corridor*, by Steve Lerner
*Dying from Dioxin*, by Lois Gibbs
*Having Faith: An Ecologist's Journey to Motherhood*, by Sandra Steingraber: www.steingraber.com
*Living Downstream: A Scientist's Personal Investigation of Cancer and the Environment*, by Sandra Steingraber: www.steingraber.com
*Patient No More: The Politics of Breast Cancer*, by Sharon Batt
*Toxic Deception: How the Chemical Industry Manipulates Science, Bends the Law, and Endangers Your Health*, by Dan Fagin & Marianne Lavelle
*An Unreasonable Woman: A True Story of Shrimpers, Politicos, Polluters and the Fight for Seadrift, Texas*, by Diane Wilson
*The Secret History of the War on Cancer*, by Devra Davis.
*When Smoke Ran Like Water*, by Devra Davis:
www.whensmokeranlikewater.com

# 26

# Plan a Winning Campaign

> I do not know what your destiny may be, but I do know the only ones of you to find happiness will be those who have found a way to serve.
>
> — Albert Schweitzer

How can a group of citizens who want to win the attention of a city council, corporation or the federal government make themselves heard? The media has the attention span of a six-year-old cub reporter on a sugar high, and our elected leaders have to deal with 50 issues every day.

A winning campaign requires careful strategy and attention to detail. Chris Rose is an experienced campaigner and author of *How to Win Campaigns: 100 Steps to Success*. In 2001 the World Wildlife Fund (WWF) in Britain asked him to devise a campaign that would make a difference in the long and bitter struggle over the European Union's proposed REACH legislation (see Solution 69), to create a much tighter framework of control for toxic chemicals that accumulate in our bodies.

The WWF needed to choose a focus that would make a clear impact and influence the vote by Members of the European Parliament (MEPs). If the campaign highlighted how dangerous the chemicals were, it would invite a quick industry response, and the debate would disappear into the merits of risk-based assessment versus the precautionary principle. Important stuff, but a big yawn for Joe and Jasmine Public.

What about a campaign on "the right to know" and the demand for clear labelling? Again, important stuff, but it would lead to a debate about the wording of the small print (yawn), and even if it succeeded, the chemicals would still be in the products.

Ask the public and businesses to sign a petition? Another yawn. The campaign needed to be visual and tell a compelling story. So they decided to search for chemicals in the human body.

The WWF set up a blood testing program, initially using their own staff. After forming an alliance with the Women's Institute (WI), the

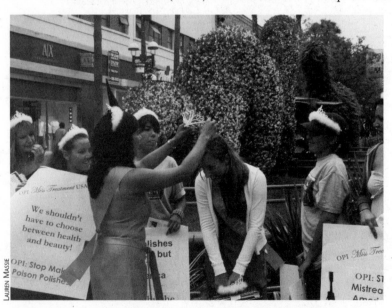

In May 2006, the Campaign for Safe Cosmetics held a Miss Treatment mock beauty pageant to protest O·P·I's use of dibutyl phthalate (DBP) – a known reproductive toxin - in their nail polish. O·P·I has since removed both DBP and toluene but they still use formaldehyde in their nail polishes.

- *Good Neighbor Campaign Handbook* (168-page guide from Ohio Citizen Action): www.ohiocitizen.org
- *How to Win Campaigns*: www.campaignstrategy.org
- Prevention is the Cure: www.preventionisthecure.org
- Rainforest Action Network: www.ran.org
- Ruckus Society: www.ruckus.org
- Women's Institute Campaign: www.nfwi.org.uk
- WWF Campaign: www.wwf.org.uk/chemicals/biotour.asp
- WWF Safer Shopping: http://safershopping.wwf.org.uk

bastion of hats and apple pie that won fame in the movie *Calendar Girls*, they extended the campaign and tested families, politicians and celebrities, gathering publicity each time, locally and nationally. When the WI chartered a bus and took the Eurostar train to lobby their MEPs in Brussels, Belgium, the "blood-tested grannies" with their blood bags, test results and photos of grandchildren made an irresistible story for the media.

The Cooperative Bank, which had recently remade itself as "the ethical bank," formed a very successful partnership with the WWF. The bank funded blood tests for 150 volunteers, including its own staff, MPs and MEPs. Every test result told the same story: people's bodies were thoroughly contaminated with dangerous industrial chemicals. Finally, they tested the umbilical cords from 30 newborn babies — and every baby's blood contained contaminants from non-stick chemicals, flame-retardants, perfumes and pesticides linked to cancer, asthma and genital abnormalities.

For building public awareness, the campaign was a huge success. Industry fought back, saying it proved nothing. The WWF followed up with a website that encourages "safer shopping," giving people the information they need to avoid some of the chemicals.

Every campaign needs to be planned carefully. Chris Rose suggests five starting points:

1. What do you want to achieve? What is the difference you want to make?
2. What do you want to communicate? What is the message you want the media to report?
3. What are the social weather conditions? What are the trends? How is the world changing relative to your campaign?
4. What resources, skills and intelligence can you draw on or attract to your cause?
5. Who are your potential allies and obstacles? Who will win — and lose — if you are successful?

It is important to remain positive. To learn how to launch protest actions that are colourful, creative and non-violent, contact the Ruckus Society. The Rainforest Action Network is also worth studying: they run some of the world's most effective, successful campaigns.

A campaign must pass the "photo test": if you can't photograph your objective, it probably isn't much use. It must have a strong visual language that people can see in their minds and on television. The bigger your audience, the simpler your message must be. Beware of preconceptions: you never know who your allies might be. Make your campaign solution-oriented. People are turned off by campaigns that simply tell us how bad things are.

You never know when your campaign may trigger a pivotal moment in history, but one thing is for sure: this moment will come.

# 27

# Work for Environmental Justice

These are the opening words (see right) of the 17 Principles of Environmental Justice that were drafted by delegates at the First National People of Color Environmental Leadership Summit (Washington DC, October 1991). There has always been environmental injustice, but for many years nobody saw it except those who lived under its pall:

- The low-income residents of communities near Louisiana's "Cancer Alley," a 100-mile stretch of the Mississippi River that is home to 150 chemical-making facilities, who drink water contaminated by vinyl chloride and other toxics.

- The families who live in fenceline communities such as Westside, Port Arthur (Texas) and Diamond (Louisiana), a stone's throw away from refineries, petrochemical plants, landfills and incinerators.

- The 30,000 people of Bhopal, India, who died in December 1984 and the years that followed, after a chemical storage tank exploded due to Union Carbide's decision to cut back on maintenance.

- The people of the Aamjiwnaang First Nation, in Sarnia, Ontario, who learnt in 2005 that the reason why puppies were being born with no eyes or ears, why girl births outnumbered boy births by 2 to 1 and why multiple miscarriages were happening lay with the chemical pollution of their water and soil by nearby petrochemical plants.

- The Siberian Yup'ik Eskimo residents of St. Lawrence Island, 100 miles west of Alaska's

**Environmental Justice affirms the sacredness of Mother Earth, ecological unity and the interdependence of all species, and the right to be free from ecological destruction.[1]**

**Environmental Justice demands that public policy be based on mutual respect and justice for all peoples, free from any form of discrimination or bias.**

coast, whose land has been poisoned by spilled fuel oil, solvents, asbestos, heavy metals and PCBs from when the US military used the island, whose blood now contains PCB levels 10 times higher than the average American's, and who find themselves stricken with cancer.

- The Asian workers and their families who are being poisoned by toxic solvents and lead from the semiconductor industry in California's Silicon Valley.

- The residents of Wagner's Point, Baltimore, Maryland, who after a long campaign were finally relocated away from the chemical manufacturing plants and petroleum storage tanks they lived beside.

- The Mexicans and their families who work in the factories of Tijuana, along the US border, where the air and water are fouled by toxic emissions and untreated industrial waste from the thousands of foreign corporations that operate there with minimal environmental care.

- The residents of East Austin, Texas, who live with a racist 1931 "Master Plan" that steered Mexican and black minorities towards a section of town where they are surrounded by polluting industries.

The environmental justice movement was born in 1982 when the residents of Warren County, a predominantly poor, black community in North Carolina, refused to accept that

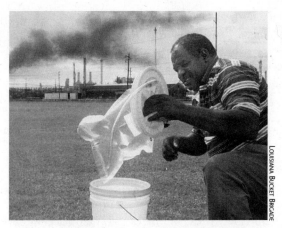

LOUISIANA BUCKET BRIGADE

A community a bucket brigade training session.

they should live next to a PCB-laden landfill, and where 532 people were arrested after six weeks of peaceful civil disobedience. In the aftermath, studies found that 75% of landfills in the US southeast are located in communities of color; that Superfund offenders pay 54% lower fines in communities of color than in white communities; that people of color are more likely to live in a polluted neighborhood; and that Latinos and blacks are much more likely to develop — and die of — diseases related to pollution.

After 20 years, the Warren County landfill was finally decontaminated and restored. The question environmental justice asks is, "If the landfill had been among the leafy farms of Vermont or the heritage homes of Ottawa, how long would it have taken for justice to be done?"

Although the environmental justice movement is becoming organized, the very people who are affected by dirty industry and bad zoning laws also need the jobs the most; therefore, we need to insist that economic development can co-exist with a clean environment.

One tool that has been developed by the Bucket Brigade to help communities protect themselves is a $75 version of the $2,000 canister that government and industry use to

- Bucket Brigade: www.bucketbrigade.net
- Communities for a Better Environment (CA): www.cbecal.org
- Community Coalition for Environmental Justice (WA): www.ccej.org
- Deep South Center for Environmental Justice: www.xula.edu/dscej
- *Diamond: A Struggle for Environmental Justice in Louisiana's Chemical Corridor*, by Steve Lerner, MIT Press, 2005
- Environmental Justice Support Center: www.ejrc.cau.edu
- EPA's Environmental Justice Site: www.epa.gov/compliance/environmentaljustice
- Indigenous Environmental Network: www.ienearth.org
- Louisiana Bucket Brigade: www.labucketbrigade.org
- *Principles of Environmental Justice*: www.ejnet.org/ej/principles.html
- Refinery Reform Campaign: www.refineryreform.org
- Sierra Club Environmental Justice: www.sierraclub.org/environmental_justice
- Southwest Network for Environmental and Economic Justice: www.sneej.org
- WE ACT West Harlem: www.weact.org
- Wilma Subra: www.commondreams.org/ headlines01/1021-03.htm

check air quality. With a little training and a simple bucket, residents can prove (for instance) that there is benzene, toluene and carbon disulfide in the air, as the residents of Diamond, Louisiana, did when Shell Chemical had been feigning ignorance for so long. Having an award-winning scientist and activist on your side helps, as Wilma Subra does for hundreds of polluted communities along the Mississippi River.

When we all work together to support each other in our different struggles, we will move that much faster towards the goal we seek: the right to healthy, safe environments for all.

# 28

# Build Coalitions

We know that we must get to the front end of the problems, and that prevention is what is needed. Government that truly represents the best interest of its people must not be seduced by corporations that work at the back end of the problem. We are leading the way to survival in the 21$^{st}$ century. Our planet cannot sustain a throwaway society.

— Terry Swearingen, winner of the 1997 Goldman Environmental Prize for her campaign to close down a hazardous waste incinerator next to people's homes and a school in East Liverpool, Ohio

Everyone who is working towards the goal of detoxifying the world accepts that it is a large and complex task. Through the combined efforts of millions of people, however, we can achieve results that no individual or group could achieve on its own.

### Working Together Regionally

Washington State, Oregon and California all have citizen-led coalitions that represent the efforts of many smaller groups to change state legislation and establish new government policies that will protect us against toxic hazards. Alaska, Maine, Massachusetts and New York State have similar coalitions. In the South, the Deep South Center for Environmental Justice and the Louisiana Bucket Brigade serve a similar purpose.

Other groups such as the Alliance for Reducing Cancer, Northwest (www.arcnw.org), are linked to the federal Cancer Prevention and Control

initiative (www.cdc.gov/cancer) that places most of its focus on the medical side of things.

In New York State, the Citizens Environmental Coalition, representing 110 community, labor, faith-based, youth, health and environmental groups, was instrumental in securing the passage of New York's Hazardous Waste Reduction Law that required industry to substantially reduce its toxic waste, and it led the campaign that stopped a huge radioactive waste dump from being given a permit. Over the years, its members have helped communities stop the siting of more than 80 hazardous waste landfills and incinerators. Without their efforts, most of these projects would now be releasing toxins and dioxins (www.cectoxic.org).

Most of North America's 62 states and provinces, however, do not have any such citizen protection. There's a lot of work to be done.

### Working Together Nationally

The Science and Environmental Health Network, led by Carolyn Raffensperger and Ted Schettler, provides leadership for the campaign to persuade governments to embrace the precautionary principle as the basis for environmental and public health policy (see Solution 67) (www.sehn.org).

The Coming Clean coalition serves as an incubator for new campaigns and strategies. It was formed following the groundbreaking

Breast Cancer Action activists protest a corporate face on public health documentary, *Trade Secrets: A Bill Moyers Report*, that shows how the chemical industry has produced thousands of chemicals that have never been tested for their effects on public health and safety. It is developing a nationwide campaign around our growing body burden of chemical toxins, and it leads the Campaign for Safe Cosmetics (www.safecosmetics.org).

The Collaborative on Health and the Environment is a network of over 400 organizations and 2000 individuals who are concerned about environmental contaminants and their links to disease. It has working groups on cancer, EMF and other topics, and regional groups in Washington, Oregon, Alaska and Pennsylvania (www.healthandenvironment.org).

The Center for Health, Environment and Justice (CHEJ) was founded in 1981 by Lois Gibbs, who led the struggle to get the residents of Love Canal, near Niagara Falls, New York, relocated after they learned they were living on top of 20,000 tons of dumped hazardous wastes. Lois established CHEJ to help other communities deal with similar toxic hazards, responding to thousands of calls for help every year. They also run three campaigns: BE SAFE works with hundreds of groups across the country to build a national movement to promote the precautionary principle; Child Proofing Our Communities works with other groups to educate and empower communities to protect children from toxic exposures; and the Green Flag Schools Program for Environmental leadership provides a framework for schools to engage in environmental advocacy. (www.chej.org)

- Alliance for a Healthy Tomorrow (Massachusetts): www.healthytomorrow.org
- Canada's PIRGs: www.pirg.ca
- Environmental Health Strategy Center (Maine): www.preventharm.org
- Military Toxics Project: www.miltoxproj.org
- Northwest Coalition for Alternatives to Pesticides: www.pesticide.org
- Oregon Toxics Alliance: www.oregontoxics.org
- Pesticides Action Network: www.panna.org
- San Francisco Breast Cancer Action Network: www.bcaction.org
- Silicon Valley Toxics Coalition: www.svtc.org
- US State PIRG campaigns: www.uspirg.org
- Washington Toxics Coalition: www.watoxics.org

In Canada, Prevent Cancer *Now* has set its sights on the complete elimination of hazardous chemicals nationwide by 2020 and the adoption of legislation similar to that in Europe (www.preventcancernow.ca). The Toxics Caucus of the Canadian Environment Network brings groups together to work on legislative and regulatory reforms (www.cen-rce.org).

The heroic Dr. Samuel Epstein, who has campaigned to stop cancer since the 1960s and is author of *Cancer-Gate: How to Win the Losing War on Cancer* spearheaded the Cancer Prevention Coalition (www.preventcancer.com), and there's more. The network of state Public Interest Research Groups (PIRGS) based on campuses across the US is running a wide-ranging Safe from Toxics campaign (www.safefromtoxics.org); Greenpeace USA also runs a continuing toxics campaign (www.greenpeace.org/usa/campaigns/toxics).

Is this enough? No, of course not. Which is why we need more local groups and community engagement. Which is why we need *you*.

# 29

## Create New Legislation

> It is difficult to get people to understand something when their salary depends upon them not understanding it.
>
> — Upton Sinclair

At the end of the day, most grassroots campaigners find themselves saying "We need proper legislation, to protect us from harm."

Drafting legislation and getting it passed, is a matter of learning the ropes and applying your efforts to the goal. This includes understanding that you may encounter opposition from groups such as the American Chemistry Council and being organized to mobilize the public to defend your proposal. Here are some great pieces of legislation that should be introduced in every community.

### Toxics Use Reduction Legislation

In the late 1980s, in Massachusetts, a coalition led by the National Toxics Campaign and the Massachusetts Public Interest Research Group wanted to see certain chemicals restricted or banned, while a business coalition wanted to make sure the legislation would not cause companies to leave the state. The two sides were encouraged to talk, and as a result, the groundbreaking Toxics Use Reduction Act was passed unanimously by both houses of the State Legislature in 1989 (see Solution 72). The Act has been a stunning success, causing a 90% reduction in toxic releases to the environment by 2001, with further reductions since. (www.turi.org)

### Local Right to Know Legislation

In 1996 the citizens of Eugene, Oregon, drafted the US's only right to know law that requires local manufacturers to produce a yearly ledger sheet of their toxic inputs and outputs, showing how they balance. It was passed 55% to 45% by local initiative and written into the City's charter, where City Council cannot alter it. The law has worked very well, but the American Electronics Association and Oregon Associated Industries were so upset that they persuaded the Oregon Legislature to pass a law that prevents any other Oregon community from doing the same. This so frustrated the campaigners that it led to the formation of the Oregon Toxics Alliance (www.ci.eugene.or.us/toxics).

### Toxics Phase-out Legislation

In the late 1990s, the Washington Toxics Coalition built a good relationship with the Director of the Washington State Department of Ecology, which led to a statewide strategy to phase out persistent bioaccumulative toxics, including dioxin and mercury. The Coalition then linked up with other environmental, faith-based, civic, medical and labor groups and launched several initiatives to build public support for the phase-out, including running public meetings, forming a People's Plan for eliminating persistent pollution, running a full-page advertisement, organizing a letter from Washington doctors and holding meetings with legislators. Their efforts were successful, and the legislation was approved in 2004 (www.watoxics.org and www.toxicfreelegacy.org).

### Canada's Pesticide Bylaws

In Canada over 70 cities and towns have passed bylaws restricting or prohibiting the use of pesticides for cosmetic purposes. The entire province of Quebec now has a Pesticide Code that bans the use of many chemicals in areas where children may be exposed. It all started in 1990 with a

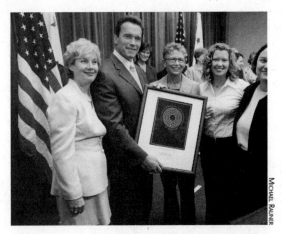
Michael Rauner

Breast Cancer Fund staff present Gov. Schwarzenegger with a Tibetan prayer flag after the signing of Senate Bill 1379 — the California Environmental Contaminant Biomonitoring Program which enacted the US's first statewide program to measure human exposure to chemicals linked to cancer.

- Berkeley *Stop Cancer Where It Starts*: www.bcaction.org/ Pages/TakeAction/BerkeleyResolution.html
- Legislative Steps: www.come-clean.org/stepslegis.htm
- Municipal Pesticide Bylaws: www.cche-info.com/Bylaws.html
- Oregon's Pesticide Use Reporting Program: www.pesticide.org/PUR.html
- Pesticide Free Ontario: www.pesticidefree.ca

small group of activists in the town of Hudson (pop. 4,786) who persuaded their town council to pass a bylaw. It was challenged by two lawn care companies, Chemlawn and Spraytech, but it was upheld in the local court, in the Quebec Superior Court and in Canada's Supreme Court, which ruled that such a bylaw was "consistent with international law's precautionary principle, which states that it is better to be overly cautious than to create a potential risk to the environment." A coalition of groups formed Pesticide Free Ontario, which led to many bylaw campaigns across the province.

### California's Safe Cosmetics Law
Passed in 2005, California's Safe Cosmetics Law requires companies to report any ingredients linked to cancer and birth defects and allows the State to regulate products to protect salon workers if there is a safety risk. This is the first such legislation of its kind in North America. The success followed a two-year campaign by Breast Cancer Action, the Breast Cancer Fund and the National Environmental Trust and tough opposition from cosmetics companies including Mary Kay, Avon, Estée Lauder, L'Oreal, Neutrogena, Proctor and Gamble and Johnson and Johnson. Twenty California cosmetics manufacturers supported the bill, and 200 companies have signed the Compact for Safe Cosmetics, pledging to replace hazardous ingredients with safer alternatives within three years (www.safecosmetics.org).

### More Important Legislation for Cancer Prevention
- Europe's REACH legislation (see Solution 69)
- Oregon's Pesticide Use Reporting Program
- Massachusetts' Safer Cleaning Products Bill: www.healthytomorrow.org
- Massachusetts' Safer Alternatives to Toxic Chemicals Bill: www.healthytomorrow.org
- British Columbia's Workers Compensation Board's toxics substitution clause (see Solution 73)
- Berkeley's *Stop Cancer Where It Starts* measures (see Solution 24)
- San Francisco's ordinances/by-laws on mercury and dioxin
- Solutions 66 to 85 include many more important legislative suggestions.

# 30

# Learn the Art of Advocacy

> If you don't exist in the media, for all practical purposes, you don't exist.
>
> — Daniel Schorr, National Public Radio

As we build the work to prevent cancer, we need to learn how to deal with governments, politicians, the media and the general public.

## Pass Local Resolutions

When Breast Cancer Action decided to ask the City of Berkeley to pass a resolution declaring October Stop Cancer Before It Starts month (see Solution 24), they did a lot of homework. They formed a coalition with like-minded groups and made a list of practical actions they wanted Berkeley to take, such as eliminating PVC plastic in building construction. They approached Council members who were sympathetic to discuss what might be achieved, and asked them to sponsor the resolution. As the vote drew near, they contacted other councillors and developed a media strategy. You never know how the vote will go, so preparation of this kind will increase your chances. Student governments are also good places for resolutions.

## Learn the Art of Advocacy

To get legislation passed, you will need a strategy to win the attention of your legislators and build good relationships with the staff. When the Washington Toxics Coalition wanted to bring in Toxics Phase-out legislation, it was their relationship with the Director of the Washington State Department of Ecology that was important. They also piled on the pressure with letters and e-mails from the public.

## Build Public Support

All political initiatives need public support. For their campaign against toxic phthalates in cosmetics, the Not Too Pretty coalition created an Internet flash movie that directed people to their website (www.nottoopretty.org/images/Poison_Small.mpg). A good website can do wonders to inform people and encourage them to write letters. Individually written letters carry much more weight than form letters and e-mails.

## Learn from RESULTS

RESULTS, one of North America's most effective nonprofit societies, works to create the public and political will to

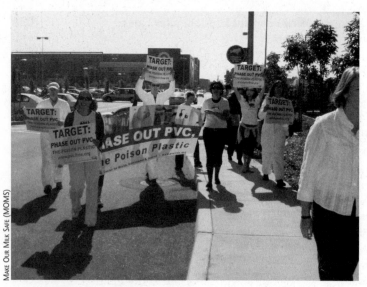

Make Our Milk Safe (MOMS)

PVC Day of Action in October 2006, organized by BE SAFE and Make Our Milk Safe (MOMS).

end world hunger and the worst aspects of poverty. Each month, members meet at someone's home to study a particular issue, write to their MPs or Congressmen and submit letters and op-ed pieces to local and national papers. They follow up with personal meetings. This builds the political will for change and leads to increased government funding to fight diseases like TB and malaria. In Canada in 2004, for every $1 that a supporter donated, RESULTS leveraged $72 in increased funding from the government. RESULTS' methods are clear, focussed and effective. *Reclaiming Our Democracy: Healing the Break Between People and Government*, by RESULTS founder Sam Daley-Harris, is a very inspiring read.

**Learn from the Rainforest Action Network**

The Rainforest Action Network (RAN) is another group we can learn from. Its goal is to protect forests and the rights of their inhabitants by campaigning to break America's oil addiction, promote sustainable logging and bring green ethics to Wall Street. RAN's campaign to persuade the giant finance bank Citigroup to adopt progressive environmental and human rights policies included television spots with Hollywood celebrities cutting up their Citibank credit cards, a full-page ad in *The New York Times* and a super-sized banner across the street from their midtown New York offices. After years of campaigning by countless volunteers, Citigroup, Bank of America and JPMorgan Chase adopted policies that safeguard old-growth and endangered forests, curb investments in climate change and protect the

- 20/20 Vision Resources: www.2020vision.org
- The Art of Advocacy: www.ccednet-rcdec.ca/en/docs/pubs/AdvocacyHandbook-FIN2.pdf
- Developing Relationships with Reporters: www.spinproject.org/downloads/Reporters.pdf
- Electronic Advocacy Tools for Canadian nonprofits: www.actionworks.ca
- Electronic Activists Toolkit: www.onenw.org/bin/page.cfm/secid/5
- Guidelines for Legislative Lobbying: www.renewamerica.us/handbook/helps.htm
- How a Bill Becomes a Law: www.environmentalleague.org/BILL2LAW.html
- Legislative Testimony, A Guide for Citizen Activists: www.environmentalleague.org/Testimony.htm
- Media Advocacy Manual: www.apha.org/about/news/mediaadvocacy.htm
- News Releases: www.spinproject.org/downloads/PressReleases.pdf
- Results: www.results.org
- Activists' Milestones and Toolkit: www.results.org/website/article.asp?id=1745
- The Spin Project: www.spinproject.org
- You, Too, Can Be an Effective Health Advocate: www.healthyamericans.org/community/guides/advocacy.pdf

rights of indigenous peoples. RAN is very feisty, and they make it work for them. (www.ran.org).

**Learn from Internet Activism**

It is safe to assume that almost everyone in your group has access to the Internet, which you can use to deliver newsletters, action reminders and reports, and encourage your members to talk to each other, and discuss strategy. There are many toolkits to help, but don't think that an e-mail is as good as personal contact. Personal meetings and good relationships will always be the backbone of good activism, whether with the media, politicians or the public.

# 31

# Champion Public Health and Environmental Justice

S tudy after study has shown that economic inequality is a major source of health problems, including cancer.[2] Wealthy people are healthier. They can afford the best of everything, including medical care, nutritious food and healthier environments that people on lower incomes can't. And while it *is* true that toxic substances trespass virtually everywhere, the worst pollution is experienced by poor and poorly served communities, with ethnicity being a significant factor. Environmental degradation adds insult to the injury of poverty.

The growing gulf between rich and poor, along with the overwhelming focus on treatment rather than prevention, is sapping already weakened public health systems and failing citizens in both Canada and the US.

The core principles of public health — prevention, precaution and equity in health status for all — are being swamped by urgent medical

- American Public Health Association: www.apha.org
- Canadian Health Network: www.canadian-health-network.ca
- Canadian Public Health Association: www.cpha.ca
- Center for Healthy Environments and Communities (PA): www.chec.pitt.edu/mambo
- Community Outreach and Education Program: www.niehs.nih.gov/external/outreach.htm
- Environmental Health links: www.neetf.org/Health/links.htm
- Harvard School of Public Health: www.hsph.harvard.edu

The US spends more (per capita) on health than any nation in the world, yet it continues to have some of the poorest health outcomes in the industrialized world, especially in communities of color and low-income populations.

— Thomas Milne[1]

demands that a properly funded public health system could have alleviated. "It's been the tyranny of the acute," explained Canada's minister of public health in 2004. "The urgent took over the important and we focused on repair shops in a 'sickness care' system. We forgot that we must focus on both health *and* health care."[3]

What can health care professionals do under these circumstances?

### Advocate for Public Health

Income disparities demand both political *and* economic solutions, leading Dr. Peter Montague of *Rachel's Environment & Health Weekly* to strongly endorse public health activism. "If economic inequalities are a major source of public health problems, then public health specialists have a professional obligation to work to reduce inequalities, and to speak openly about the problem."[4] All health professionals who are committed to the "First, do no harm" credo must stand up for effective public health systems in both Canada and the United States — and for the funding to achieve them.

### Go Beyond "Lifestyle"

Public health institutions that focus on cancer must embrace more than the narrowly defined personal "lifestyle" factors that are commonly identified — smoking, diet, alcohol, exercise and sun sense. They must also address the underlying social, economic and environmental injustices that play an important role in cancer incidence. Here are some inspiring examples:

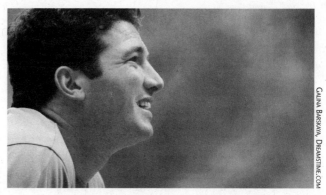

Meet 'Reference Man', the hypothetical adult Caucasian male, 20-30 years old and 5' 7" tall. He is used widely to set standards for radiation and toxic exposures, and in the name of public health, he should be retired. Instead, federal agencies need to protect all at risk, including pregnant women, fetuses and embryos, infants and children, the weak and aged.

- The National Institute of Environmental Health Sciences sponsors a Community Outreach and Education Program (COEP) that helps schools of public health to develop environmental health education and action strategies in partnership with poor communities. The Columbia University School of Public Health Outreach Program, for instance, works with a Harlem environmental justice group, WE ACT, to address a wide range of toxics issues, including cancer. In 2004 COEP's activities included an environmental health and justice leadership training program.

- In 2005 a working group of the National Environmental Justice Advisory Council (NEJAC) produced recommendations for actions to address the complex problems of environmental racism in US communities. They concluded that the EPA's 2003 Frameworks for Cumulative Risk Assessment, combined with a collaborative problem-solving approach, "is the fastest and surest way to bring about tangible and sustainable benefits for disproportionately impacted communities and (Native Indian) tribes."[5]

- In Toronto the South Riverdale Community Health Centre has developed many accessible resources on environmental health since its inception in the 1970s, in consultation with local partners and residents. Its primer, *Making Environmental Health Happen in the Community!*, is available at www.healthycommunities.on.ca/publications/misc/southriverdale_healthmanual.pdf.

## Offer Environmental Health Education

The National Environmental Education & Training Foundation (NEETF) is a coalition of over 20 leading US health organizations. Recognizing the shortcomings of professional training in environmental health, in late 2004 its members recommended several initiatives, including:

- Adopt environmental health education and practice standards so that health care providers learn about environmental exposures in clinical, educational and preventive health care.

- Use validated tools and resources to recognize, manage and prevent health effects from environmental exposures.

- Appoint an environmental health faculty champion at each medical and nursing school to ensure that environmental health considerations are integrated into the medical and nursing school curricula.[6]

# 32

# Promote Healthy Parenting Before Conception and Birth

Consider this: A compulsory education program for health professionals called *Cancer Prevention Before Conception*.

Yes, it may sound bizarre at first, but a growing body of evidence links childhood cancers with hazardous substances that parents are exposed to before conception occurs, as well as during pregnancy, especially at work.[2] Many preconception and *in utero* risks also lead to birth defects, asthma, allergies and low birth weights. Add these up, and it makes sense for health care professionals responsible for healthy babies to offer preconception *and* prenatal health guidance to prospective parents — including information about exposures to toxic substances.

Infertility itself is a problem. The National Center for Health Statistics estimates that about 10% of the population of childbearing age — six

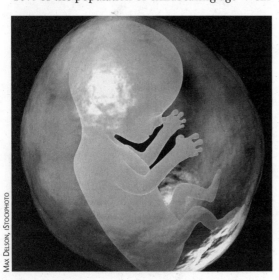

MAX DELSON, iSTOCKPHOTO

When research data from well baby clinics from before World War I were analyzed, it became readily apparent that health outcomes for life are determined not only by what happens while in utero, but — even more importantly — by the state of health our mother and father were in 100 days prior to conception.

— Dr. Allan Lieberman[1]

million couples in the US alone — experiences infertility; others say it's as high as 15%. One reason is that many women now delay pregnancy until their thirties or early forties, which significantly lowers fertility rates. Environmental factors also appear to play a role. Exposure to agricultural pesticides has been linked to declining sperm counts, as has exposure to chemicals such as styrene, formaldehyde and toluene.[3] The main medical response to date has been to intervene with a wide array of costly and often complex reproductive technologies.

Most preconception care, when it is practiced, mirrors the approach of the mainstream cancer establishment, focusing on lifestyle issues such as smoking, healthy diet, exercise and personal factors such as age, prescription medications and family histories of disease. Environmental and occupational hazards are rarely examined.

The Center for Occupational & Environmental Medicine in South Carolina offers preconception care that does consider the toxic world we live in. Dr. Allan Lieberman, the Center's medical director, credits the British pioneer Belinda Barnes, who had no medical degree, with a "remarkable record of pregnancy outcomes that no medical establishment has ever accomplished":

- No premature births
- No miscarriages
- No birth weight below 5lbs., 2oz.
- No congenital malformation
- No need for neonatal intensive care.

- Center for Occupational & Environmental Medicine, *Preconception Care*: www.coem.com/preconception.asp
- *Health Professionals' Guide to Preconception Care,* by Dr. Marilyn Glenville: www.foresight-preconception.org.uk/booklet_healthproguide.htm.
- *Planning for a Healthy Baby,* by Belinda Barnes and Suzanne Gail Bradley (Vermillion): www.foresight-preconception.org.uk/books_planninghealthybaby.htm

Belinda Barnes's book, *Planning for a Healthy Baby: Essential Preparation for Pregnancy*, offers a practical program of health care that includes advice on nutrition, family planning, common illnesses and diseases, and toxic substances to be avoided.

At the Foresight Preconception Clinic in the UK, the preconception program focuses on the following, based on the work of the nutritional therapist Marilyn Glenville:

- Nutrition
- Tobacco, alcohol and street drugs
- Food additives
- Food allergies/malabsorption
- Organophosphate pesticides
- Drinking water
- Mineral analysis, toxic metals and supplementation/cleansing
- Contraception
- Genitourinary infections
- Other areas of concern, including electromagnetic radiation.

The same approach could be adopted by naturopaths, midwives and other complementary and alternative health practitioners. Dr. Sat Dharam Kaur's book *The Complete Natural Medicine Guide to Women's Health* is an excellent resource.[4]

The impact of preconception and in utero exposures to a wide range of toxic substances presents a forbidding challenge to science and public health, as Dr. Ted Schettler concluded in his report *Infertility and Related Reproductive Disorders:*

Human studies designed to examine these questions (of infertility) are complex, difficult to carry out and expensive. Studies that measure fetal exposures to substances of interest and then follow offspring as they mature and attempt to reproduce require decades and consistent, close follow-up.[5]

In 2005 the American government scuttled a major children's health study slated to monitor a wide range of health indicators including contaminants in umbilical cord blood and other toxic substances. Even if the study had gone forward, complete results would not have been available for more than two decades. Dr. Schettler makes a strong case for using the evidence that's already in hand, even if it's partial and imperfect:

A central question requiring public discussion and policy decisions is the extent to which the results of animal testing, wildlife observations and limited information about human health trends should be used now for protecting the reproductive health of humans and wildlife.

We will say more bluntly what Dr. Schettler implies: We can't afford to wait for more studies. Cleansing and detoxifying our world — which will eliminate common environmental hazards such as dioxins and trace solvents from crossing the placenta — is the only way to proceed. The first environment for developing infants must be safe, protective and pollutant-free.

# 33

## Ensure a Safe Childhood

**People who wouldn't dream of abusing a child think nothing of giving their children and grandchildren an environment that has been abused.**

— Richard J. Jackson, MD, Director, National Center for Environmental Health

By the time you read this, basic training in children's environmental health may finally be making its way into undergraduate medical and nursing education programs and pediatric residencies. Continuing education programs on this subject for MDs and nurses may also be growing. But by early 2007, most of these notions were still a gleam in the eye.

According to a multi-disciplinary American expert group on children's health:

**Pediatric medical and nursing education currently lacks the environmental health content necessary to appropriately prepare pediatric health care professionals to prevent, recognize, manage and treat environmental-exposure-related disease. Leading health institutions have recognized the need for improvements in health professionals' environmental health education. Parents are seeking answers about the impact of environmental toxicants on their children.**[1]

### Educational Resources

While basic training may still be waiting in the wings, good print and Web resources are increasing steadily.

**Pediatric Environmental Health**, American Academy of Pediatrics (2003), covers many preventable environmental hazards, such as water pollution, pesticides, lead and mercury, gasoline, food irradiation, nickel, manganese and chromium. Chapters include "Environmental Health Advocacy" and "Environmental Threats to Children's Health in Developing Countries" (www.aap.org):

**Children's Environmental Health Project,** Canadian Association of Physicians for the Environment (CAPE), is an on-line resource that introduces doctors to the fundamentals of children's environmental health, with a unit on cancer and immune functioning. Covers environmental history-taking, and offers a commentary on the physician's role in the primary prevention of environmental health problems among children (www.cape.ca/children).

**Child Health and the Environment: A Primer,** Canadian Partnership for Children's Health and Environment (2005), is suitable for a wide range of readers, including women of child-bearing age, new and prospective parents, teachers, health care and child care practitioners and environmental and health policy developers. Covers cancer, environmental exposures, research, political action, regulation and the precautionary principle (www.healthyenvironmentforkids.ca).

**Children's Environmental Health: Reducing Risk in a Dangerous World,** by Dona Schneider and Natalie Freeman, American Public Health Association (2000). Clear, understandable information about the environmental threats and what we can do to prevent them (www.apha.org/programs/additional/mch/programsResourceCenter.htm).

**Child Health and the Environment,** by Donald T. Wigle, Oxford University Press (2003). This "first textbook to focus on environmental threats to child health" covers children's environmental health issues, including the health effects of metals, PCBs, dioxins, pesticides, hormonally active agents, radiation, indoor and outdoor air pollution and water contaminants. Also covers the role of environmental epidemiology and risk assessment in child health protection; the susceptibility of the fetus and infant to environmental toxicants; the importance of modifying factors; uncertainties surrounding environmental exposure limits; and the importance of timely intervention (www.mclaughlincentre.ca).

**The Pediatric Environmental Toolkit,** Greater Boston Physicians for Social Responsibility (2006) is one of several excellent environmental health resources produced by this group.

"Incorporating Environmental Health into Pediatric Medical and Nursing Education," *Environmental Health Perspectives*, 112(17), Dec. 2004: www.ehponline.org/realfiles/ members/2004/7166/7166.html.

**Training Manual on Pediatric Environmental Health: Putting It Into Practice,** Children's Environment Health Network was designed to assist health care faculties to incorporate pediatric environmental health into their teaching programs. Includes case studies, discussion questions and suggested assignments for students, medical residents and colleagues: www.cehn.org/cehn/manual-front.htm.

**Resources for Nurses**
- *EnviRN* is a virtual resource for environmental health and nursing from the University of Maryland, Baltimore, School of Nursing: www.envirn.umaryland.edu
- *RN No Harm*, American Nurses Association: www.nursingworld.org/coeh/rnnoharm
- Children's Health, Environmental Health, American Nurses Association Online Continuing Education: www.nursingworld.org/ce

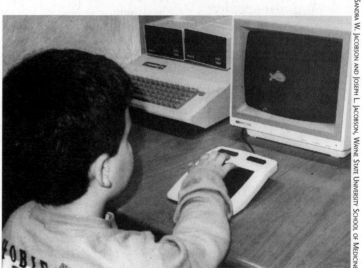

SANDRA W. JACOBSON AND JOSEPH L. JACOBSON, WAYNE STATE UNIVERSITY SCHOOL OF MEDICINE

Since 1980, Joseph and Sandra Jacobson, psychologists at Wayne State University have studied 242 children whose mothers frequently ate salmon and lake trout contaminated with PCBs, noting lower IQs, among other deficits. It will probably take many more years to find out if the higher exposure to PCBs, a probable carcinogen, increases cancer risk for these children.

# 34

# Solutions for Cancer Organizations

It's rare to hear words like "carcinogen," "chemical risk," or "radionuclide" in the hallways and inner sanctums of most cancer agencies and hospitals. Tobacco, yes. Diet, yes. Alcohol and exercise, yes. But personal care products? Air pollutants? Contaminants in food and water? Not very often.

**The Center for Environmental Oncology of the University of Pittsburgh Cancer Institute (UPCI)** is a world leader when it comes to the environmental links to cancer. It embraces traditional "lifestyle" factors such as smoking, alcohol, diet and exercise, but it also includes cancer hazards in the air, water, soil and food, as well as ingredients in personal care products. The whole health profile of people living in Pittsburgh depends on their neighborhoods, their work conditions, their racial and ethnic origins and their income levels.

While most cancer institutions focus on crusades for the cure, the Center for

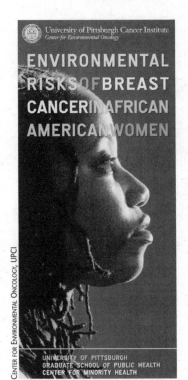

Cover of the Center for Environmental Oncology's information brochure.

**Medical, patient, public health and environmental groups that share some of the same concerns too often have not worked together toward common goals ... Everyone concerned — health-affected groups, scientists, health professionals and environmental organizations — can serve as resources for each other in collaborations that will help reduce public exposure to environmental toxicants.**

**— Philip R. Lee, MD, Chairman,
Collaborative on Health and the Environment**

Environmental Oncology of the UPCI, by contrast, synthesizes the blizzard of data about the environmental links to cancer and converts positive associations into public policy and patient education programs, with an emphasis on primary prevention and precaution.

Dr. Devra Davis, author of the award-winning book, *When Smoke Ran Like Water*, and *The Secret History of the War on Cancer*, is the driving force behind the center, which opened in 2004. She writes: "Given enough knowledge and the ability to make changes, individuals can take action to avoid at least some of the known cancer-causing agents or carcinogens in their daily lives, thus lowering personal risks of getting cancer during their lifetimes."[1]

One example: It is well established that African-American women under 40 have a higher risk of breast cancer than other categories of women. It's also known that the more estrogen a woman is exposed to during her lifetime, the greater her risk of contracting breast cancer. In 2005 the center followed up a study of African-American girls who had developed breasts and pubic hairs as toddlers. The study identified one common factor among these young girls — all of their mothers had used creams containing hormones to style their children's hair. The girls stopped developing breasts when their mothers

- Canadian Cancer Society: www.cancer.ca. Search "prevention" and "advocacy"
- Center for Environmental Oncology: www.environmentaloncology.org
- Collaborative on Health and the Environment: www.healthandenvironment.org
- Ontario College of Family Physicians: www.ocfp.on.ca

stopped using the hair creams.[2] A simple, basic example of the precautionary principle in action.

Many shampoos, styling gels and cosmetics targeted to African-Americans contain chemicals known to act like estrogens when applied to the scalp or body. And while there's no conclusive proof that these hair products are linked to breast cancer, there's enough evidence to warrant concern. The Pittsburgh center offers consumer-friendly information about the issue — and on specific products — in its Guide to Green Living website: www.environmentaloncology.org/green_living.htm.

Another departure from the mainstream is the public stand taken in 2002 by the **Canadian Cancer Society** (CCS) against "ornamental" pesticides containing known or probable carcinogens used in public places and gardens. It was CCS's first major step into the toxics-use fray following its formal adoption of the precautionary principle as a core belief. This CCS position has proved valuable to dozens of Canadian municipalities that are working to restrict or ban lawn and garden pesticides, a cause that was further strengthened when the Ontario College of Family Physicians released its *Pesticides Literature Review* in April 2004.[3] In 2005 CCS took another stand for precaution by endorsing a strong advocacy statement on occupational exposure.[4]

The **Collaborative on Health and Environment** (CHE), based in California with members mainly in the US and Canada, is a diverse partnership of health professionals, scientists, concerned individuals and organizations working together to address concerns about links between environmental factors and human health, including cancer. Underlying CHE's activities are commitments to strong, uncompromised science and to the precautionary principle when compelling evidence of potential for harm to human health and the environment exists.

Their resources include:

- *Environmental and Occupational Causes of Cancer: A Review of Recent Scientific Literature.*
- CHE Toxicants and Disease Database, a searchable database summarizing links between chemical contaminants and approximately 200 diseases or conditions.

Goals of the Center for Environmental Oncology, UPCI, include:

- Building links from basic research to clinical studies of avoidable carcinogens, including hormonally mediated agents
- Developing and applying state-of-the-art technology to the identification of carcinogenic exposures
- Pilot-testing institutional interventions to modify cancer risks consistent with "greening" facilities, and providing healthy options regarding exercise, nutrition and avoidable chemical exposures
- Educating and training health professionals and communities
- Informing patients, their families and communities about cancer risks and ways to reduce their chance of recurrence.

# 35

# Practice Health Care Without Harm

It sounds so obvious. Hospitals and health clinics *ought* to be places where patients have the best chance to recover from their illnesses and injuries. The irony is that too many "health care" centers have the potential to make people even sicker by exposing them to dioxins, phthalates, PVC, mercury and volatile organic compounds (VOCs).

Hospitals, like other large institutions, take their toll on the environment — they're major users of water, energy, building products and ongoing goods and services — but not all "good" from a health standpoint. They also pose unique challenges, including environmentally significant precursors and potentially toxic bodily by-products of medications, complex and hazardous solid, air and water emissions and toxic, infectious and radioactive wastes.[2]

**Health Care Without Harm** (HCWH) was founded in 1996 in response to a disturbing US EPA report that cited hospital incinerators as the

**Imagine if cancer centers were built without materials linked to cancer; if pediatric clinics used no asthma-triggering chemicals; if hospitals offered healthy food and rooms with views.**
— Health Care Without Harm[1]

leading source of dioxin, a potent carcinogen. HCWC is now an international coalition of hundreds of organizations in more than 50 countries, with a mission to transform the health care sector to become ecologically sustainable, and no longer a source of harm to people and the environment.

HCWH's goals include:

1. Creating markets and policies for safer products, materials and chemicals in health care, and promoting safer substitutes, including products that avoid mercury, polyvinyl chloride (PVC) plastic and brominated flame retardants.

2. Eliminating incineration of medical waste, minimizing the amount and toxicity of all waste generated and promoting safer waste treatment practices.

3. Transforming the design, construction and operations of health care facilities to minimize environmental impacts and foster healthy, healing environments.

4. Encouraging food purchasing systems that support sustainable food production and distribution, and providing healthy food at health care facilities.

*The Green Guide for Health Care* is helping to transform the health care profession from the ground up. Developed in the US by a team of architects, engineers, health care professionals and public health advocates, it is a "best-practice tool for the design, construction, operation and maintenance of health care facilities." While geared primarily toward new construction, it also

**The Continuum Center for Health and Healing** is part of Manhattan's Beth Israel Medical Center. All of the building materials and installation methods in this integrative health center were chosen to optimize indoor air quality and environmental responsibility. All flooring, paint, adhesives and cabinet substrates eliminate use of formaldehyde and VOCs. The use of carpet is minimized, and major flooring materials are cork and linoleum — natural, biodegradable products. The fabrics contain recycled and compostable fibres. All materials were selected for easy maintenance with natural cleaning products, in order to preserve a high level of indoor air quality.[4]

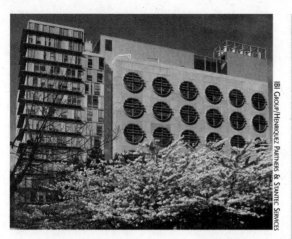

IBI GROUP/HENRIQUEZ PARTNERS & STANTEC SERVICES

BC Cancer Agency Research Centre, a LEED Gold green building in Vancouver with very high energy and water efficiency, fresh air, natural daylight, and very low emissions from paints and finishes.

- Canadian Centre for Pollution Prevention Health Care Environet: www.c2p2online.com
- Canadian Coalition for Green Health Care: www.greenhealthcare.ca
- Continuum Center for Health and Healing: www.healthandhealingny.org
- Green Guide to Health Care: www.gghc.org
- Green Health Care Practice: www.teleosis.org
- Health Care Without Harm (includes *Going Green: A Resource Kit for Pollution Prevention in Health Care*: www.noharm.org
- Hospitals for a Healthy Environment: www.h2e-online.org
- Sustainable Hospitals Project: www.sustainablehospitals.org

addresses renovations and expansions and includes a section on operations. By 2006, the *Green Guide* had 84 projects on the go, representing more than 20 million square feet of construction.

**The Hospital for Sick Children** in Toronto targeted biomedical waste as a key part of the first-ever comprehensive pollution prevention (P2) plan for a hospital in Canada. Sick Children's reduced the biomedical waste from its lab and patient care areas by 35%, which resulted in the shutdown of its incinerator, saving 50% of the hospital's annual $1.2 million waste management budget.[5]

Tracy Easthope of The Ecology Center in Ann Arbor, Michigan, takes the vision of sustainable hospitals and health care several steps farther:

**An ecologically integrated system would be a model of reciprocity. It would understand its location in a particular place, within a particular ecosystem. It might buy organic food from local, small farms in the surrounding community, supporting not only a local green belt,** **farmland preservation, and local scale activity, but a gradual restoration of the local ecosystem as well. It might provide for the transportation of its staff and visitors to and from its doors, to minimize impacts. It might decentralize. It might restore native habitat in its surrounding area, and work to revive streams or lakes or soils in its midst ... It would also work to change the social systems — political and economic — that threaten health.** [6]

And that notorious hospital food? Thanks to HCWH and others, it, too, is undergoing a transformation. At the **Dominican Hospital in Santa Cruz**, California, for example, executive chef Deane Bussiere offers organic, sustainably grown, in-season food dishes that sound more at home on a high-class restaurant menu than on a patient's dinner tray or in the hospital cafeteria. Dominican Hospital has its own organic produce garden tended by local high-school students, and Bussiere also buys from a nonprofit community-based organic farm in nearby Salinas.[7]

# 36

# Create a Cancer Prevention Action Plan

Inside the problem of cities lies the solution. The city — always the place of greatest dynamism and creativity — may also present the greatest opportunity for a greener, healthier future.

— Vanessa Baird, Green Cities[1]

For the first time in Earth's history, over half of all humanity now lives in cities, a trend that will accelerate over the next two decades. Seoul, Korea and 20 other large urban centers have populations of 10 million or more, a stunning figure when you realize that 200 years ago, London was the only city with a population greater than 1 million. Even in 1900, just 15%

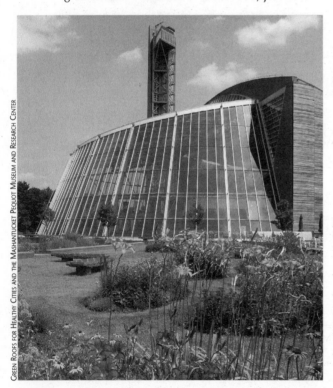

GREEN ROOFS FOR HEALTHY CITIES AND THE MASHANTUCKET PEQUOT MUSEUM AND RESEARCH CENTER

Green roofs aren't just beautiful, they contribute to less toxic run-off, a serious problem in asphalt-laden cities. Green Roofs for Healthy Cities: www.greenroofs.org.

of the globe's population was urban. What a difference a century makes!

The challenges facing cities are colossal. "No precedent exists for feeding, sheltering, employing or transporting so many people. No precedent exists for protecting the environment from the pollution and resource consumption required by such multitudes," said Janice E. Perlman of the Mega-Cities Project in the US.[2]

Then there's cancer. Comparing the incidence of cancer in cities versus rural areas is complicated by a lack of data, but the statistics that do exist appear to confirm what most people suspect — that cancer rates are higher in cities. One thing is certain: urban centers bear the overwhelming responsibility for cancer care and treatment, given their lopsided portion of health care resources, including major hospitals.[3] And as cancer rates explode in the 21st century, cities of all sizes are racing just to keep up with record numbers of new cases.

Toronto has decided to grab hold of the problem. Fiona Nelson, the colorful and outspoken chair of the Toronto Cancer Prevention Coalition (TCPC), points out that she grew up during World War II, when everyone rallied to plant Victory Gardens, and electricity, gasoline and food was rationed. "We mobilized to kill people back then," she said bluntly, "so why can't we mobilize now to save them?"

How *does* a city take on cancer, especially in these days of meager public health funds? Toronto set out to meet the challenge by creating an official cancer prevention plan based on the premise that the right combination of motivated citizens

- Toronto Cancer Prevention Coalition:
  www.toronto.ca/health/resources/tcpc
- Green Cities: www.newint.org/issue313/keynote.htm

and health experts could create the best blueprint for action, under the guiding hand of the city's public health department.

TCPC got off the ground in early 1998 at a daylong conference at the University of Toronto. Labor leaders, city officials, health and safety specialists, physicians and nurses, cancer survivors, grassroots health organizers, environmental NGOs and others came together to focus on the substance of Ontario's landmark 1995 task force report, *Recommendations for the Primary Prevention of Cancer*. Over the next two years, this fledgling coalition grew to embrace 60 partners across Greater Toronto (population 5 million). Members are as diverse as a former Ontario health and environment minister, the Clean Air Partnership, the Toronto District School Board and labor unions including the Canadian Auto Workers and the United Steelworkers of America, as well as the Canadian Cancer Society.

The coalition established eight subgroups to identify the needs and the priorities for action. They then developed "frameworks for implementation," to show how the proposed prevention strategies could become a viable part of public health policy and practice.

Early on, two of the working groups — representing Occupational and Environmental Carcinogens — merged to generate more clout, knowing that, by themselves, these risk factors are often marginalized. This group has since become the most outspoken of the coalition. Among its recommended strategies are the phase-out of eight priority carcinogens in the city: benzene, diesel exhaust, perchlorethylene,

methylene chloride, asbestos, pesticides, polycyclic aromatic hydrocarbons (PAHs) and dioxins. It is also championing a citywide right to know bylaw.

In late 2002, Toronto City Council voted in favor of the TCPC's joint action plan, which made its way to council through the Board of Health. Several strategies have already been adopted and integrated into the City's policies and practices, and while it's too early to know if this work has begun to reduce Toronto's cancer burden, the coalition has had an impact on several City policies, including:

- A phase-out of cosmetic pesticides on public and private property
- The use of sun-protective clothing by all City employees
- A bylaw to protect trees on private property in all neighborhoods
- Action to achieve "quality daily physical activities" for Toronto citizens.

Toronto has shown that it's possible, opening the door for other cities to follow suit. There are four components needed for success, for this or any city initiative:

1. An initiative by local activist groups working together
2. A champion on council who will be your lead contact
3. A majority on council who will vote for the proposals
4. A supportive staff who will give the proposals priority.

# 37

# Become a Green Community

It's the flock, the grove, that matters.
Our responsibility is to species, not to
specimens; to communities, not to
individuals.

— Sara Stein, author of *Noah's Garden*

While most of this century's urban explosion will occur in developing countries, Western cities are Earth's worst eco-gluttons. All told, urban dwellers in the West consume 75% of the world's resources. They produce most of its waste, and they draw food, water and fuel from far outside their city limits, making enormous footprints on the hinterlands and beyond.[1] A good portion of this excessive consumption yields toxic by-products that in turn yield more cancer.

A green, sustainable community is a place where the air is pure and always breathable. Drinking water is safe, clean and way more palatable than the bottled kind. Food is fresh and organic. The city's waste is minimal, manageable and non-toxic — part of the solution, not the problem. Urban growth is measured and dense where it occurs, not absurdly out of control. There are green spaces aplenty, including rooftops and community gardens.

While San Francisco deserves full credit as a green community leader, the city of Santa Monica, just down the California coast, is also worthy of attention. Though small by mega-city standards with a population of just 90,000, Santa Monica's Sustainable City Plan, adopted in 1994, is big league. It all began when Santa Monica calculated its eco-footprint, a shocking reality check that triggered action and a plan that focuses on eight key issues, including transportation, housing and resource conservation. When you scratch the surface, it becomes clear that all eight have cancer prevention aspects, such as the use of green building materials, alternatives to cars for transport, and the promotion of organic, vegetarian diets for all citizens. In the Environmental and Public Health area, one of Santa Monica's sustainability goals is to "minimize and where possible eliminate the use of hazardous or toxic materials" not just in the City's operations, but by residents and businesses as well.

Brian Johnson, Santa Monica's Environmental Programs Coordinator, says, "I'm not a cancer prevention guy, or even a public health guy. I'm an environment guy. But we do have acres of common ground." In 1993 Johnson and his colleagues evaluated the city's

## San Francisco First US City to Adopt the Precautionary Principle

Every San Franciscan has an equal right to a healthy and safe environment...

San Francisco is a leader in making choices based on the least environmentally harmful alternatives, thereby challenging traditional assumptions about risk management. Numerous City ordinances, including the Integrated Pest Management Ordinance, the Resource Efficient Building Ordinance, the Healthy Air Ordinance, the Resource Conservation Ordinance and the Environmentally Preferable Purchasing Ordinance, apply a precautionary approach to specific City purchases and activities. Internationally, this model is called the Precautionary Principle.

— From San Francisco's landmark Precautionary Principle Policy declared June 17, 2003 [3]

- Curitiba, Brazil:
  www3.iclei.org/localstrategies/summary/curitiba2.html
- Global Ecovillage Network: www.ecovillages.org
- Santa Monica: www.santa-monica.org/epd/scp
- Sustainable Communities Network: www.sustainable.org

custodial building maintenance needs and the chemicals used for cleaning. They learned that many products, such as graffiti remover, presented unnecessary and unacceptable risks, including carcinogens. The next step was to develop health and environmental criteria to be used as the city standard. Some criteria required a detailed scoring and ranking system, while others, such as carcinogenicity, became fundamental screens with a simple pass/fail standard. "If you have carcinogens in your product, we will not buy it," Johnson says. Some vendors warned that Santa Monica was too small, and there would be no bidders, but there have always been over a dozen competitors for its cleaning products contracts. Another bonus: "We're saving about 5% on the cost of more toxic products. We're not spending more money, we're spending less."

Designing and implementing sustainable city programs isn't simple or easy, despite Santa Monica's success over the past decade, Johnson says. "These programs are resource intensive; they require oversight, encouragement and a lot of hand holding. But get used to it — that's the nature of change, both for individual behavior and for collective institutional traditions." In its 2005 Report Card, Santa Monica gives itself a B+ in the "Environment and Public Health" area.

Efforts by local environmental organizations and regulations at the local, state and federal level have all combined to help reduce sources of pollution to Santa Monica Bay and to reduce mobile and non-mobile sources of air pollution. Santa Monica residents have excellent access to locally grown, organic foods. Under city programs, use of toxic chemicals in parks and public buildings has plunged. Some gaps remain: The city is short of meeting its targets for reducing beach closures and pollution, regional air pollution is on the rise again after decades of improvement, and persistent toxic chemicals remain common products that Santa Monicans use daily.

Johnson and his staff have gone the distance in researching, digging and evaluating their programs over the years, and the work is paying off for other cities too. "I don't do programs just for Santa Monica. Our models are helping to reduce the workload that used to scare managers of other cities away."[2]

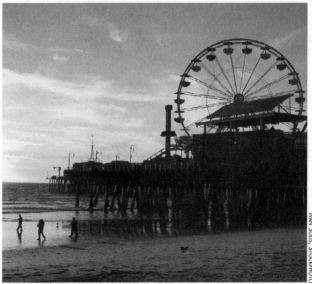

The Santa Monica Pier at sunset.

# 38

# Clean the Air

**Remember all that grime we had on the cars, how
we had to drive with our headlights on in the
afternoon? How the sun didn't shine for days at a
time? .... Look, today they might call it pollution.
Back then it was just a living.**

— Jean Langer Davis[1]

M ost city skies *look* a lot brighter these days
than the smudgy, sooty air of Donora,
Pennsylvania, in the mid-1940s, as described by
author Devra Davis's mother, Jean. But looks can
be deceiving. City air is still dirty — and deadly.

In 2002 the report *Toxic Beginnings* found
that, in just 12 days, a baby born in Los Angeles
would breathe enough air pollutants to exceed
its lifetime acceptable risk for cancer, the overwhelming majority of which comes from diesel
particulate matter and four chemicals: 1,3 butadiene, benzene, carbon tetrachloride and
formaldehyde.

The worst polluters of city air are gas and
diesel engines, from the smallest two-stroke leaf
blowers and lawn mowers to cars, SUVs, buses,
heavy construction equipment and jet aircraft.
Coal-fired power plants are major sinners in the

- American Forests: www.americanforests.org
- Car Free Cities: www.carfree.com
- Centre for Sustainable Transportation (Canada):
  www.cstctd.org
- Green Power Partnership: www.epa.gov/greenpower
- Location Efficient Mortgages: www.locationefficiency.com
- Pedestrian and Bicycle Planning, A Guide to Best
  Practices: www.vtpi.org
- Toxic Beginnings:
  www.net.org/health/ toxic_beginnings.pdf
- Tree Canada Foundation: www.treecanada.ca
- Walkable Communities: www.walkable.org

air-fouling department; so are steel plants and
other heavy industries where they still exist in
North American cities. Toxic chemicals from factories, dry cleaners and pesticide applications all
contribute their share.

## Practice Teamwork

In 1969 the US federal government concluded
that Chattanooga, Tennessee, had the most polluted air of any city in the United States. There
were a lot of Donora days back then.[2] Enough
was enough, and Chattanooga mobilized to
clean up its act. The key to the turnaround was
teamwork: citizens' groups, local government,
the medical community and industry came
together to take action. New air-quality standards and monitoring techniques were put in
place, and industries led the way by curtailing
their toxic emissions. The downtown was transformed into a magnet for rejuvenated housing,
with new, cleaner businesses and a sparkling
network of parks, galleries, museums and entertainment venues along the riverfront. Electric
buses, locally built and free to ride, provide
downtown transit. Today, Chattanooga is once
again the focus of widespread attention, but this
time for its progress in reversing air pollution
and becoming a vibrant, livable city.

## Plant a Forest

Urban forests in North America have suffered
acutely from disease, sprawl and neglect, but
they're making a comeback in many cities —
and just in time. Trees not only prevent skin
cancer by providing an abundance of shade;

they also reduce urban heat, curb air pollution, reduce the need for storm-water treatment and air conditioning and delight our senses. American Forests helps communities of all sizes to re-leaf themselves, using urban ecosystem analysis technology to calculate the dollar savings that trees provide in any given locale. The Tree Canada Foundation does the same.

### Buy and Generate Green Power

In 1999 Santa Monica led the way by announcing that all of its public buildings, street lights and traffic signals would be powered by 100% renewable energy from solar, wind, biomass and geothermal, in order to reduce fumes from coal-fired power plants. Initially, the green power cost 2% more than the dirtier variety, but now it costs less. Since then, 20 other cities have followed suit, including Los Angeles, Seattle, Chicago and Boston.

### Move Faster on Public Transit

The city of Boulder, Colorado, has shown that it is possible to increase transit ridership even in the land of sprawl. By rethinking how their service worked, and moving to small, smarter buses where the drivers get to choose their onboard music, Boulder increased ridership threefold, and even has teenagers riding the bus. The cost of an annual Neighborhood EcoPass is just $50 to $115. Conventional diesel buses contribute 20% of the urban air pollution in the US, so getting off diesel is crucial. Boston, Houston, Los Angeles, Miami and Portland were first on the natural gas bandwagon; hybrid and electric

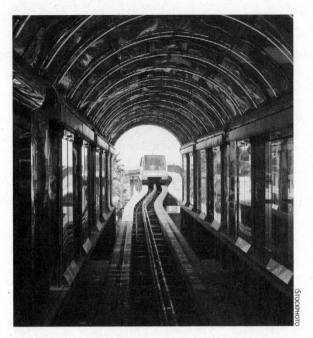

Walk, bike or take the train!

buses have been introduced in New York, Toronto and other cities, while Chicago and Vancouver are experimenting with fuel cell buses.

### Encourage More Walking and Cycling

There are many ways that a creative city can encourage more people to walk and use their bikes. A bicycle-friendly city has bicycle lanes on all major roads; priority bicycle routes through quiet residential streets; bike racks on all the buses; bicycle-controlled traffic signals; cycling maps; bicycle deliveries; cycling education programs; free electric charging stations for electric bikes; and an active cycling advocacy group. A walkable city puts care into the design of its pedestrian routes, widens the sidewalks, builds sidewalk bulges at intersections, creates open-air pedestrian shopping centers and encourages pedestrian advocacy groups. A cycling and walking city is a healthier, quieter, safer, cleaner, more affordable, climate-friendly, people-friendly city.

# 39

# Stop Incinerating Waste

Incineration. Oh my goodness. What a
dumb thing to do. To take every single
material that you consume in society,
convert it into tiny little pieces, then
blow them out of a spout and let them
settle out in our lungs, on our food and
so on.[1]

— Dr. Paul Connett

The good news is that both incineration *and* landfilling can be eliminated forever as a way of handling all those mountains of city "garbage." The tougher — but by no means "bad" — news is that getting rid of mega-tonnes of trash does require planning, commitment, hard work and cooperation. There is no magic bullet, but the payoffs from *not* incinerating and *not* dumping can be huge, both for the local economy (an

abundance of new jobs) — and for the community (no more dioxins escaping from incinerators, or toxic stews leaching from landfills).

Call them what you will — energy-from-waste mass burners, gasification units — the new generation incinerators are still not the answer to waste. Although they have reduced toxic emissions, including carcinogens, far lower than their predecessors, they still demolish vast quantities of valuable resources.

As Dr. Paul Connett and Bill Sheehan explain so clearly in *Citizens' Agenda for Zero Waste*, stopping incineration makes recycling possible, and recycling makes economic development possible — with the caveat that the recovered materials are made into value-added, finished products within the local community. The same goes for landfilling. There is no sense in trading off an incinerator for a huge new landfill site.

Zero waste is the best way to transform our garbage problem into a productive, positive solution, but it can only happen with a solid partnership between the community and the producers. The community sorts, reuses, repairs, recycles, composts and removes hazardous materials from the resource stream. The producers work to phase out toxic product ingredients and redesign their products and packaging to eliminate all but the most necessary wrapping. At the end of the stream, industry transforms the waste resources into jobs and profits.

Sheehan and Connett identify eight steps for communities to get to zero waste:

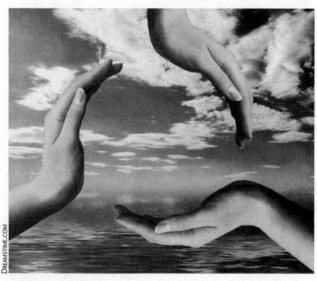

What can we learn from nature? As the Zero Waste Alliance says, "Natural cycles function without producing waste...From a systems viewpoint, the sun provides the energy for the system. The sun's energy drives the photosynthesis processes that order atoms and molecules to higher value such as forest and food products. Dead matter is processed by microbes in the soil to become food for the next cycle. A popular expression of this concept is that 'Waste = Food.'"

Nature recycles everything. Nature rewards cooperation. Nature banks on diversity. Nature demands local expertise. Nature curbs excesses from within. Nature taps the power of limits.

— Janine Benyus, author of *Biomimicry: Innovation Inspired by Nature*

- Designate a target year, usually 15 to 20 years ahead. This allows the collective mindset to shift from discarding wastes to managing resources in a realistic, doable, time frame.

- Include the whole community — businesses, citizens, educators, money managers, elected officials and students.

- Ban key items from the landfill or incinerator. Keep out all compostable organic material, all current recyclables and all hazardous waste.

- Place a surcharge on material to be landfilled or incinerated. This will help finance other important parts of the zero waste program.

- Offer incentives for recycling to stimulate new businesses to collect, process, reuse, repair or recycle materials in the waste stream.

- Encourage waste audits. Pillsbury's baking operations in Eden Prairie, Minnesota, divert 96% of their waste.[2]

- Stimulate take-back programs for bottles and containers.

- Convert the old landfill site into an industrial eco-park that uses materials from both the community's source-separated materials and its discard stream, as Berkeley's Urban Ore Eco-Park does in California.

Communities large and small worldwide are getting aboard the zero waste bandwagon. Canberra, Australia, was the first in 1996, and many more have made the commitment — San Francisco, Buenos Aires, New York City, Thunder Bay, Ontario — the list grows. They all plan to be no-waste communities by as early as 2010 (Canberra) and at the latest by 2024 (New York).

The staff of the Del Norte County, California, Solid Waste Management Authority, the first municipality in the United States to adopt a comprehensive zero waste plan, agree that terminology can be a difficult barrier. When developing their zero waste plan, they had to convince local leaders that they weren't talking about foisting a 100% recycling mandate on a rural, economically depressed county ... Far beyond setting up recycling programs, Del Norte's definition of zero waste includes building community partnerships and new job-creating enterprises, and advocating for changes in public policy and corporate behavior to significantly decrease the amount of material the county is asked to dispose of each year.

— *Rachel's Precaution Reporter*, No.16, December 2005

- Dioxins Homepage: www.ejnet.org/dioxin
- Global Alliance for Incinerator Alternatives: www.no-burn.org
- Zero Waste Community: www.grrn.org
- *Incineration and Human Health*, Greenpeace: http://archive.greenpeace.org/toxics/reports/euincin.pdf
- Institute for Local Self-Reliance: www.ilsr.org
- *Rachel's Precaution Reporter* No.16, "Zero Waste": www.precaution.org
- Successful Re-Use and Recycling: www.ciwmb.ca.gov/LGLibrary/Innovations
- Zero Waste California: www.zerowaste.ca.gov

# 40

# Grow Organic Food and Forests

Since the ornamental use of pesticides has no countervailing health benefit and has the potential to cause harm, we call for a ban on the use of pesticides on lawns and gardens.
— Canadian Cancer Society

A funny little story called "Winterize Your Lawn" made the rounds of the Internet a few years ago. It featured God complaining to St. Francis of Assisi about all the fuss humans make about a ground cover with no nutritional value or aesthetic appeal (at least not in Her opinion). "Frank," God grumbles, "You know all about gardens and nature. What in the world is going on down there in the Midwest? What happened to the dandelions, violets, thistles and stuff I started eons ago? I had a perfect, no-maintenance garden plan …. I expected to see a vast garden of colors by now. But all I see are these green rectangles."[1]

Green rectangles indeed. North Americans seed, sod, fertilize, water and mow over 30 million acres of lawn — more than the entire acreage devoted to wheat or corn.[2] The US Environmental Protection Agency estimates that gas-powered mowers, trimmers and blowers account for over 5% of urban air pollution.[3]

Lawns may look innocent, but not when they're doused with more than 80 million pounds of pesticides every year. Although regulators say the risk is "acceptable" when home and garden pesticide products are used "as directed," there are plenty of reasons to just say no — including cancer. The US Physicians for Social Responsibility and the Ontario College of Family Physicians have released reports describing links between pesticide exposure and cancers in both children and adults.[4]

Cities can promote backyard and rooftop gardens that yield a hefty percentage of fresh, organic food for local needs and flourish with native gardens. Urban forests will thrive again as city dwellers learn to prize the many benefits of trees, trees and more trees.

## Ban the Cosmetic Use of Pesticides

In 1991 the small town of Hudson, Quebec, passed Canada's first bylaw restricting "cosmetic" (non-agricultural) pesticide uses on public and

Dandelion FESTIVAL
Sunday
May 15 2005

Falstaff Family
Centre 1 - 4 pm

Join us for the
6th Annual Celebration
of the Dandelion!

- The Grandest Taproot Competition
- Expert Lawn Care Advice
- Gardening with Mary Carrington Dominic Franken, MC
- Plant Exchange:
  Bring a plant, take a plant
- Live Music for the entire family
- Children's Craft and Activity Tent
- Build the Longest Dandelion Chain
- Eat Dandelion Ice Cream,
  Pizza and more
- Herbalist Kerry Hackett

ground
swell

Dandelions are nutritious too!

## TREES, TREES, TREES!

Andy Lipkis, a teenager in the early 1970s, was obsessed with organizing a tree-planting project in his native Los Angeles — and not growing out of it. By now, the Tree People have planted millions of trees — to hold back erosion, to offer shade from the heat, to provide fruit for hungry people. And they've planted millions of seeds — of ideas about what might be possible, sprouting in the minds of an entire generation of Angelenos who have been through their school programs or seen the green pleasure of their groves.

— Bill McKibben, "Sustainability: Planet at the Crossroads," *YES! Magazine*, Spring 2006

- Backyard and Urban Agriculture: www.panna.org/resources/panups.html
- Chicago City Farm: www.resourcecenterchicago.org/70thfarm.html
- Halifax Pesticide Bylaw: www.halifax.ca/pesticides
- Homeless Garden Project: www.infopoint.com/sc/orgs/garden
- Lawn and Garden Pesticides — Reducing Harm (video): www.cape.ca
- Pesticide Bylaw Resources: www.sierraclub.ca/atlantic/programs/healthycommunities/pesticides/index.htm
- Toronto Food Policy Council: www.city.toronto.on.ca/health/tfpc_index.htm
- Toronto Pesticide Bylaw: www.toronto.ca/pesticides

private property. Two chemical spray companies fought the ban all the way to the Supreme Court of Canada. In 2001 the Court ruled that "permitting the town to regulate pesticide use is consistent with international law's precautionary principle."[5] In late 2005 the Supreme Court threw out the chemical industry's challenge to Toronto's bylaw. By 2007, nearly 200 (see p. 107) Canadian communities had adopted pesticide bans, with one of the best in Perth, Ontario. In Halifax, Nova Scotia, there has been a 98% reduction in the use of pesticides since its bylaw came into force.

### Grow Organic Food, Not Grass

A healthy lawn is a pesticide-free lawn. Many gardeners replace grass with low-maintenance clover or native plants. Urban food gardens are springing up everywhere — in city parks, on factory rooftops and apartment balconies, even under railway tracks in one south Philadelphia neighborhood.

In downtown Chicago, four urban farms have taken root and flourished on once derelict lots, growing a variety of organic produce that's sold at farmers markets and to restaurants and nearby residents. "With local ownership, the whole neighborhood has a stake in each farm's success, and the whole neighborhood is lifted," says Ken Dunn, who sowed the first seeds of Resource Center Farms in the mid-1970s and now watches it thrive.[6]

In Santa Cruz, California, the Homeless Garden Project raises vegetables, herbs and flowers on 3.5 acres. Its 25 workers eat a daily lunch made from the garden's produce. The remainder is sold wholesale, distributed to their community-supported agriculture subscribers and donated to a soup kitchen and an AIDS project.[7]

### Start a Food Policy Council

This is one of the best steps a city can take to inspire creative solutions to urban food problems, particularly the lack of access to nutritious food by low-income people. If poverty is a carcinogen, as the Harvard School of Public Health maintains, one of the root causes is the failure of our food systems to nourish everyone, rich and poor. The Toronto Food Policy Council offers a fresh and lively model.

# 41

# Create Safe, Green Schools

For too long, policy-makers have retrospectively pleaded, "If only we had known earlier what we know now."

— Dr. Roberto Bertollini,
World Health Organization

Most people are shocked to learn that indoor air is often far more polluted than just about anyplace outside. And it's not just our homes, schools and workplaces. It's practically *all* interiors — even cars. (Yes, our cherished vehicles are highly toxic, especially when they're fresh off the dealer's lot. Bumper-to-bumper traffic also cranks up toxicity inside vehicles.)

Since children are more vulnerable to toxic substances than adults, it is unacceptable that a great number of school buildings in Canada and the US flunk the health test. The Coalition for Healthier Schools says a significant number of public school buildings in America are notoriously unhealthy: "Polluted indoor air, toxic chemical and pesticide use, growing molds, lead in paint and drinking water, and asbestos are factors that impact the health of our nation's students and school staff." Indoor problems are worse if schools are sited near polluting industries or on abandoned landfills and toxic waste dumps.[1] Think Love Canal, in Niagara Falls, New York, where the school was built right on top of a chemical waste disposal site.

Until recently, the majority of buildings focused solely on energy savings, which made sick buildings even sicker. Airtight construction stopped most indoor pollutants from escaping.

Grades are improving for many public education facilities. Today's high-performance schools are no longer prone to sick building syndrome, and they do address a wide range of environment and health issues.

**A high performance school is healthy; thermally, visually and acoustically comfortable; energy, materials and water efficient; safe and secure; easy to maintain and operate; has an environmentally responsive site; is a building that teaches; a community resource; is stimulating architecturally; and is adaptable to changing needs.[2]**

Healthy means as non-toxic as possible; it means reducing or eliminating hazardous chemicals such as pesticides, industrial cleaners containing carcinogens, exhaust from idling vehicles, radon gas leaks, asbestos insulation and playground equipment made from arsenic-treated wood.

- Building Green Schools:
  www.nesea.org/buildings/greenschoolsresources.html
- Chicago Center for Green Technology:
  www.ci.chi.il.us/Environment/GreenTech
- Citizens for a Safe Learning Environment, Halifax:
  www.chebucto.ns.ca/education/CASLE/casle.html
- Evergreen: www.evergreen.ca
- Green Buildings:
  www.smartcommunities.ncat.org/buildings/gbintro.shtml
- Healthy Schools Network: www.healthyschools.org
- Indoor Air Quality Toolkit:
  www.epa.gov/iaq/schools/toolkit.html
- LEED: www.usgbc.org & www.cagbc.org
- www.onlineethics.org/environment/lcanal/
- Portland's Green Building Resource:
  www.green-rated.org

Toronto's Real Food for Real Kids' goal is to ensure that children in daycares and schools are fed healthy, organic sustainably produced food at snack and lunchtime. RFRK has won several City of Toronto 2006 Awards of Excellence for its contribution to healthy food for children.

The Coalition for Healthier Schools urges municipalities and school board officials to act boldly to make their schools healthier:

- Adopt and support the use of best environmental practices, including training for school officials and staff for pest control, and the selection of least-toxic materials and cleaning products.
- Adopt the US EPA's IAQ Tools for Schools and Design Tools for Schools to improve indoor air quality and to design healthy, productive learning environments.
- Adopt an integrated pest management program to reduce or eliminate the use of toxic pesticides.
- Provide parents and employees with right to know information about chemicals and environmental hazards at school.[3]

Schoolyards also need attention, given the long history of pesticide use and playground areas chock-full of pressure-treated wooden equipment. In 2001 the Toronto District School Board and Evergreen launched a School Ground Greening Initiative to provide schools with the support to create and sustain healthy, diverse, naturalized school grounds.[4] The project runs interactive, hands-on workshops and offers professional design consultations to help school grounds go green.

Most cities have some carrots and sticks they can use to provoke toxic schools to get fixed, but impoverished municipalities and boards of education simply can't go it alone. Jonathan Kozol's 2005 book, *The Shame of the Nation: The Restoration*

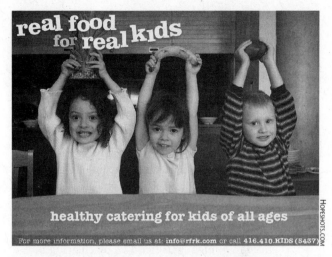

real food for real kids

healthy catering for kids of all ages

For more information, please email us at: info@rfrk.com or call 416.410.KIDS (5457)

HOPESHOTS.COM

*of Apartheid Schooling in America*, described continuing and often worsening segregation in US public schools, where the environmental conditions are as abysmal as the educational standards. In countries as wealthy as the United States and Canada, higher levels of government must ensure that indeed no child is left behind, or sickened by shabby, unhealthy schools.

The Leadership in Energy and Environmental Design (LEED) Green Building Rating System standard has become a benchmark for excellence for green building that many school boards are adopting. Studies show that students taught in classrooms that are lit by sunlight or full-spectrum lighting are healthier, happier, have higher attendance rates and perform better on tests. In New Jersey, the Governor wants the more than 400 new or substantially renovated schools to incorporate the LEED guidelines.

It's not just schools, either. Municipal public building sites such as the Chicago Center for Green Technology and the City of White Rock's Operations Building, near Vancouver, BC, have achieved the highest LEED standards. Some municipalities such as Chicago and Portland offer tax incentives for businesses to build LEED certified structures.

# 42

# Curb Electromagnetic Radiation

Pope Urban VII led the Roman Catholic Church for just 13 days in September, 1590 — the shortest papacy in history — but he gave the world its first known public smoking ban. Urban called for the excommunication of anyone who "took tobacco in the porchway of or inside a church, whether it be by chewing it, smoking it with a pipe or sniffing it in powdered form through the nose."[1]

Four hundred years passed before the next major smoking ban was declared, but this time, it was a city that led the crusade. San Luis Obispo, California, launched the first municipal smoking ban in 1990, despite worrying about possible economic damage. Once that concern proved groundless, smoke-free bans spread like wildfire across the United States, Canada and Europe. In the US, 2,103 cities and 5,700 municipalities had

> Because [EMR] effects are hard and costly to detect through population studies, people look for causal relationships and mechanisms. You know, the kinds of relationships and mechanisms that apologists for businesses ... and power companies always demand.
>
> — From a parent on an EMR blog

passed some kind of smoking restriction by 2006,[2] and many were totally smoke-free. City crusades against the evil weed continue boldly as we write...

Just a few decades ago, smoking was alleged to be safe. So were other products and practices that later proved to be undeniably dangerous, such as DDT, nuclear bomb tests, asbestos and x-rays of pregnant women.

Over the past decade, a new alarm has been sounded about cellphones and other wireless devices. Many scientists — and the wireless industry — say research has vindicated the technology, but other experts continue to call for precaution and "prudent avoidance" until wireless has proved safe over a much longer period.

Based on the precautionary principle, we urge cities and communities of all sizes to apply caution in the siting of cell towers and antennas, and to refrain from blanketing heavily populated areas with Wi-Fi (wireless fidelity) networks. These applications expose everyone — users and non-users alike — to levels of electromagnetic radiation (EMR) that may prove, over time, to be the second-hand smoke of the 21st century.

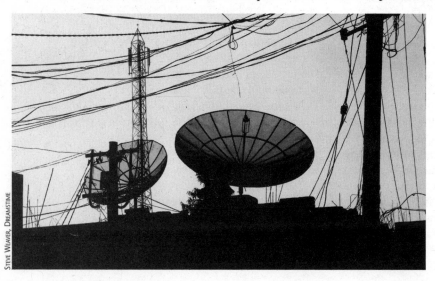

STEVE WEAVER, DREAMSTIME

## Mandate the Right to Know

In the case of cellphone antennas, detailed information about siting is available free on the Internet in several European countries; this should be universal. The Office of Communications in Great Britain maintains the Sitefinder database, which shows the location of each mobile-phone tower, along with its height, frequency, output power and operating company.[3] One site in the United States (www.antennasearch.com) provides antenna locations within an eight-mile radius from any continental US address.

## Offer Alternatives to Wi-Fi

The San Francisco Neighborhood Antenna-Free Union isn't opposed to universal Internet access, but it supports a wired, fiber-optic-based network that raises none of the health issues of Wi-Fi and would provide faster and more secure connections. The fiber optic cable could be easily included in the city's water-main replacement program.

## Protect Students and Everyone

In February 2005, the Vancouver School Board passed a motion preventing the installation of cell towers on any school buildings or school grounds regularly used by students. It amended its Incompatible Land Uses Near Schools Policy so that cell towers cannot be installed within 305 meters (1000 feet) of schools, and it requires notification of any potential installation near a school. Such a policy should also apply to residences, health care facilities, day cares, senior centers, playgrounds, places of worship and other inappropriate locations.

## Canadian University Stands On Guard Against Wi-Fi

While Toronto announced plans to forge ahead with citywide Wi-Fi networks in 2006, a small university in northern Ontario decided instead to rely on its fiber optic network for Internet access. Lakehead University in Thunder Bay said it would continue to monitor research on wireless technology on an ongoing basis and re-evaluate the university's position at an appropriate time.

The jury is still out on the impact that electromagnetic forces have on human physiology. Some studies have indicated there are links to carcinogenetic occurrences in animals, including humans, that are related to energy fields associated with wireless hotspots, whether those hotspots are transmissions lines, whether they're outlets, plasma screens, or microwave ovens that leak.

— Fred Gilbert, Lakehead University President

- Americans for Non-Smokers' Rights: www.no-smoke.org
- Associated Bioelectromagnetics Technologists: www.emfbioeffects.org
- California EMF Program: www.dhs.ca.gov/ehib/emf
- Cell Towers and Schools: www.protectschools.org
- Council on Wireless Technology Impacts: www.energyfields.org
- Don Maisch's EMF Consultancy: www.emfacts.com
- EMR Network: www.EMRNetwork.org
- Microwave News: www.microwavenews.com
- San Francisco Neighborhood Antenna-Free Union: www.antennafreeunion.org
- Smoking Bans: www.Tobacco.org

# 43

## Clean the Water and Sewage

When someone flushes a toilet in Baima, a city of six million in southeastern China, the waste spills into a 50-mile network of open canals, where it joins industrial effluent and storm runoff to flow into a major river system. The canals are a health risk not just to the people of Baima but also to communities and fisheries downstream. The discharge is fetid and toxic — fairly typical of sewage "treatment" in many developing world cities.

Are we so much better? Cities in North America dispose of raw sewage more discreetly. We channel human waste and other effluents via underground sewers to treatment facilities positioned beside rivers, lakes and oceans. The fluids are separated from the solids, and the liquid wastes are treated with aerobic bacteria, disinfected with chlorine compounds, ozone, ultraviolet light or hydrogen peroxide and discharged into the same river, lake or ocean.

### Stop Fluoridating Tap Water

Boys who drink tap water containing fluoride at levels considered safe by federal US guidelines are five times more likely to acquire a rare, often fatal bone cancer than boys consuming unfluoridated water, concluded a Harvard study in *Cancer Causes and Control*, May 2006.[1] Many organizations, including the Washington-based Environmental Working Group (EWG), urge communities to stop fluoridating water until proven safe and advise parents not to give it to children, particularly bottle-fed infants. Fluoridated toothpaste applied directly to teeth is fine, EWG adds.[2]

And the "solids"? After settling, digesting and reducing the sludge, most urban sewage treatment facilities donate tons of the newly minted "bio-solids" to farmers, gardeners and nurseries for use as an organic soil amendment. Not always, however. Some cities, such as Victoria, BC, still discharge their sewage straight into the ocean; some incinerate sludge; and others — when the sludge is particularly toxic — bury it in hazardous waste sites.

Storm-water runoff sounds like the least of a big city's problems. But the Natural Resources Defense Council (NRDC) says it's time to wake up: "Storm-water runoff rivals or exceeds discharges from factories and sewage plants as a source of pollution throughout the United States." Combine precipitation with impervious surfaces, including asphalt, then add plenty of petrochemicals, fertilizers, pesticides and heavy metals and "what started as a friendly rainfall is now a serious polluter."[3]

Many cities, including municipalities around the Great Lakes, draw their drinking water from the same source where the discharged waste water is dumped. Despite best available technologies, the chlorine mixes with leaves and other natural organic materials, producing trihalomethanes and haloacetic acids, which can cause cancer and reproductive problems. Arsenic, radon, the rocket fuel perchlorate and other carcinogens are also common contaminants, along with household chemicals, pharmaceuticals and biogenic hormones that often pass directly through the wastewater treatment process.[4] The Canadian Cancer Society notes that "studies suggest that

- *A Safe and Sustainable World: The Promise of Ecological Design*, by Nancy Jack Todd (Island Press)
- Eco-Machines: www.oceanarks.org
- Report on Drinking Water:
  www.nrdc.org/water/drinking/uscities.asp

10% to 13% of bladder and possibly colon cancers in Ontario may be attributable to long-term exposure to by-products of chlorination in household water supplies."[5]

Putting urban sewage and drinking water on a sustainable, non-toxic footing is a huge challenge, but we can learn from some inspiring examples.

In Baima butterflies and sweet-smelling air are returning to a heavily polluted 600-meter stretch of the city's sewer-canal. In 2002 John Todd, creator of a natural sewage treatment system called the Eco-Machine, installed a 500-meter linear "restorer" in the canal. The floating apparatus supports 12,000 plants of 20 native species and works with beneficial bacteria and fine-bubble aeration to cleanse the canal's sewage. Known as Solar Aquatics in Canada, this system is being applied in the Municipal Sewage Treatment Plant in South Burlington, Vermont, the Adam Joseph Lewis Center for Environmental Studies at Oberlin College in Ohio and numerous other locations.

Gathering and applying "night-soil" (human feces) to cropland is an ancient and venerable practice, but today's pristine sounding "bio-solids" are a problem. Prescription drugs join toxic chemicals and industrial poisons in our sewer pipes and end up on farmland. In 2002 the National Academies of Science concluded that the EPA regulation of sludge applied to agricultural land was based on "outdated science."[6] The solution, says the Organic Consumers Association, is to "strictly separate our residential sewage from industrial sewage, creating a closed loop for industrial wastes, then composting human waste."[7]

For its highly toxic urban runoff, Santa Monica has constructed the world's first urban runoff treatment facility. Known as SMURRF, the Santa Monica Urban Runoff Recycling Facility captures 90% of the city's urban runoff (500,000 gallons a day) and runs it through a four-stage treatment process. The final stage uses UV radiation, not chlorine, to kill pathogens, and the city sells the end product as irrigation water to large landscaped areas throughout Santa Monica.[8]

The real bottom line, of course, is the need for pollution prevention throughout the entire water, food and waste cycle. All life on our precious blue planet depends on it.

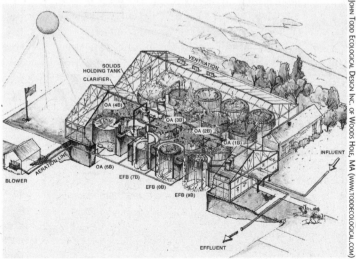

JOHN TODD ECOLOGICAL DESIGN INC. OF WOODS HOLE, MA (WWW.TODDECOLOGICAL.COM)

Diagram of natural wastewater treatment plant designed by John Todd.

# 44

# Get Smart: Fight Poverty, Stop Sprawl

If we are going to thrive as a city, we must be a healthy city.
— Detroit Mayor Kwame M. Kilpatrick

At first glance, it would not seem that poverty, urban sprawl and cancer are connected. But many of the world's big metropolises are experiencing a sharp, double-edged sword: rampant poverty at the core, and unchecked development at the outer edges. Both can lead to cancer.

Low-income areas in cities are frequently disadvantaged by inferior services and shoddy schools. They are also deliberately targeted by tobacco, liquor and junk food outlets. Smoking + low quality fatty food + too much alcohol = excess cancer. Added to the mix are far more polluting industries and toxic waste sites than are ever found in the lush, leafy neighborhoods outside the core. When you top it off with the higher exposure of blue-collar workers to carcinogens on the job, being poor in the city increases the risk of several cancers, especially tumors of the lung, cervix and stomach.[1] "Socioeconomic disparities in cancer are large, persistent and possibly widening. Twenty-five years after President Richard Nixon declared war on cancer, it is increasingly evident that fighting cancer also requires war on poverty." (Harvard Center for Public Health, 1996)[2]

Meanwhile, on the outskirts of town, urban sprawl is having its own powerful and negative effects on health through increased asthma, obesity — and cancer. Obesity is more common in the suburbs than the city and more commonly associated with heart disease and diabetes. In August 2004 *Nature Reviews Cancer* reported an association between excess body weight and 12 types of cancer, including breast and colorectal, as well as uncommon malignancies such as esophageal cancer.[3] The Sierra Club, citing a wide range of peer-reviewed, published research, concluded in 2004 that relying on gas-powered vehicles to get people to and from their sprawling suburban neighborhoods put them at higher risk for cancer. The main culprits? Regular exposure to diesel particulate matter (soot), volatile organic compounds such as benzene and formaldehyde, and PAHs (polycyclic aromatic hydrocarbons).[4]

What can be done? On the poverty front, cities face huge challenges. In both Canada and the US, upper levels of government have often cut budgets for city programs to deliver vote-winning personal and corporate tax cuts instead. At the same time, they have been eliminating or downloading health, education and social programs to the next level. It is critical to restore these responsibilities to higher levels of government. In spite of this, many cities are moving creatively to address the hazards of poverty.

- BedZED: www.peabody.org.uk/bedZED
- Community-Based Brownfield Redevelopment: www.smartgrowth.org/library/articles.asp?art=2298
- Dockside Green: www.docksidegreen.ca
- SeaGreen: www.seattle.gov/housing
- Smart Growth America: www.smartgrowthamerica.org
- Smart Growth Canada Network: www.smartgrowth.ca
- Smart Growth Scorecards: www.epa.gov/dced/scorecards/municipal.htm

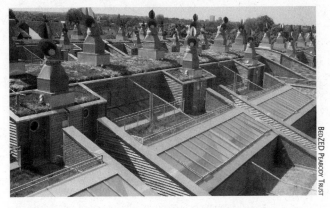

BedZED Peabody Trust

The Beddington Zero Energy Development (BedZED), outside London, UK

## Build Green, Affordable Housing

Cities have a major role to play in creating healthy, low-cost housing. Imagine a development that has been constructed from sustainable, non-toxic resources. It uses no fossil fuels, produces no net $CO_2$, recycles its household wastes, provides a daycare facility, sports club and solar-powered electric cars for use by the residents and includes a portion of affordable units.

Such a development already exists in the Beddington Zero Energy Development (BedZED) outside London, England. A similar project is emerging in Canada at Dockside Green, Victoria. Elsewhere, Toronto is transforming its notorious Regent Park social housing project "to replace the squalor of the neighborhood with a modern, car-free, spacious and pleasant environment,"[5] and Seattle is developing a SeaGreen project for the city's affordable housing.

## Healthy Inner-City Edibles

There are some superb examples of organic gardens and food programs in the US and Canada (see Solution 35), but Western cities have much to learn from economically poorer urban dwellers in the developing world. In Accra, the capital city of Ghana, 90% of the city's fresh vegetable consumption comes from production within the city.[6]

## Sprawl: The Smart Answer

The term "smart growth" was popularized by former Maryland governor Parris Glendening, who launched the Smart Growth and Neighborhood Conservation Program in 1997. There are now civic organizations and government agencies promoting smart growth policies and sprawl reduction programs all across North America and beyond.

Portland and Vancouver are leaders of the smart growth pack. As environmental writer Alan Durning describes Vancouver:

> **[It's] a continent-wide leader in arresting sprawl — with inward rather than outward growth. The West End, a tree-lined square mile of residences, offices and shops between downtown Vancouver and Stanley Park, is the Northwest's best model of urban livability. Most of North America has sought to provide access through greater mobility. The West End had provided it through greater proximity.[7]**

What is the connection to cancer? Smart growth developments reduce the need to drive, which improves the air quality, and encourage people to walk and cycle, which improves personal health and helps fight obesity. They also foster a stronger sense of community, which is good for everything. For an inspiring before-and-after visual presentation of how ugly, sprawling urban areas can be transformed into inviting, people-friendly streetscapes, see the Urban Advantage web page at www.urban-advantage.com.

# 45

# Work with Other Cities

Mayors [of the world's cities] are emerging as the most powerful and flexible agents of change. They are able to respond quickly to environmental issues and are uniquely accountable to their citizens. Their enormous purchasing power is shaping markets and making environmental sustainability a manufacturing consideration. They are tackling the globe's most challenging environmental issues, and their visionary solutions provide inspiration and serve as models to all sectors of society.[1]

— San Francisco's invitation to World Environment Day meetings, 2005

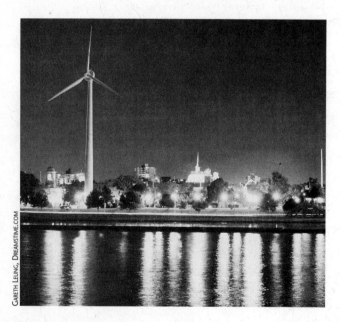

GARETH LEUNG, DREAMSTIME.COM

In Bogota we chose to build a city for people, not for automobiles. Cities built for cars' mobility suffer from congestion and unsafe street conditions and leave many residents with poor access to jobs. Instead of these problems, we gave our citizens enjoyable public spaces and unprecedented mobility.[2]

— Enrique Penalosa, former mayor of Bogota

It is almost impossible to grasp that every week, one million people on our planet will move to cities from surrounding rural areas. Mayors will surely need all the vision, power and flexibility they can muster to tackle the problems of their cities, while accommodating the masses of newcomers flooding into cities for decades to come.

City leaders are stepping up, however, where other levels of governments have failed to act. During the December 2005 International Climate Conference in Montreal, the World Mayors and Municipal Leaders Declaration of Climate Change called for a 30% reduction in greenhouse gases below the 1990 levels by 2020 and an 80% reduction by 2050. In the US over 200 mayors signed another Declaration, committing their cities to reduce their greenhouse gas emissions. The necessary shift away from fossil fuels to achieve these goals will also remove the benzene, diesel fumes and smog that are big contributors to cancer.

On World Environment Day in June 2005, more than 50 mayors from around the globe launched the Urban Environmental Accords in San Francisco. These are not just rhetoric. The goal is for each city to pick 3 actions to adopt each year from the 21 that were ratified in San Francisco, and to achieve as many as possible by World Environment Day in 2012, being recognized with a graded "green star" award for doing so. Some examples:

- Establish a policy to achieve zero waste to landfills and incinerators by 2040.
- Every year identify one product, chemical or compound that is used within the city that represents the greatest risk to human health and adopt a law and provide incentives to reduce or eliminate its use by the municipal government.
- Promote the public health and environmental benefits of supporting locally grown organic foods. Ensure that 20% of all city facilities (including schools) serve locally grown and organic food within seven years.

Local organic food, toxics reduction, clean water, better air quality and walking/bikeable neighborhoods are all included in these healthy urban accords. They are all vital to cancer prevention.

In what is now the developed world, the cities of the 19th century were dirty, dangerous, smelly, miserable places to live, without sewers or clean water. In contrast to the filth and crime, the suburban dream that appeared after World War II shone like a garden of peace and calm.

The suburbs, in turn, have been responsible for more air pollution and the abandonment of older city centers. The new vision that is uniting city leaders around the world is of a vibrant urban life that is healthy and exploding with growth of the green kind, where people can enjoy the pleasures of community without the noise and stress of excess traffic and pollution from cars and dirty industry.

It is a vision that can unite us, while also helping to prevent cancer.

- International Council for Local Environmental Initiatives, Local Agenda 21: www.iclei.org/index.php?id=798
- Local Government Commission, Building Livable Communities: www.lgc.org
- Precautionary Mister Rogers: a 3-part series on how to apply the precautionary principle at the local level: www.rachel.org (search "Precautionary Mister Rogers").
- Resources for Exuberant Cities: www.yesmagazine.org/article.asp?ID=763
- San Francisco Urban Environmental Accords: www.wed2005.org/3.1.php
- UN Sustainable Cities: www.unhabitat.org/categories.asp?catid=369

## Bogotá, Colombia

During the years 1998 to 2001, Mayor Enrique Penalosa transformed Bogota, a city of seven million people, from a hopelessly congested "repulsive mess" — as one journalist bluntly described it — into one of the world's leading models for sustainable urban development.

Under Penalosa's leadership, Bogota:

- Created the Trans-Milenio, a bus rapid transit system which now carries half a million passengers daily on special bus lanes that offer most of the advantages of a metro at a fraction of the cost.
- Established or refurbished 1,200 parks and playgrounds.
- Reclaimed the sidewalks from motorists, who often used them as either passing lanes or parking lots.
- Established 300 kilometres of cycleways.
- Created the world's longest pedestrian street (17 kilometres).
- Reduced traffic by 40%, with a system where motorists must leave cars at home during rush hour for two days a week.
- Inaugurated weekly car-free Sundays.
- Planted 100,000 trees.

# 46

# Educate and Organize

> For most chemicals, we're still living in the Wild West. Anything goes.
>
> — *Rachel's Democracy & Health News*[1]

Workers in at least 60 occupations have higher death rates from cancer than the general population.[2] Blue-collar workers bear the brunt — especially the non-unionized — but chemotherapy nurses, chemists, dentists and many others also experience higher rates of cancer.

Getting organized is tough work in the Canadian and American labor movements these days. Unions in the United States, and to a lesser extent Canada, have lost both ground *and* political clout since corporate-driven international trade deals have triggered the exodus of highly paid manufacturing jobs.[3]

It's tragic enough to lose good jobs across international borders, but losing tens of thousands of *lives* every year to preventable, work-related cancers is devastating. Over the past decade, several labor groups have said "Enough!" and gathered the inspiration to take action.

Bud Jimmerfield was a machinist, or "grinder," for 31 years, exposed every working day to cancer-causing metalworking fluids at an auto parts plant in Amherstberg, Ontario, near the Canada-US border cities of Windsor and Detroit. He contracted esophageal cancer in 1996 and died 18 months later at age 49, leaving his wife Diane and eight children.

The poignant sequences of Jimmerfield in the 1997 documentary film *Before Their Time*, which focuses on workers facing premature death from occupational cancers, spurred his union, the Canadian Auto Workers (CAW), to launch the first major Canadian labor campaign against cancer.

The CAW held three Canada-wide cancer prevention conferences on occupational health, environmental health and workers' compensation. The educational aspect of their campaign emphasized in-depth training for health and safety representatives that focused on workplace carcinogens, substitution with less hazardous substances and filing Workers' Compensation claims on behalf of members with cancers that might be related to toxic exposures at work.

In 2005 the CAW launched a new phase of its campaign, stepping up the pressure for a worldwide ban on asbestos, joining many international labor organizations under the umbrella of the International Ban Asbestos Secretariat. Exposure to asbestos directly causes mesothelioma, a lung cancer that is indeed a Canadian-made epidemic, as the CAW asserts. One of the most striking tools in the CAW's kit is *Pure White: Asbestos, A Canadian Scrapbook*, a book of photographs exposing the nonchalance and negligence of the asbestos industry, especially as it affects unprotected workers and their families who have no notion how deadly asbestos is.

Pictures are worth a thousand words when it comes to inspiring people to take action for cancer prevention. Films and videos can be even more persuasive. Look closely at the photo on this page, then meet Bud Jimmerfield in the video *Before Their Time*. It's a powerful, moving experience.

## Tools for Your Workplace Cancer Prevention Kit

- The Canadian Labour Congress, with over three million members from 90 public and private sector unions in Canada, held a cancer

Bud Jimmerfield, left, passed away in January 1998 from cancer of the esophagus caused by exposure to metalworking fluids at his workplace.

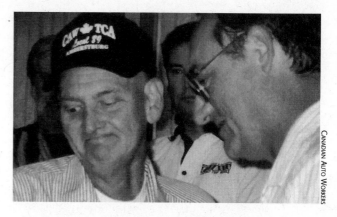

CANADIAN AUTO WORKERS

prevention symposium in 2003 that drew labor Health and Safety activists from across Canada to discuss and develop strategies to eliminate workplace carcinogens. Its excellent toolkit, *Preventing Cancer: A Campaign for Workers*, is available at www.canadianlabour.ca.

- The US National Council for Occupational Safety and Health (a.k.a. National COSH) doesn't specify cancer as a target disease. But the "Workers' Toolbox" and "Hazards Info" sections of its website have many resources on right to know legislation, American health and safety legislation, workers' rights and links to information on hazardous materials in English and Spanish. National COSH is a federation of 23 local and statewide non-profit COSH groups that coordinate national advocacy campaigns, share educational training materials and spearhead strategies for improving workplace health and safety conditions (www.coshnetwork.org).

- The Workers' Health & Safety Centre, Toronto, has two video documentaries, *Before Their Time* and *Never Walk Alone*, that focus on cancer as an occupational disease and the critical need for prevention (www.whsc.on.ca).

- *Dying for a Living. It's a Crime* is a booklet co-produced by the United Steelworkers (USWA) of Canada and the Workers Health & Safety Centre (www.whsc.on.ca/yw/day_mourn.cfm).

- The Canadian arm of the Steelworkers' Union has numerous cancer resources. Search "Workplace Carcinogens" at www.uswa.ca.

- Occupational Health Clinics for Ontario Workers (Sarnia-Lambton) list of Occupational Carcinogens (www.whsc.on.ca/pdfs/OHCOW_OccCarcinogens.pdf).

- NIOSH Pocket Guide to Chemical Hazards (more than carcinogens) (www.cdc.gov/niosh/npg/default.html).

- *Prevent Cancer Campaign: Devil of a Poison*, a booklet on occupational cancers by the Canadian Auto Workers (www.caw.ca/whatwedo/health&safety/pdf/cawcancer.pdf).

- *Pure White: Asbestos, A Canadian Scrapbook*, Canadian Auto Workers (www.caw.ca/whatwedo/health&safety/pdf/purewhite.pdf).

- *Corporate Corruption of Science*, Special Issue of the *International Journal of Occupational and Environmental Health*, Volume II, No. 4, Oct/Dec 2005 [4] (www.joeh.com).

- "Trade Secrets," transcript of the PBS *NOW* documentary with host Bill Moyers (www.pbs.org/tradesecrets/transcript.html).

- The British Columbia Federation of Labour and the Labour Environmental Alliance held *Toxins in the Workplace* workshops throughout BC in 2005-06 to help worker activists from scores of Health and Safety committees audit their worksites and then enforce the province's substitution regulations (www.leas.ca/Workplace-toxins.htm).

# 47

# Agitate and Compensate

Our goal must be to protect all communities
and workers — whether they are organized
in their own defense or not — from chemical
exposures that can compromise their health.
— Louisville Charter for Safer Chemicals

Simple arithmetic reveals the ugly truth about occupational cancers. If just 5% of cancers are linked to workplace exposures — a modest estimate — then 75,000 Canadians and Americans are diagnosed with job-related cancers annually. If the ratio of incidence to death is the same as for Canada and the US as a whole, 30,000 workers, mainly blue-collar, die from cancer — every year.

The actual number is probably much higher. The National Institute of Occupational Safety & Health (NIOSH) and the National Institute of Environment Health Sciences (NIEHS) have calculated that 20% to 40% of all cancers are related to occupational exposures. This ratchets up the worker deaths to between 120,000 and 240,000 annually.

This is shocking enough, but equally tragic is the fact that only a tiny fraction of work-related cancers are ever compensated.

The tide is slowly turning. Spearheading the charge are unions and worker health clinics that have mobilized to identify job-related cancers and to pursue financial settlements relentlessly.

What does compensation have to do with cancer *prevention*? It's simple: when employers are forced to pay compensation premiums for cancers in their workplaces, they're more likely to fix the problem. There are precedents — chemicals in the rubber and dye industries, benzene, vinyl chloride monomer, asbestos, hardwood dusts. Compensating workers for occupational cancers also shifts the huge cost of health care from the public to the employers, who are ultimately responsible.

## Persistence Pays

In the late 1960s, two Italian workers recognized, investigated and documented a cancer epidemic in their workplace, the Ipca dye factory in Cirie near Turin. "Over one hundred workers had died in a bladder cancer outbreak missed by scientists, medics, the company doctor, the factory's owners and managers," the magazine *Hazards* reported in 1999. "Detective work by the two workers led to massive compensation payouts, fines and jail sentences in the late 1970s for the factory owners, managers and even the company doctor," who was also complicit.[1]

The deaths of individual workers can help make the case for improvements to an entire workplace, even a whole industry. Months before grinder Bud Jimmerfield died from work-related esophageal cancer in 1998, the Canadian Auto Workers (CAW) helped him file a compensation claim. He lost the first round days before his death, but his union appealed on behalf of the family and won, setting a precedent that has helped many others across Canada.

In 1995 an employee at the Owens Corning fiberglass plant in Sarnia, Bud Simpson, took a list of 34 co-workers who had died or were ill with cancer to his union, the Energy and Chemical Workers. The CEP, as the union is now known, referred Simpson to the Occupational Health Clinic for Ontario Workers (OHCOW) in nearby Windsor. In 1998 Bob Clarke, the first CAW health and safety representative for the Holmes Foundry in Sarnia, and later union plant chairperson, sounded his own health alert. He reported that dozens of workers who had been

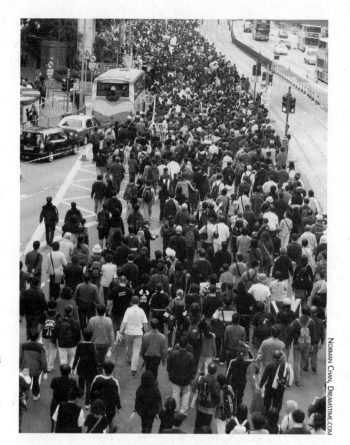

exposed to asbestos fibers in three Holmes factories — all closed by 1991 — were sick or had already died from cancer. In both cases, OHCOW and the two unions collaborated to set up worker intake clinics. Simpson and Clarke succumbed to their own workplace-related cancers, but the clinics they inspired assisted hundreds of Sarnia-area workers and their families to receive compensation.

### Agitate Locally

In Ontario's Chemical Valley, where Sarnia is located, community and union activism grew swiftly in late 1999 when the Ontario Federation of Labour (OFL) launched its campaign, A Job to Die For. Family survivors organized under the banner Victims of Chemical Valley, bolstered by the OFL and CEP, and staged a successful demonstration and sit-in at the head office of the Ministry of Labour. The group secured a commitment from the ultra-conservative Ontario government then in power for some of world's lowest exposure limits for workplace chemicals.

In 2005 the firefighters of Manitoba and British Columbia won hard-fought campaigns to get work-related cancers scheduled in compensation legislation.

### Agitate Globally

Large corporations often intimidate local labor campaigns by threatening plant closures — sometimes following through — or by declaring bankruptcy. They can't necessarily do this worldwide, but as *Hazards* explained: "James Hardie Industries [in Australia] was a global giant, highly respected and highly profitable. Then the company crossed the unions by trying to evade its asbestos compensation liabilities." Facing an unrelenting international campaign, "the company gave in and signed a deal for what is believed to be the largest personal injury settlement in Australia's history."[2]

Creating a well-organized ruckus clearly pays off in campaigns for cancer prevention. But health and safety activists are fighting on many fronts, not solely cancer. Hence, it's crucial for activists to insist — at the very least — on rigorous application of existing regulations, including occupational exposure limits, and the right to refuse dangerous work.

# 48

# Negotiate, Legislate and Enforce the Rules

**The important thing is you never let up.**
— British Columbia union member

On paper, Canadian and American workers are well protected against carcinogens and other hazardous substances. Occupational health and safety laws in both countries have enshrined several fundamental rights:

- The right to know about hazards in the workplace, including carcinogens.
- The right to participate in identifying and removing hazards through joint health and safety committees.
- The right to refuse unsafe work.
- Mandatory labeling of workplace chemicals.
- Right to access and training on use of Material Safety Data Sheets(MSDS) under Workplace Hazardous Materials Information System (WHMIS) legislation.[1]

In practice, however, many state and provincial jurisdictions have grossly inadequate occupational exposure standards. Even where more stringent limits have been won, these can fly out the window when a pro-business government takes power or when public debt triggers spending cutbacks. Protective measures may continue to exist in law and regulation, but the resources supporting them may be crippled, enforcement can evaporate and organized labor may be left to haggle over issues such as "acceptable" levels of toxicity for hazardous substances measured by old standards having little to do with health protection.

Contemporary European workplace legislation has much to teach Canadian and American lawmakers. The European Union is putting into practice what virtually all workers here know in theory but remains beyond their legal grasp — that the best way to eliminate cancer-causing substances from the workplace is to oblige employers to adopt two key measures:

- Replace carcinogens and other hazardous substances with the safest possible alternatives, and
- Restrict the use of carcinogenic substances to zero emissions or zero exposure in closed systems.

The European Union's *Occupational Carcinogens Directive* and its REACH initiative (see Solution 69) also embrace the precautionary principle. If current scientific knowledge cannot establish a level below which health risks cease to exist, this precautionary logic says, any reduction in exposure to carcinogens will reduce the risk.[2]

There are some promising steps on this side of the Atlantic:

- British Columbia's landmark Health and Safety Regulation (Section 5.57) requires that, whenever a workplace carcinogen is in use, "the employer must replace it, whenever practicable, with a material that reduces the risk to workers." When substitution is not practical, "the employer must implement an exposure control plan to maintain workers' exposure as low as reasonably achievable below the exposure limit"[3] (www2.worksafebc.com).
- In early 2006 California labor activists were close to achieving landmark "close the gap" legislation to protect workers from carcinogens

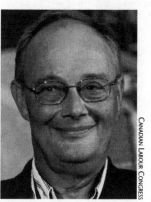

Dick Martin worked his way up through labor movement ranks to finish his career as Secretary-Treasurer of the Canadian Labour Congress. He was a highly respected advocate for health and safety, who died in 2001 at age 57 of colon cancer.

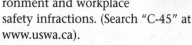

and reproductive hazards. Lawyer Amanda Hawes, who represents chemically exposed workers with cancer in lawsuits against employers, helped draft Bill AB 815 (a.k.a. Equal Protection for Workers Against Toxics). The goal of the legislation is simple: to close the gap between what is legal on the job and what good science says California must do to protect citizens against the same substances in the general environment. Updates on AB 815 appear at www.worksafe.org. For background, see *Take Immediate Action to Protect Communities and Workers* at the Louisville Charter for Safer Chemicals (www.louisvillecharter.org).

## More Steps to a Less Carcinogenic Workplace

- **Whistleblower protection** is essential in collective agreements and labor legislation, to balance the loyalty that employees owe their employers against their right to freedom of expression and disclosure in the public interest and for worker safety.

- **Make corporations criminally responsible**. In 2003 Canadian steelworkers (USWA) lobbied vigorously and led the charge for successful federal legislation that is more far-reaching than any other occupational health and safety legislation in North America. As part of the Canadian Criminal Code, Bill C-45 packs a powerful punch by imposing a legal obligation on employers — and all those who "direct work" — to take reasonable steps to protect employee and public safety or else face hefty fines, probation, even jail time. The 2004 law, inspired by the 1992

Westray mine disaster in Nova Scotia, applies to all offences, including crimes against the environment and workplace safety infractions. (Search "C-45" at www.uswa.ca).

- **Bargain away carcinogens**. Several unions have effectively bargained or worked through Joint Health and Safety Committees to reduce or ban cancer-causing substances. In one recent collective agreement reached with Ford Motor Company and General Motors of Canada, the CAW successfully negotiated to eliminate several carcinogens including asbestos, carbon tetrachloride, PCBs and vinyl chloride.[4]

- **Registries for occupational disease**. An important tool in identifying workplace cancers is the occupational health registry. The Occupational Health Clinic for Ontario Workers in Windsor developed a prototype registry called CROME (Computerized Recording of Occupations Made Easy), with early work identifying elevated breast cancer incidence among area farm women.[5] Canadian unions are now calling for occupational registries in all provinces, and the Canadian Labour Congress is striving for a national registry similar to Finland's that tracks toxic exposures, including carcinogens, over a worker's lifetime.

Once protective laws and regulations are in place, the key for labor is to keep insisting on enforcement.

# 49

# Go for Just Transition

I f there were ever a golden opportunity to put the principles of just transition into action, it is surely asbestos.

The world is not so patiently waiting. In June 2005 Global Unions, an international alliance representing major labor organizations, kicked off an Asbestos Ban at the UN's annual International Labor Organization conference in

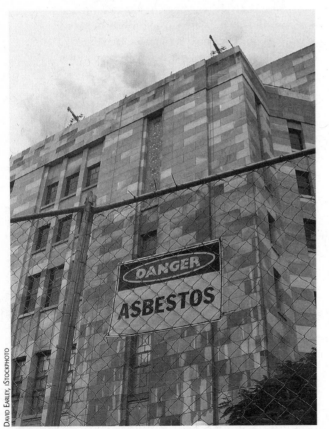

DAVID EARLEY, ISTOCKPHOTO

> I thought I was living in an age of enlightenment until I listened to Canadian government officials extolling asbestos and telling everyone what a boon it is to the Canadian economy. At that point, I realized that alchemy is alive and well in Canada.
>
> — **Paul Brodeur**, author of *Outrageous Misconduct: The Asbestos Industry on Trial*, 1986

Geneva: "We will extend our appeal to every employer, trade union and civil society organization within every country to get involved in the ban, as a matter of urgency and human decency." At that time, nearly 40 countries had already banned asbestos; 80 more still actively using asbestos were being called upon to join the prohibition.[1]

Labor activists have got it right: "There are no jobs on a dead planet." For Earth to carry on supporting life, asbestos and other unsustainable industries such as petrochemicals, nuclear energy and coal mining will need to be phased out and replaced with sustainable alternatives. Critical to success is the fair and equitable shift of workers from old, toxic industries into green jobs and a sustainable future — officially known as "just transition."

Just transition is far more than the usual safety-net supports for workers who lose jobs — unemployment insurance, social assistance and ad hoc retraining efforts. While these programs are necessary, and do soften the blow on a short-term basis, they don't eliminate job loss fears or focus on a more promising future.

Just transition embraces a set of initiatives grounded in two central principles:

1. Workers displaced for environmental reasons have a right to education, retraining programs *and* alternative employment at an equivalent level of compensation.

- Canadian Labour Congress manual on just transition: www.canadianlabour.ca
- Communications, Energy & Paperworkers Union Just Transition Policy: www.cep.ca/policies/policy_915_e.pdf
- *Hazards* magazine: sustainable jobs and just transition: www.hazards.org

2. New jobs will serve long-term ecological and community sustainability and will, therefore, be more secure than work in toxic industries.

Early and sustained government involvement is crucial. As British Columbia-based activist Delores Broten of Reach for Unbleached and Prevent Cancer Now points out, "Typically, governments have addressed transitional problems only *after* a crisis has occurred. An agency will undertake an economic diversification study after the industry in a one-industry town has been shut down, for instance. That is not the idea."[2] In addition to developing appropriate sets of transition programs, identifying where programs will be needed and applying them in an anticipatory way, governments must foster environmentally desirable initiatives that generate more green jobs, Broten explains.

Two programs that facilitate just transition are *clean production* and *extended producer responsibility* (EPR). Both are based on the principle that manufacturers must be responsible for the environmental impacts of their products through their entire life cycle, beginning with the selection of materials, including the complete production process and finishing with the environmental consequences of their ultimate recycling or disposal.

Extended producer responsibility is embedded into law in several European countries and is already creating more jobs in the auto industry, for example, where used car parts and components are refurbished and recycled instead of trashed. Many North American unions are actively involved in campaigns to implement clean production and EPR programs.

As for the Canadian asbestos sector, it is well past time that the governments of Quebec and Canada stopped using tens of millions of taxpayers' dollars to fund the Asbestos Institute to promote this deadly substance internationally. These funds, with an appropriate share from the asbestos industry, should be spent instead on cleaning up polluted Quebec communities and financing the transition to sustainable employment for workers.

For its part, Canadian labor needs to be solidly behind this just transition effort. To date, however, the asbestos issue has been extremely divisive and has undercut union efforts on the entire cancer prevention front.

**If you promise to make sustainable jobs a product of environmental protection, we will promise to make environmental protection our most important job.**

— **David Foster, United Steelworkers of America, District 11, Minneapolis**

When the gasoline additive tetraethyl lead was banned in Canada, there wasn't a living, breathing human being who said this wasn't best for our environment and our health, particularly the health of children. But in the process, 2,000 Sarnia-area petrochemical workers paid a heavy price as a direct result of the ban. Many remained unemployed years later.

— *Dying for a Living: It's a Crime*

# 50

# Link Up With Other Activists

Why is the amount of funding to investigate cancer in the workplace so disproportionately low in relation to the 'success' of confirming human causes of cancer by studying blue-collar workers?
— Dr. Peter Infante, former director of Standards for the Occupational Safety and Health Administration (OSHA)

As the last line of the grand old labor anthem goes, "The union makes us strong." While organized labor struggles to maintain memberships in Canada and the United States, many unions are linking up with new and unusual allies. With neighborhood and grassroots organizations, health professionals, scientists and cancer agencies, they are establishing cancer prevention campaigns and striving for healthier workplaces and communities beyond the plant gate.

In 1998 the **Labour Environmental Alliance Society** (LEAS) was organized in British Columbia to help defuse an ugly "jobs versus the environment" impasse between forest workers and environmentalists. Since then, Vancouver-based LEAS has successfully bridged several gaps between labor groups, environmentalists and consumers, with much of its work focused on cancer and cancer prevention.

LEAS led off with a workplace campaign called Cleaners, Toxins and the Ecosystem. Executive Director Mae Burrows explains how the program works:

"We cooperate with health and safety committees at workplaces around BC,

- Blue Green Alliance of Minnesota (one of several Blue Green alliances in the US): www.bluegreenalliance.org
- Green Labor, a project of the Public Health Institute: www.greenlabor.org
- Steelworkers & Sierra Club: Good Jobs, a Cleaner Environment, a Safer World: www.uswa.org/uswa/program/content/1922.php

reviewing all cleaning products used at a particular site and identifying ingredients that are hazardous. Then the health and safety committee works with the employer and its suppliers to replace toxic products with safer alternatives."[1]

Next LEAS produced the *CancerSmart Consumer Guide*, applying what it learned in the workplace to home pesticides, pesticide residues in food, cleaning products and plastics (www.leas.ca).

**New Jersey's Work Environment Council** (WEC) is dauntless. In a state with sky-high occupational disease rates, over 9,000 toxic waste sites and where 85% of waterways are too polluted for fishing or swimming, WEC faces huge challenges. Its goal of "safe, secure jobs in a healthy, sustainable environment" is a bold mission in a state where occupational blackmail — the threat that demanding less hazardous workplaces will kill those jobs — is very common.

Still this coalition of over 50 unions and locals and a host of community groups has achieved some impressive victories:

- Helped more than 5,000 citizens get vital information about toxic risks on their jobs and in their neighborhoods.
- Compelled the state labor department to notify 200,000 employers that they must post notices of employee rights to speak out for safety and a clean environment under the Conscientious Employee Protection Act.
- Successfully defended New Jersey's Right to Know law from industry attacks and worked

with the state health department to ensure that vital information about hazardous chemicals reaches workers, firefighters and the public.

- Helped win the US's first county Right to Know law, giving Passaic County workers and neighbors the right to conduct onsite surveys of hazardous facilities (www.njwec.org).

Back in the 1940s, President Franklin D. Roosevelt remarked, "If I were a worker in a factory, the first thing I would do would be to join a union." Until recently, that "first thing" has not been feasible for Wal-Mart "associates" or workers in thousands of small, unorganized factories. But the **United Steelworkers of America's Associate Member Program** has opened up union affiliation to workers and activists "no matter where they work or what they do — even if they are unemployed or in college." The Steelworkers Associates "join a powerful organization of 700,000 workers fighting for social and economic justice — and for a healthy environment," as well as signing up for membership benefits such as low-cost dental and vision services, prescription drugs and legal assistance (click on "Associate Member Program" under "Organizing" at www.uswa.org).

**The Alliance for Sustainable Jobs and the Environment**, Washington State. Its motto: "Where nature is protected, the worker is respected and unrestrained corporate power is rejected." The Alliance merges the goals of two movements with distinct social bases into a bloc focusing its energy on achieving "good work in a healthy community" (www.asje.org).

Canadian labor is playing a key role on the **National Environmental and Occupational Exposures Committee** (NEOEC) of the Canadian Strategy for Cancer Control. NEOEC's excellent report, *Prevention of Occupational and Environmental Cancers in Canada: A Best Practises Review and Recommendations* has prompted numerous cancer and public health agencies to pay more attention to occupational hazards.[2] In 2005 the Canadian Cancer Society adopted a position statement asserting that Canadian workers "should not be exposed to known or probable carcinogens in the workplace, [and] where exposure cannot be eliminated, it should be reduced to the lowest achievable level."[3] NEOEC is a good example of a national stop cancer alliance uniting labor, cancer organizations, national environment groups, progressive industries and academics specializing in occupation and environment issues.

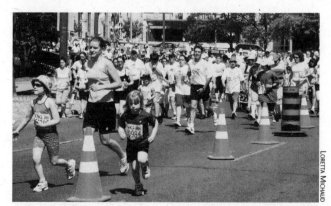

Labor, health and environmental health activists link up every year in Canada to raise funds in the Run, Walk & Roll for Cancer Prevention. (www.StopCancer.org)

# 51

# Become a Green Business

We start with the premise that you want to know how your business can contribute to the solution to cancer and other environmental health problems, while at the same time improving your bottom line.

Many of the toxic substances that are accumulating in our bodies have been developed by companies offering us new, improved products. Collectively we have embraced a non-stick, waterproof, fireproof, pestproof, dirtproof, germproof, sweet-smelling, convenient world, but the consequences of our rush to new products is becoming evident in rising cancer rates and other chronic diseases. We need to learn how to do things differently. These 15 solutions explore how businesses can contribute to the goal of a world with far less cancer.

A new vision is emerging for what makes a successful business, with a new language. Its

**Companies that do not understand toxic hazards in their products and who do not take steps to eliminate them face the risk of disruption to their supply chains, exclusion from markets, damage to their reputation, foregone profits and toxic tort litigation.**

— **Richard Liroff, Senior Fellow, World Wildlife Fund Toxics Program**

proponents speak of sustainability, clean production and a "triple bottom line" integrating financial, social and environmental benefits. They admire the efficiencies of closed-loop recycling and zero waste. They get excited about green chemistry, toxics use reduction and chemical substitution. They read papers about industrial ecology and eco-intelligent design. They're into environmental management, and many are trained in The Natural Step, a system of analysis originating in Sweden that helps a business align its operations with the fundamental laws of nature. Over the dinner table, they discuss big ideas such as biomimicry, natural capitalism and cradle-to-cradle product life cycles. More importantly, they put their ideas into action, creating value and making higher profits along the way.

Businesses are also encouraging their workers to carpool, bicycle and telecommute, and they're seeking ways to reduce their greenhouse gas emissions. They are serving healthier food in their cafeterias and supporting fitness regimes. They are exchanging their office cleaning products for non-toxic varieties and using unbleached paper. They are retrofitting their buildings to introduce fresh air and daylight and conserve water and energy.

Companies that resist this change put themselves at a disadvantage. Shareholders are already targeting corporate annual meetings to demand disclosure of risks in products. In 2006 DuPont shareholders forced a vote that would

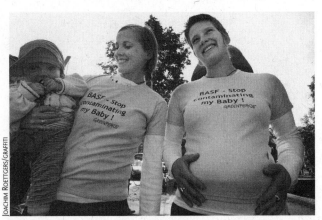

Greenpeace protest against the production of phthalate toxic chemicals, during a BASF shareholder meeting.

- Biomimicry: www.biomimicry.org
- Clean Production Action: www.cleanproduction.org
- Cleaner Production: www.cleanerproduction.com
- Corporate Environmental Strategy Journal: www.cesjournal.com
- Global Environmental Management Initiative: www.gemi.org
- GreenBiz: www.greenbiz.com
- Green Suppliers Network: www.epa.gov/greensuppliers
- International Society for Industrial Ecology: www.is4ie.org
- Natural Capitalism: www.natcap.org
- The Natural Step: www.naturalstep.org
- The Next Industrial Revolution: www.thenextindustrialrevolution.org
- SC Johnson Greenlist: www.scjohnson.com/community/greenlist.asp
- *The Sustainability Advantage*, by Bob Willard, New Society, 2002: www.sustainabilityadvantage.com
- US Green Seal: www.greenseal.org
- Zero Waste Alliance: www.zerowaste.org

have required DuPont to report on options for eliminating PFOA, the stain repellent chemical used on carpets, textiles and fast-food wrappers that has been found to be carcinogenic. Avon, Chemlawn and Dow Chemical have all faced similar shareholder resolutions demanding safe substitutes.

As the scientific evidence confirms that certain chemicals are carcinogens or endocrine disrupters, companies will eventually be forced by the public or regulators to get rid of them.

On the other hand, there are companies that make chemical safety their top priority. They assess their chemical use throughout the supply chain and comply with the strictest standards globally. They win with innovative materials and products that set them apart from their competitors, and with customers who are increasingly looking for safe, carcinogen-free products.

SC Johnson is one of the biggest manufacturers of cleaning and personal care products, makers of products such as Ziploc, Glade and Windex that have traditionally contained numerous toxic chemicals. They have created a Greenlist™ which classifies and screens the ingredients used in every product the company makes, and they use the information to score the ingredients according to their impact on health and the environment, and reduce the use of chemicals with the highest impact.

Since 1996 SC Johnson has eliminated chlorine-based packaging, including polyvinyl chloride (PVC) bottles; cut 60% of their process waste while increasing production by 50%; reduced the use of virgin materials in packaging by a third; and eliminated large volumes of solvents from their products, in pursuit of the goal of a 50% reduction in volatile organic compounds (VOCs).

The company is doing this out of a desire to integrate sustainability into their product development process, but they are also aware that when a toxic component is *not* eliminated, it has to carry the new European "Dangerous for the Environment" hazard label of a dead fish/dead tree.

No company can achieve an overnight turnaround. What matters is to get started, by setting up a management framework that integrates sustainability goals into your company's core objectives and working for steady, month-by-month progress, with indicators to show how you are doing.

# 52

# Move to Sustainability

What do most business leaders know about the chemistry of their products? Without being in any way derogatory, the usual answer is "very little." The chemicals are ordered from a chemical company, the products are manufactured and the resulting toxic by-products are considered a normal — if inconvenient — part of life. Many are found to be dangerous to health and, in some cases, cause cancer.

Take Interface. They make carpets and fabric. In 1994 their factories produced thousands of tons of solid waste, millions of gallons of contaminated water and many tons of toxic gases. Their discarded carpets filled landfills across

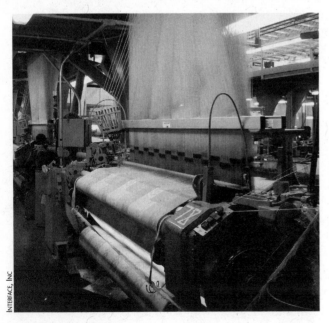

Interface Fabric loom

*For the first twenty-one years of Interface's existence, I never gave one thought to what we took from or did to the Earth, except to be sure we obeyed all laws and regulations ... Frankly, I didn't have a vision, except "comply, comply, comply." I had heard statesmen advocate "sustainable development," but I had no idea what it meant.*

— Ray Anderson, Interface CEO

North America. Their nylon carpets and fabrics, spun from petrochemicals, were bonded in fiberglass and PVC and dyed with hazardous pigments.

That same year the company's founder and CEO, Ray Anderson, was asked to deliver a speech on Interface's environmental goals. After reading Paul Hawken's book *The Ecology of Commerce* and Daniel Quinn's book *Ishmael*, he realized with pain that Interface was contributing to the assault on the world's environment and decided to take his company on a journey of environmental rediscovery.

Interface's managers called their staff together to brainstorm how to make it happen, and they started to ask some central questions. Could they make their products with less fiber? Could they design them to create less waste in the manufacturing process? Could they use materials that could be recycled? Could they put their wastes back into the loop?

Interface's goal is to become 100% sustainable by 2020. By 2005:

- Greenhouse gas emissions were down by 46%.
- Water use was down by 78% for modular carpets, 40% for broadloom carpets.
- Energy use was down by 31%; biomass and wind were being used for 12%.
- Solid wastes had fallen by 65%, saving $231 million.

- Interface: www.interfacesustainability.com
- *The Next Sustainability Wave: Building Boardroom Buy-In* by Bob Willard, New Society, 2005

- The number of smokestacks had been reduced by 33%, effluent pipes by 47%.
- The use of petrochemical materials had fallen from 87% to 80%.

Interface has now become a leader in sustainability. Its latest innovation is the development of environmentally conscious fabrics. It created the first commercial interior fabric, Terratex™, made from 100% renewable biopolymer fibers, originating from corn that is processed via fermentation. It consumes less fossil fuel, uses less water and emits fewer greenhouse gases than conventional petrochemical-based polymers. Not only is the product free of carcinogens and other chemical hazards, it is also completely biodegradable.

In order to ensure that the new fabric would not be contaminated by dyes and treatments used to finish it, Interface developed a stringent chemistry screening protocol that does not allow any chemical that is carcinogenic, mutagenic, bioaccumulative, persistent, toxic to aquatic life or sensitive to skin. Only 30 chemicals passed the test.

As Interface has shown, it *is* possible to design a business whose products and processes are nontoxic and still make a healthy profit. It starts with a plan.

1. Set up a leadership team involving every level of your company and write a mission statement. Set an agenda to become fully sustainable by 2020.
2. Identify all of the chemicals in your products. Set up a tracking system for materials from arrival to disposal, using MSDS to find out which products are harmful.
3. Create a plan to substitute or eliminate toxic chemicals.
4. Plan to reduce your greenhouse gas emissions, your wastes and your use of water and energy.
5. Design new products. Take responsibility for products from cradle to grave. Require data from suppliers on chemicals and materials used in products. Work with suppliers to create healthy ingredients. Design products to be reused, recycled or composted. Take back products at end-of-life.
6. Develop a green purchasing plan, including paper, cleaning products, fuel, ink and other basics.
7. Write green contracts in conjunction with all your staff. Provide training opportunities to encourage participation.
8. Work collaboratively with environmental advocates.
9. Link up with other companies that follow the same goals. Find ways to help each other.
10. Support policies and laws that promote green chemistry and the elimination of toxic chemicals.

Many companies are following Interface's lead, including companies as diverse as Patagonia, IKEA, Marks and Spencer and even Wal-Mart. The challenge that our planet faces is for *all* businesses to get on board, so that we can face our grandchildren without shame when they ask, "What did you do to help protect the environment, Grandpa?"

# 53

# Reduce Your Emissions to Zero

Everyone thinks of waste as an environmental issue. That's a natural mistake. Waste is .... the biggest opportunity North American manufacturers have ever had to increase their profits.

— Charles Rooney, Orr and Boss

To a traditional business, leftover chemicals are just another waste disposal problem. North America is full of landfills, industrial ponds, lagoons, rivers and underground injection wells where industry's unwanted chemicals have been dumped. From there, they migrate, leak, evaporate and infiltrate our lives.

Smart companies, realizing that the way they buy chemicals makes no sense, are asking, "How can I reduce my wastes, my costs and my chemical footprint?" Through process changes, product reformulation, materials substitution and investing in clean technology, wastes can be drastically reduced.

**Aim for Zero Emissions and Zero Discharge**
Herman Miller, a Michigan-based manufacturer of commercial office furniture, is going for zero — zero landfill, zero hazardous waste and zero air and water emissions. In 1991 their Environmental Quality Action Team made zero landfill its first environmental goal, and it is close to reaching it. Their signature office chair is designed for reuse and recycling so that no part of it needs to be landfilled. The company developed a special corn-based fabric that is biodegradable, and to avoid toxic chemicals that would end up as hazardous waste, they have a cradle-to-cradle design protocol that replaces brominated flame-retardants and PVC with safer earth-friendly materials.

Zero water emissions was the goal for Millar Western in Alberta when they installed the technology for their Meadow Lake pulp mill, the first mill in the world to successfully implement zero-liquid effluent discharge technology. While other pulp mills treat and release their waste water, Meadow Lake cleans and reuses all waste water, discharging none to the environment. The mill is designed as a chlorine-free closed-loop water system with no dioxins, furans or other organics contaminating its water.

Small businesses can reach zero too. Perchloroethylene (perc) is a suspected carcinogen that has been the solvent of choice for most dry cleaners, but governments are working to phase it out. In Los Angeles, perc cannot be used in any new cleaning operations. Dry cleaners are investing in alternatives such as wet cleaning and citrus-based cleaners. Carriage Trade Cleaning Centre, in Oshawa, Ontario, was one of the first Canadian cleaners to adopt wet cleaning. Although the investment was expensive, the company has saved on drastically reduced electric and water bills and by not having to buy perc.

**Substitute with Non-Toxic or Less Hazardous Substances**
Substitution is also a way forward for companies that want to reduce their toxic chemical use. Domfoam, a Montreal manufacturer of polyurethane foam, replaced dichloromethane, a suspected carcinogen, with a non-toxic water-based glue that did the same job. Many printing companies have replaced solvent-based inks with less toxic water-based ones.

A landmark study in 2006 by the Massachusetts Toxics Use Reduction Institute found that industries could save money by replacing hazardous chemicals with cheaper

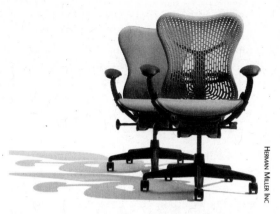

Herman Miller sustainable designed Mirra chairs, 96% recyclable by weight; no PVC; 42% recycled content; 69% green chemistry composition.

alternatives. They found feasible alternatives for lead, formaldehyde, perchloroethylene, hexavalent chromium and the phthalate DEHP, all known or suspected carcinogens. [1]

### Sign up for Chemical Service Programs

In a traditional relationship, a business buys chemicals from a number of suppliers. The sales reps want to sell as much as they can to maximize their bonuses, while the companies want to minimize their costs while getting the best performance from their chemicals. This often leads to an adversarial relationship.

The full cost of using chemicals might be 10 times the actual cost, including procurement, delivery, inventory, testing, insurance, health and safety, environmental compliance, use, contamination, misapplication, waste collection, waste treatment and disposal. If a company spends $7 million a year on chemicals, it might spend $70 million on associated costs. [2]

One solution is chemical servicing, or "shared savings chemical management." Instead of paying different companies, you pay one company to manage all your chemical needs with a guaranteed annual contract. If they

- Canadian Centre for Pollution Prevention: www.c2p2online.com
- Center for Clean Products and Clean Technologies: http://eerc.ra.utk.edu/ccpct/index.html
- *Chemical Management: Reducing Waste and Cost Through Innovative Supply Strategies* by Thomas Bierma and Francis Waterstraat, Wiley, 2000
- Chemical Strategies Partnership: www.chemicalstrategies.org
- Clean Production Action: www.cleanproduction.org
- Green Profit: www.greenprofit.net
- Journal of Cleaner Production: www.elsevier.com/locate/jclepro
- Lowell Center for Sustainable Production: www.sustainableproduction.org
- National Pollution Prevention Roundtable: www.p2.org
- *The Non-Toxic CEO*, by Mark Wysong: www.nontoxicceo.com
- Pollution Prevention Resource Exchange: www.p2rx.org
- Pollution Prevention World Information Network: www.p2win.org
- PollutionWatch, Canada: www.pollutionwatch.org
- Pulp Mills Zero Discharge: www.rfu.org/cacw/production.html#ZeroDischarge
- Southwest Network for Zero Waste: www.zerowastenetwork.org
- Toxics Release Inventory: www.epa.gov/tri
- Zero Emissions Forum (UN): www.unu.edu/zef
- Zero Emissions Research Institute: www.zeri.org

reduce your chemical needs, they share in the savings. Instead of thinking adversarially, their managers help you to become more efficient in your use of chemicals.

When Chicago-based Navistar International, which makes diesel engines for trucks and buses, made the change, its chemical service provider installed a new process to clean and rinse its grinding-fluid wastes, reducing chemical usage by 50% and wastes by 90%.

# 54

# Embrace Green Chemistry

**If chemists direct their strengths to contributing to a sustainable civilization, chemistry will become more interesting and compelling to people, and may lose its "toxic" image[1].**

— Terry Collins, Thomas Lord Professor of Chemistry, Carnegie Mellon University, Pittsburgh

Evolution has taken place over billions of years, but the science of chemistry is barely 250 years old. It is still in its infancy, and there is a reason why many of the processes that industry uses result in pollution - and cancer.

When a company decides to develop a new product, its chemists work to create a set of chemical reactions to produce it. Typically, they take carbon from fossil fuels and a lot of elements from the periodic table, and use relatively simple reagent designs to achieve the reactivity they want. The process often results in substances and contaminants unknown to nature. Many persist as toxic pollutants and end up contributing to cancer, reproductive failures, birth defects and other health problems. They even attack the planet's ozone layer, threatening all life on Earth.

Nature works the other way around. It takes a handful of common elements and uses a huge range of elaborate biochemical processes to achieve its ends. It applies a lot of intelligence, which has evolved over millions of years, and the result is zero pollution.

That is what green chemistry is learning from nature: how to create the products we need with more intelligence, fewer elements and no toxic waste. By embracing green chemistry, and using only those chemicals that are found inside the human body (carbon, oxygen, hydrogen, nitrogen and iron), businesses can leave behind the dirty past and step into a clean, sustainable future.

## Green Chemistry in Practice

- Instead of using heavy metals such as cadmium and lead to make paint, green chemists are making paints from vegetable oils. They are making water-repellent coatings that mimic the way a lotus leaf works and developing colors based on the biochemistry of butterfly wings.

- Instead of using chlorine-based bleaches in the pulp industry, which leave many toxic chlorinated residues like dioxins and furans, green chemists are whitening paper using the catalytic reaction of oxygen or hydrogen peroxide, nature's principal oxidizing agents.

- Instead of making plastics from oil, green chemists are making bio-plastics from bio-based polymers and fermented corn sugars.

- Instead of using harsh solvents in cleaning processes, with their high off-gassing of volatile organic compounds and toxic waste streams, green chemists are developing solvents that use supercritical carbon dioxide, ethyl lactate made from corn, and room temperature ionic liquids.

- Instead of using chemical agents to reduce vat dyes in the textile industry, green chemists

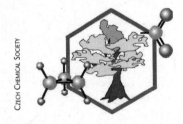

CZECH CHEMICAL SOCIETY

The Czech Chemical Society's Green Chemistry logo. www.csch.cz/green.htm

are using electrons, resulting in less use of chemicals, water and wastewater treatment.

- Instead of making glues from neurotoxins such as toluene or methyl ethyl ketone, green chemists are making super-strong fibers from protein and water that mimic the way a silkworm makes silk. They have also discovered that common blue mussels use the iron in seawater as a super-bonding agent when they cling to rocks.

Green chemistry has gone from an idea to a multi-million dollar business in 15 years, but it needs help to proceed further. Universities are quickly establishing green chemistry courses and starting to train young chemists in environmental principles.

Regulations that ban lead, cadmium and brominated flame-retardants are driving the trend in Europe. The European Social Investment Forum reported in 2005 that "over the next 5 to 10 years, green chemical innovation could be a significant source of competitive advantage for companies manufacturing chemicals used in consumer products, particularly in markets where brand or product differentiation based on green credentials is a key component of value for the final customer."[2]

In California, a special report on *Green Chemistry in California*, written for two Senate and Assembly environmental committees, has called for a comprehensive chemicals policy, embracing green chemistry, to place California on the path to a sustainable future.

> Green chemistry represents a primary, long-term solution to many of the chemical problems facing California. It is a key element of an industrial development strategy that is environmentally, socially, and economically sustainable.
>
> — Green Chemistry in California

- Canadian Green Chemistry Network: www.greenchemistry.ca
- Center for Green Chemistry, University of Massachusetts Lowell: www.greenchemistry.uml.edu
- EPA Green Chemistry Program: www.epa.gov/greenchemistry
- Green Chemistry Group, University of York (UK): www.york.ac.uk/res/gcg
- *Green Chemistry in California*: http://coeh.berkeley.edu/FINALgreenchemistryrpt.pdf
- Green Chemistry Institute (US): www.chemistry.org/greenchemistryinstitute
- *Green Chemistry* Journal: www.rsc.org/greenchem
- Green Chemistry Network (UK): www.chemsoc.org/networks/gcn
- GreenBlue: www.greenblue.org
- *Greenlist* (weekly): www.turi.org
- Institute for Green Oxidization Chemistry: www.chem.cmu.edu/groups/Collins
- Leeds Cleaner Synthesis Group (UK): www.chem.leeds.ac.uk/People/CMR
- Twelve Principles of Green Chemistry: www.epa.gov/greenchemistry/principles.html

# 55

# Phase Out Toxic Chemicals in Products

We will not sell products if they contain chemicals which are harmful to customers.

— Marks & Spencer, UK

How is a hardworking cosmetics executive to respond? It's a great morning, and your quarterly results look good. You are proud of your company's efforts to make your business more sustainable.

But then your secretary tells you there's a group of women at the front entrance carrying signs and claiming that their bodies are contaminated with dibutyl phthalate, a chemical your company uses to make nail polish. Dibutyl phthalate has been linked to developmental problems and liver and kidney damage. They're very upset.

What are you to do? The public has become alarmed by the increased incidence of cancer and the disturbing evidence of chemicals in their bodies. Even the Disney Corporation was targeted when Greenpeace found that PVC-embossed Mickey Mouse and Princess T-shirts were leaking hazardous chemicals into the bodies of the children who wear them.

Some chemicals simply have to go. It was true in the past for DDT, and it's true today for the persistent organic pollutants that are being phased out under the global Stockholm Convention, including nine pesticides, PCBs, dioxins and furans (see Solution 93).

It is also true for a whole new parade of troubling chemicals, including brominated flame-retardants like PDBEs (used as fire-retardants in foams, furniture and computers); perfluorinated compounds (used to make everything from Teflon-coated cookware to stain- and water-resistant coatings for bedspreads, furniture, shirts, handbags and other common products); bisphenol A (a hormone-mimicking chemical used in plastic food packaging, cans

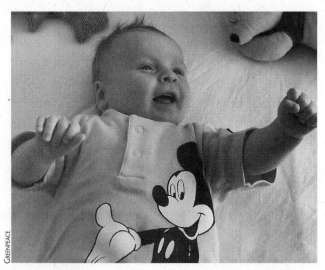

GREENPEACE

Disney children's wear often contains toxic chemicals. However, some retailers have pledged to avoid toxic chemical in their products.

We should be able to trust industry not to make dangerous chemicals, and manufacturers not to use them. But this toxic toy story shows us that they won't clean up their acts unless we force them to. We can all make a difference by shopping wisely and choosing environmentally sound products, but only by demanding tougher laws can we be sure that all hazardous chemicals are replaced with safer alternatives.

— Nadia Haiama-Neurohr, Greenpeace

and hard clear plastic baby bottles); formalde-hyde (used in pressed wood shelving, cupboards and plywood); various pesticides; and phthalates (used to soften plastic, in everything from cosmetics to baby toys). In time it will be true for all chemicals whose toxic and bio-accumulative effects cannot be contained.

The European Union (EU) is leading the drive to clean up, as it moves to a tighter system of chemical regulation (see Solution 69). There are 600 substances used in cosmetics in North America that can no longer be used in Europe, including any compound linked to cancer, genetic mutations or reproductive effects. The EU has banned all use of lead, mercury, cadmium, hexavalent chromium, polybrominated biphenyls and PBDEs in electrical and electronic equipment. It has also banned the use of six phthalate chemicals in children's toys such as the Teletubbies and rubber ducks, but only after a long and bitter eight-year battle with the chemical and toy industries.

There is a better way. After seeing its name listed in red in a Greenpeace report called *The Chemical House*, Samsung Electronics became the first electronics company to substitute safer chemicals in all its products, and it phased out brominated flame-retardants by the end of 2005.

In creating its SD Video Camera, Panasonic designed it to be easily recycled and to use no hazardous materials, following a 40-step process that carefully reviewed all materials it was using. Through its Green Plan 2010, Panasonic's parent company, the Matsushita Electric Group, set a

- Campaign for Safe Cosmetics: www.safecosmetics.org
- *The Chemical Home*: www.greenpeace.org.uk Click on "Campaigns" then click on "Toxics".
- Computer Take Back Campaign: www.computertakeback.com
- Database of POPs Alternatives: http://dbserver.irptc.unep.ch/irptc/owa/ini.init
- IKEA: www.ikea.com.sg/about_ikea/environment.asp
- Marks & Spencer: www.marksandspencer.com/csr
- Panasonic Sustainability Report: www.panasonic.net/eco/index.html
- Persistent Organic Pollutants: www.chem.unep.ch/pops
- PFCs Report: www.ewg.org:16080/reports/pfcworld
- Rethink: Fresh Ideas for a Cleaner World: http://rethink.ebay.com

goal to exclude hazardous materials from all its products worldwide, including PVC.

IKEA, the Swedish furniture maker, has also phased out the use of PVC in all products (except the isolating plastic on electric cables), as well as its azo-dyes, used to color textiles, leather and natural fibers. Azo-dyes can be carcinogenic to people working with the dyeing process over many years and can cause skin problems for consumers.

The major British retail chain, Marks & Spencer, has developed a special code of conduct for the suppliers who are dyeing, printing and finishing the 300 million items of clothing that it sells each year. It has banned the use of 56 harmful chemicals in textiles including phthalates and nonylphenol ethoxylates, known hormone-disrupting chemicals. It has also banned PVC from its children's wear and food packaging. The company's policy is "to phase out chemicals that they believe to be harmful to customers, production workers or the environment, and to support substitution by safer chemicals."

# 56

# Phase Out Most Uses of Chlorine

PVC is one of the most environmentally hazardous consumer materials ever produced.

— Joe Thornton, Professor of Biology, University of Oregon, author of *Pandora's Poison*

When the universe was born, it contained 92 fundamental elements, including chlorine, from the Greek word *chloros*, meaning "pale green." It is a poisonous greenish-yellow gas that combines easily with many other elements, most commonly found as the relatively benign sodium chloride, known as salt.

In the 1890s, Herbert Dow developed a way to harvest chlorine from salt using electrolysis on brine found in central Michigan, where an ancient inland sea had left large underground salt deposits. He combined the chlorine with other elements, and Dow Chemical was off and running as the early leader in chlorine chemistry.

Today there are 15,000 chlorinated compounds in commercial use. Chlorine is used to disinfect swimming pools, bleach paper and make a myriad of products such as pesticides, pharmaceuticals, resins, detergents, solvents and plastic PVC. The global production of chlorine is about 40 million tons a year.

Many of these products are toxic enough. But there is another dark side to chlorine chemistry. When chlorine or its waste materials are released into the environment or burned, they create many accidental and very toxic by-products, including the family of chemicals known as dioxins and furans, among which is the most deadly dioxin, known as TCDD (tetra-chloro-dibenzo-p-dioxin). Dioxins and furans often escape into air and water where they bioaccumulate and biomagnify up the food chain and eventually reach our bodies. There they accumulate mainly in our fatty tissues, where they can be implicated in cancer and birth defects. Along with dioxins and furans, chlorine by-products combine with organic matter (the carbon-based "stuff of life") to create a long, very problematic list of chlorinated organic pollutants.

Over half of the 362 toxic compounds found in the Great Lakes are chlorinated organic chemicals, and many fish in them are no longer safe to eat, especially for children and pregnant mothers.[1] The International Joint Commission, the US-Canadian body that oversees the Great Lakes, has called for chlorine to be phased out as

Make Our Milk Safe (MOMS)

PVC Day of Action at the Target store in Albany, CA, urging them to phase out PVC from their packaging and products, organized by BE SAFE, Make Our Milk Safe (MOMS), and the Ruckus Society.

a feedstock for other chemicals and in plastics. In 1993 the American Public Health Association urged industry to stop using chlorine.

The biggest source of dioxins is polyvinyl chloride (PVC), used in pipes, tubing, windows, vinyl siding, flooring, wiring, packaging and consumer goods. Producing PVC is a risky occupation, in spite of industry cleanup, and the danger continues when PVC burns in a municipal waste incinerator, when a building catches fire or when a plant explodes, as Formosa Plastics' PVC plant did at Illiopolis, Illinois, in April 2004, causing four towns to be evacuated.

Chlorine has been used to make DDT, chlordane and dieldrin — the pesticides Rachel Carson sounded the alarm about in her 1962 bestseller *Silent Spring* — as well as the herbicide Agent Orange, used extensively in Vietnam and implicated in multiple cancers of Vietnam veterans and Vietnamese civilians. Another dioxin-contaminated pesticide, 2,4,5-T, was also used as a herbicide to spray Canada's Maritime forests until citizen opposition stopped it.

Chlorine is also used to produce chlorofluorocarbons (CFCs), once used widely in coolants and aerosols, that came close to destroying the Earth's protective ozone layer. Millions of cases of skin cancer, and millions yet to come, can be laid at the feet of chlorine.

There are replacements for 90% of the industrial processes that use chlorine, and Greenpeace lists the many alternatives on its comprehensive website. The pulp and paper industry has already moved to using chlorine dioxide instead of elemental chlorine in the bleaching process

- *Blue Vinyl* (the film): www.bluevinyl.org
- Dioxins and furans: www.epa.gov/opptintr/pbt
- *Dying from Dioxin,* by Lois Gibbs et al., Black Rose Books, 1997
- Euro Chlor Sustainability Goals: www.eurochlor.org/index.asp?page=179
- *Health Effects of Dioxin,* by Ted Schettler: www.greenaction.org/zerodioxin/healtheffects.shtml
- The Legacy of Agent Orange: www.heureka.clara.net/gaia/orange.htm
- *Pandora's Poison : Chlorine, Health, and a New Environmental Strategy* by Joe Thornton, MIT Press, 2001
- PVC Alternatives: www.healthybuilding.net/pvc/alternatives.html
- PVC Alternatives Database: http://greenpeace.org/toxics/pvcdatabase
- PVC Information: www.pvcinformation.org
- PVC Phase-out: www.acereport.org/pvc1.html
- PVC, The Poison Plastic: www.pvcfree.org
- Scientific Facts on Dioxins: www.greenfacts.org Search "dioxins"
- *Trespass Against Us: Dow Chemical and the Toxic Century* by Jack Doyle, Common Courage Press, 2005

for most of its products. Natural linoleum makes a perfectly adequate flooring substitute for PVC. Playmobil phased PVC out of its toys 20 years ago, and Lego has almost completely eliminated it. Reebok has eliminated PVC from its running shoes, and Sony has plans to remove PVC from its electronic products.

Terrence Collins, Director of the Institute for Green Oxidation Chemistry at Carnegie Mellon University, believes that the use of PVC should be "restricted to those uses where uncontrolled combustion cannot occur," such as buried piping.

In Europe the chlorine industry has established 14 sustainability benchmarks. Between 1985 and 2001, it achieved a 94% reduction in emissions to water and 90% to air; a 2010 target is set for a further 75% reduction to water and 50% to air.

# 57

# Protect Your Workers

> It's quite incredible. If other companies took this kind of a lead, we'd be a much better society.
> — Anthony Hannem, Husky worker

Husky Injection Molding Systems, based in Ontario, has 3,000 employees worldwide. It is one of the world's leading suppliers of injection molding equipment and services to the plastics industry, and spends over $4 million a year on employee benefits, including on-site aerobics classes, a fitness center, daycare center, naturopath, masseuse, doctor, physiotherapist, smoking-cessation program and a cafeteria that serves organic, vegetarian food and has eliminated fries and all meat except chicken and fish. When employees walk or cycle to work, drive a fuel-efficient car or do community service, they earn shares in the company through Husky's GreenShares program. All this pays off financially. Compared to other companies in the same industry, Husky has far lower rates of employee turnover and absenteeism, and its injury claims are 80% below average.

## Exposed to Carcinogens at Work

| | |
|---|---|
| Aluminum Smelter Workers | Metal Workers |
| Asbestos Workers | Miners |
| Auto Workers | Paint Sprayers |
| Chemical Workers | Pathologists |
| Diesel Truck Drivers | Pharmaceutical Workers |
| Dry Cleaners | Plastics and Rubber |
| Electrical Workers | Workers |
| Farmers | Pulp and Paper Workers |
| Firefighters | Steel Workers |
| Hairdressers | Textile Workers |
| Iron Workers | Wood Workers |
| Lab Technicians | ... and many other |
| Mechanics | occupations[3] |

Since you have paid to hire and train workers and win their loyalty, protecting them against serious health problems like cancer surely makes sense.

Husky not only encourages a healthy lifestyle for its workers, it also tries hard to protect their health by ridding its operations of carcinogens and other toxic chemicals. Since 1997 Husky has eliminated the annual use of 250,000 liters of trichloroethane by converting to water-based washers; stopped using more than 4,000 liters of toluene and naphtha a year; eliminated the release of 86 tonnes of VOCs by converting its painting processes to water-based; eliminated all use of herbicides, pesticides and chemical fertilizers; and reduced the number of hazardous chemicals used by 40%.[1]

In 1978 the US National Institute of Occupational Safety and Health estimated that 20% to 40% of all cancers were occupational in origin. There are at least 60 occupations where workers are exposed to carcinogens, and therefore suffer higher cancer rates (see box). The World Health Organization reports that cancer accounts for 34% of all global work-related mortalities.[2] Some of the toxic substances are passed onto workers' children, causing cancer in the next generation, while others cause brain damage, liver and kidney damage, sperm loss, infertility, birth defects and reproductive disorders.

## Substitute for Carcinogens and Other Hazardous Chemicals

A common response by many businesses has been to push the issue under the carpet, or supply

- MSDS National Search: www.msdssearch.com
- MSDS Index: www.hazard.com/msds
- National Whistleblowers Center: www.whistleblowers.org
- Ten Ways to Find Safer Cleaners: www.turi.org
- Where to find MSDS Sheets: www.ilpi.com/msds

personal protective equipment and improve the ventilation. However, the real solution is to reduce or eliminate the problem. In some places like British Columbia, legislation gives workers the right to substitute less hazardous materials for carcinogens. This gives companies and workers the chance to work together on alternatives.

*Step 1*: Raise the issue with your joint company-worker Health and Safety Committee, and agree on a process to identify possible carcinogens. Analyze the Material Safety Data Sheets (MSDS) for every chemical, and create an inventory of known and possible carcinogens. (The MSDS should be no more than three years old.) It always pays to involve your employees; they know all about workplace hazards and have a personal interest in making the workplace safer.

*Step 2*: Use toxics reduction, clean production and green chemistry knowledge to research possible substitutes. Massachusetts companies that have to comply with the Toxics Use Reduction Act have saved millions. Invite occupational health professionals like the Occupational Health Clinics for Ontario Workers (OHCOW) into the workplace to assess the toxic hazards and give advice on reduction or substitution.

*Step 3*: Plan to eliminate all your carcinogens over time, including from your cleaning products. Develop a substitution strategy, with goals and a timetable.

*Step 4*: Do regular air testing while the toxins are still in use, and use all the necessary safety systems, such as ensuring that your employees never go home in contaminated work clothes.

*Step 5:* Where there is evidence of illness, work with your employees to develop a workplace epidemiology map, or pay for health studies of the most threatened. If one worker has a headache, it's just a headache. If many workers do, it's an occupational health problem that should be addressed sooner rather than later.

*Step 6*: Put an end to secrecy, and guarantee that whistleblowers who raise concerns about environmental harm or worker health will be protected from recrimination or firing. In the long run, they could save you an enormous amount of grief.

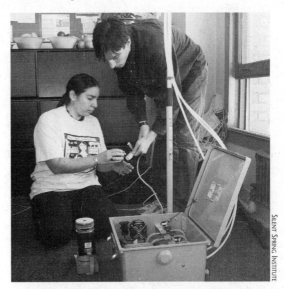

Members of the Silent Spring Institute team up with Communities for a Better Environment to answer community questions about how much pollution enters homes near an oil refinery and major highway.

# 58

# Protect Your Neighbors

In the course of one generation, we have contaminated virtually all of Earth's biological systems. Every day, we expose millions of people to chemicals and chemical mixtures for which the toxicity is unknown.

— Michael Wilson, Center for Occupational and Environmental Health, U of C, Berkeley

As a business, you have neighbors. If you operate a small dry-cleaning business, downtown gas station, or car-repair shop that releases gases into the air, your fumes may be entering your neighbor's lungs and settling in their bodies.

If you run an oil refinery or a chemical complex, people who live in the neighborhood may breathe your emissions when your valves leak or when you spill unwanted chemicals into the air. They may be at risk when your trucks move through their communities. They may be poor or minorities, who can't easily buy homes elsewhere. The book *Diamond: A Struggle for Justice in Louisiana's Chemical Corridor* conveys a powerful sense of what it means to live in a fenceline community.

Diamond

A Struggle for
Environmental Justice
in Louisiana's
Chemical Corridor

STEVE LERNER
foreword by Robert D. Bullard

MIT Press

Your neighbors may live five miles away but take their drinking water and the water their children play in during summer from a source that has been contaminated with your wastes. Years ago an employee may have been told to dump unwanted wastes into a pit, pond or deep well that is now leaking, like the hexavalent chromium from the power utility PG & E that leaked into the residents' water supply at Hinkley, California. How quickly can you say "Erin Brockovich"?

Your may also have other neighbors — frogs, birds and fish that live in a nearby creek, pond or stretch of farmland. If you are careless, they will swim in toxic water, breathe toxic air and get cancer, too.

**Talk to Your Neighbors**
Hold an annual open house or a community meeting. Give your neighbors good, clear, open information. They have a right to know what chemicals you are using and the risk that your emissions pose. Don't wait until they come knocking on your door — go and meet with them in their homes, halls and churches. They may be angry. They may demand to have the air tested. They may want you to change the way you do things. Sit and listen, and then work with them to see what can be done.

**Sign a Good Neighbor Agreement**
The goal is to lay your mutual needs down on paper. In the US, 67 million people breathe air that has been polluted by oil refineries. In the mostly African-American community of Richmond, California, in the 1990s, the

Chevron Richmond Refinery signed a Good Neighbor Agreement with the West County Toxics Coalition representing community groups. After negotiations, Chevron agreed to:

- Install 350 leakless valves in a new project and retrofit 200 to 400 valves in their existing refinery.
- Continue to reduce their toxic emissions beyond the 60% achieved from 1988 to 1992.
- Provide job skills training to 100 local residents.
- Contribute $2 million to a local health center.
- Install sirens and computers, train emergency workers and establish and fund a city Emergency Services coordinator for 5 years.
- Redirect $5 million in corporate philanthropy to local communities, over 5 years.
- Spend $100,000 over 3 years to restore native vegetation along bayshore property.
- Work with the local parks department to complete a feasibility study for constructing a bike trail.

## Don't Hide Behind Single Chemical Analysis

If you know you are releasing multiple chemicals, be willing to talk about cumulative impacts and synergistic effects. Don't hide behind the language of individual chemical analysis and "acceptable risk." There are many resources that you can use to find creative solutions and safe, green alternatives.

- *Diamond: A Struggle for Justice in Louisiana's Chemical Corridor*: www.commonweal.org/pubs/diamond.html
- Eco-Efficiency Centre: www.dal.ca/eco-burnside
- EnviroClub, Quebec: www.enviroclub.ca
- Erin Brockovich: www.lawbuzz.com/famous_trials/erin_brockovich/erin_brockovich_ch1.htm
- Good Neighbor Agreements: www.cpn.org/topics/environment/goodneighbor.html
- Responsible Care: www.responsiblecare.org
- Responsible Care Canada: www.ccpa.ca/ResponsibleCare

## Create a Green Business Program

If you run a small business, take advantage of local green business programs to identify how you can make your business more sustainable. If there is no such program, encourage your Chamber of Commerce or local government to develop a green business program to help you and your fellow businesses go green, as they are doing in Arizona, Anchorage (Alaska), Halifax (Nova Scotia), the San Francisco Bay Area (see Solution 65) and in Quebec, with its successful EnviroClub. Your staff will appreciate it and enjoy the process of becoming a healthy neighbor.

## Establish a Care Organization in Your Community

In Canada the chemical industry has established a Responsible Care program. Under the program, companies agree to give information about their chemicals to the community and to discuss chemical safety with them. They keep the communities regularly updated through meetings or ads in local newspapers, and their plants are audited regularly by a group that includes independent auditors and at least one community member. This model has now been adopted worldwide.

# 59

## Stop Sabotaging the Solutions

Our wombs are no place for poisons.
Our babies have the right to be born
toxin-free.

— Laurie Valeriano, Washington Toxics
Coalition, and mother of three

For decades, whenever new information has arisen about the toxicity of a product, or an attempt has been made to regulate a chemical for public health reasons, some companies have responded by denying the information, undermining the science and attacking the proposed regulations.

The tobacco companies led the way in the 1950s, when health advocates first warned that smoking caused lung cancer. Corporate CEOs and hired scientists were willing to assert, often under oath, that nicotine was not addictive and there was no conclusive evidence of harm. For

Deformed snapping turtle hatchling contaminated with PCBs.

decades they profited while sowing doubt in the public's mind, making it very hard for public health protectors to do their work.

As long ago as 1961, DuPont knew that the perfluorocarbons (PFCs) they used to make Teflon accumulated in the body. Their tests showed that it did not break down in the environment and that it caused cancer, liver damage and birth defects in animals. By 1981 they had evidence pointing to the risk of children being born with birth defects. By 1984 they knew that the tap water in Little Hocking, near DuPont's Teflon plant at Parkersburg, Ohio, was contaminated with PFOA. No-one was told until 2002, when town officials petitioned the government to perform tests that detected the chemical. In 2005, after 3M had decided to phase it out, DuPont was still insisting that PFOA was safe.

Corporations use four strategies to fight new regulations. They campaign against the public's right to know. They manufacture doubt by hiring scientists to come up with opposing studies, while labeling their opponents' studies as "junk science." They hire product-defense companies to try to defeat "hostile" legislation, and lobby, lobby, lobby in Washington and Ottawa. And in the US, they buy political favors by contributing to the campaign funds of politicians. (In Canada, since 2006, no company or individual can donate more than $1,000 to a political party.) They have used these methods to deny the adverse health effects of killers like tobacco, DDT, PCBs, asbestos, beryllium, lead, mercury, vinyl chloride, chromium, benzene, benzidine, dioxins, perchloroethylene, nickel, MTBE additives in gasoline, formaldehyde and numerous pesticides.

In 1986 two things caused the chemical industry to worry. First, California voters approved Proposition 65, a citizens' initiative that requires companies to label their products for ingredients that might cause cancer or reproductive toxicity. Second, the US Congress approved the Community Right to Know Act, establishing the EPA's Toxics Release Inventory. Both initiatives were successful, causing companies to change their product formulations and reduce their emissions rather than be listed among the worst pollution offenders.

The Chemical Manufacturers Association (now the American Chemistry Council) was furious. After developing a war plan to raise $70 million, they used their resources to successfully battle a Massachusetts 1989 toxics use reduction initiative,[1] California's 1990 Big Green initiative,[2] a 1992 Ohio right to know initiative[3] and a 1992 Massachusetts initiative to prohibit corporate contributions to ballot campaigns.[4] The American Chemistry Council has fought every citizens' attempt to write the precautionary principle into law, which it sees as "a threat to the entire US chemical industry." It also organized to fight Europe's REACH legislation, the best safe chemicals policy initiative in the world until it was weakened by European and US corporations (see Solution 69).

At the time of writing (summer 2006), Republicans in the US Congress were pushing legislation that would wipe out the ability of California and other states to ban or strictly

- ACC Memo to fight the precautionary principle: www.cbgnetwork.org/351.html
- California's Proposition 65: www.oehha.ca.gov/prop65.html
- Cancer Prevention Declaration: www.preventcancernow.ca
- Center for Progressive Reform: www.progressiveregulation.org
- Chemical Industry Archives: www.chemicalindustryarchives.org
- Louisville Charter: www.louisvillecharter.org
- PFCs: www.ewg.org:16080/reports/pfcworld
- Project on Scientific Knowledge and Public Policy: www.defendingscience.org
- *Toxic Deception*, by Dan Fagin and Marianne Lavelle, Common Courage Press, 1999
- *Trade Secrets*, with Bill Moyers: www.pbs.org/tradesecrets

limit the use of pesticides and toxic industrial chemicals that jeopardize human health.[5]

What is the solution? Call off the attack dogs and step back to reconsider the options, as IKEA, Interface, Nike, Samsung, Panasonic, Husky and others have done. "Responsible Care" is not enough. With the discovery in 2005 that newborn babies have 200 chemical contaminants in their blood, business leaders must surely wake up and realize that there is a juggernaut of public outrage and liability suits coming down the road. How many mothers are going to say, "I care more about my non-stick frying pan than my baby's health"?

If need be, break away from business associations that persist with deceit and denial. Form new business alliances that endorse the principles of sustainability and the public's right to know. Sign pro-health declarations such as the Louisville Charter for Safer Chemicals and Canada's Cancer Prevention Declaration. Join the movement to prevent cancer and other toxic-induced health hazards, instead of fighting it.

# 60

# Solutions for Transport Companies

The fuels we use for travel, as well as the tires and the interiors of new cars, all contribute to the rise in cancer.

You've probably stood next to a bus or a truck when it spewed thick, black diesel smoke. "This can't be good for me or my kids," you might have muttered. You were right. Diesel fumes threaten you and your child with a risk of lung cancer that is seven times higher than the combined total cancer risk from all other air toxics.

Diesel and gasoline fumes, soot, particles of old tires as they wear away and volatile chemicals off-gassing from plastics and glues in new cars all contribute to a higher cancer risk. An American study of 500,000 people found that the death rate from lung cancer caused by particulates in air pollution increases steadily as the air grows dirtier.[1]

Cars and trucks also pollute the air with three more carcinogens: benzene, 1,3-butadiene

- Diesel and Health in America: www.catf.us/goto/dieselreport
- Electric Vehicle World: www.evworld.com
- Peak Oil: www.peakoil.net
- Plug-In Hybrids: www.calcars.org
- *Plug-in Hybrids: The Cars that Will Recharge America* by Sherry Boschert, New Society Publishers, 2006.
- *Stormy Weather: 101 Solutions to Global Climate Change* by Guy Dauncey with Patrick Mazza: www.earthfuture.com/stormyweather
- *Taking Our Breath Away: The Health Effects of Air Pollution and Climate Change*: www.davidsuzuki.org

> Our children and grandchildren are going to be mad at us for burning all this oil. It took the Earth 500 million years to create the stuff we're burning in 200 years. Renewable energy sources are where we need to be headed.
>
> — **Jack Edwards, Professor of Geology, University of Colorado**

and polycyclic aromatic hydrocarbons (PAHs). Large vehicles with more than two axles, such as buses, motor homes, and tractor trailers, produce 60 times more PAHs, 32 times more 1,3-butadiene and 9 times more benzene than a smaller vehicle with two axles.[2]

A Denver study found that children who live within 1,500 feet of a busy street carrying 20,000 vehicles an hour have a sixfold increased risk of cancer, including leukemia.[3] Living close to a major road increases your risk of asthma, emphysema and heart attack.

So what are the solutions? How can a bus, truck, car, taxi or shipping company contribute to the solutions to cancer? The short-term solutions include:

- Replace mufflers with particle filters or oxidation catalysts.
- Purchase and manufacture vehicles that use cleaner alternative fuels or ultra-low sulfur diesel, which produces 90% fewer emissions.
- Install closed crankcase ventilation systems to stop diesel fumes from escaping into school and transit buses.
- Train your drivers to switch off, instead of idling.
- Equip long-haul truck stops with electric cables to power the rigs overnight.
- Plug cruise ships into the grid when they dock, instead of burning non-stop diesel to generate electricity.

- Design vehicles with interiors and plastics that don't release VOCs and other toxic gases, as the Japanese Automobile Manufacturers Association is doing.
- Ask your suppliers to produce tires that do not release PAHs and 1,3-butadiene as they wear down.
- Design cleaner engines for garden equipment and outboard motors, using overhead valve technology and fuel injection.

The long-term solutions involve thinking beyond diesel and gasoline. Global warming makes it essential that we stop burning fossil fuels. It is also a reality that, as we pass the halfway mark in the world's oil supply, what's left will become increasingly expensive until it is all gone. Now is a very good time to take action.

The most rational source of power for future vehicles is electricity. You can run a small electric vehicle for $10 to $20 a month, and the world has an ample potential supply of sustainable green electricity from the sun, wind, tides, waves, geothermal, microhydro and other non-nuclear sources, combined with conservation and efficiency, if we put our minds to it.

For longer trips, the emerging "plug-in hybrid" technology, adds extra batteries to a gas-electric hybrid vehicle, enabling it to operate as an electric vehicle for all local trips, while using a limited amount of biofuel (ethanol or biodiesel) for longer distances.

For a permanent solution to both global warming and peak oil, our global civilization needs to embrace a new sustainable energy revolution, just as it embraced oil, gas and automobiles 100 years ago. We will see cities being redesigned to encourage more walking and cycling and more use of fast, efficient transit systems, powered by electricity and biodiesel. We will see community car-sharing and ride-sharing and much more use of railways for freight.

One very welcome benefit of this revolution will be that air pollution will gradually disappear, along with the cancers it causes. The noise and stress of city life will disappear too, because electric vehicles are silent, and our grandchildren will look back from their green, peaceful, clean-air cities and wonder how we tolerated all the noise and smog.

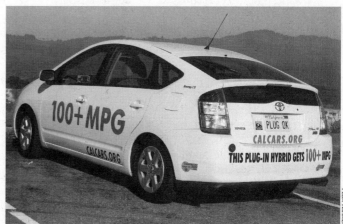

Plug-in Hybrid Electric Vehicle.

# 61

# Solutions for Power and Mining Companies

> Nearly all negative social and environmental aspects (of mining) are avoidable if companies would operate according to the best possible standards.
>
> — International Council on Mining and Metals

### Solutions for Power Companies

Coal-fired power plants are the leading toxic air polluter in North America, releasing mercury, dioxins and other chemicals that contribute to asthma and cancer, as well as being a major contributor to global climate change.

The incineration of garbage is another bad idea that keeps trying to resurrect itself. When you burn plastic you get dioxins and furans that are the most potent synthetic chemicals ever tested. Then there's nuclear power that increases the risk of cancer in nearby communities and among nuclear workers. (see p. 52) If coal, nuclear and garbage are off the table, how should power companies proceed?

### Efficiency

The cheapest source of new power is efficiency. All power companies should invest in rebates and programs designed to double the efficiency of every building, light, appliance and piece of equipment, as Seattle Light and Power is doing. All governments should ramp up their efficiency standards for appliances, as California did 20 years ago. The short-term potential is for everything to become twice as efficient; in the long-term, things could be 10 times as efficient.

### Wind and Solar Energy

A 2005 Stanford study showed that the world has five times more land-based wind energy potential than we use for all purposes.[1] North Dakota alone has enough wind to provide one third of all America's power needs — two thirds, if everything was twice as efficient. In 1980 solar photovoltaics (PV) cost $76 a watt. Today it costs $3.50. When it falls to $2, everyone will want to buy. Japan, Germany and California are leading the way, and the market is growing by 25% a year. We can also obtain safe, sustainable power from geothermal, microhydro, tidal, wave and biogas energy and forest and agricultural wastes. Worldwide, these sources could provide 8 times more energy than we currently use; 16 times more if everything was twice as efficient. The world would be not only cleaner, but safer and healthier.

### Solutions for Mining Companies

Mining has always been one of the most hazardous occupations, whether for asbestos, gold or other minerals. Miners have long had to contend with lung diseases and cancer, as well as the dangers of explosions and rockfalls.

Mining companies have often walked away from closed mines, leaving a toxic mess and a huge cleanup bill. In the beautiful Silver Valley in Idaho, the old mining town of Wallace is contaminated with lead from mining facilities that

- Global Alliance for Incinerator Alternatives: www.no-burn.org
- National Campaign Against Dirty Power: www.cleartheair.org/dirtypower
- *Stormy Weather: 101 Solutions to Global Climate Change*, by Guy Dauncey with Patrick Mazza, New Society Publishers, 2001: www.earthfuture.com
- World Information Service on Energy: www10.antenna.nl/wise

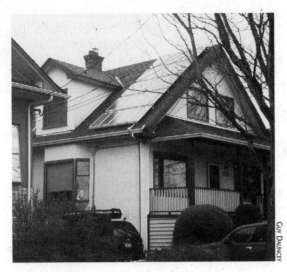

Solar PV house in Victoria, Canada.

- Diesel Emissions Evaluation Program: www.deep.org
- Framework for Responsible Mining: www.frameworkforresponsiblemining.org
- Good Practice Mining: www.goodpracticemining.org
- Haber Gold Process: www.habercorp.com
- International Council on Mining and Metals: www.icmm.com
- Mines and Communities: www.minesandcommunities.org
- MiningWatch Canada: www.miningwatch.ca
- Westerners for Responsible Mining: www.bettermines.org

spewed lead, arsenic, cadmium and other toxic pollutants into the area. It is now America's largest Superfund site, and its residents have the highest rates of cancer and attention deficit disorder in Idaho — both associated with heavy-metal poisoning.[2]

There are numerous studies that show higher rates of cancer and other diseases among miners and in mining communities,[3] and there are 500,000 abandoned mines across the US. In 2001 alone, the hard-rock mining industry released 2.8 billion pounds of toxic waste.[4] Globally, the picture is appalling.

What is to be done? Asbestos mining should be banned worldwide because of its health aspects (see Solution 96). Uranium mining should also be banned because the whole nuclear cycle is so dangerous. (see p. 53). Coal mining should be severely cut back due to its role in global climate change.

For the other kinds of mining, the International Labor Organization's long-term goal is "to ensure that without exception, an individual can devote a lifetime to a mining career and emerge healthy and unharmed."[5]

Can it be done? The answer is quite encouraging. In 1998, after years of harmful practices, the mining industry started out on a new journey. A multi-stakeholder review process, known as the Global Mining Initiative, was launched, culminating in the formation of the International Council on Mining and Metals (ICMM), with a mandate to promote sustainable development within the sector. This led in 2003 to commitments to embrace a Sustainable Development Framework, including Ten Principles for Sustainable Development, and in 2005 to join the Global Reporting Initiative with "an unprecedented level of transparency."

Other positive initiatives are also brewing. The new non-toxic Haber Gold Process can replace the use of cyanide to dissolve gold ores; the Canadian mining industry is supporting an initiative to reduce miners' exposure to underground diesel exhaust; and ICMM members are developing a program to manage the chemicals they use more sustainably. Even in the dirty world of mining, companies can contribute to stopping cancer.

# 62

# Solutions for Builders

> Green building is the next wave, and it's here to stay.
> — Kenneth D. Lewis, President of Bank of America

You may not know it, but North America is in the middle of a green building revolution. It's an exciting time to be a builder, developer, architect or engineer. You have a prime opportunity to show leadership, while crafting a world that will be a better place for your children and grandchildren.

In a peaceful, sustainable world, the buildings we live and work in will be healthy and safe. In order to start, we have first to eliminate a number of building products and practices that make us sick and contribute to the increased risks of cancer.

**Asbestos** is the most blatant example of a building product that has turned into a disaster. Asbestos dust causes a rare kind of lung cancer, mesothelioma, and yet it has been used all over North America in insulation, roofing shingles, asbestos cement, and heating and ventilating systems. In the US, 35 million homes and thousands of schools were insulated with vermiculite

ALEX ZIMMERMAN

Canmore's LEED Silver Civic Centre, Alberta.

contaminated with asbestos from the W.R. Grace mine in Libby, Montana, which also exposed its own workers. Asbestos-related diseases are killing 10,000 Americans a year; 75,000 will die by 2015. The situation is similar in Canada, where asbestos-contaminated insulation materials were widely sold. Worldwide, the asbestos cancer epidemic may take 10 million lives before asbestos is banned worldwide and exposures are brought to an end.[1] (See Solution 96)

**Pressure treated wood** infused with chromated copper arsenate is another toxic building material. Thanks to a campaign led by the Healthy Building Network, it is no longer legal to manufacture or sell it. Arsenic is a known carcinogen, yet the green telltale treated lumber is still in our fences and decks where children play, getting the arsenic-contaminated dirt on their hands. Independent research found that a typical area of arsenic-treated wood the size of a four-year-old's hand contains 120 times the amount of arsenic that the EPA allows in a six-ounce glass of water.[2] A Quebec company, Pluri-Capital, has developed a new type of wood that has been treated only with heat to preserve it.

**Plywood, particleboard and composite wood products** used for shelving, cupboards and building are made using glues that contain urea formaldehyde, a probable carcinogen that carries a risk of nasal cancer.[3] These gases contaminate indoor air. California is moving to virtually eliminate formaldehyde from wood products. Again, there are other good choices available.

We need to stop using **paints, varnishes and adhesives** that give off high levels of volatile organic compounds (VOCs), many of which are known or suspected causes of cancer, along with many other toxic additives. If it smells bad, it is bad. There are plenty of safe alternatives: just google on "non-toxic paint" or "green building supplies."

**PVC (vinyl)** is another big concern. It is used in everything from pipes and cables to windows and carpets. Polyvinyl chloride plastic is very hazardous to make and very toxic when it burns, releasing dioxins that cause cancer, endocrine disruption, birth defects and immune system damage. There is a movement to get rid of it altogether, led by the Healthy Building Network, and some excellent databases of alternatives that help with the switch.

Basements in large areas of central and eastern North America need to be protected from **radon**, a naturally occurring radioactive gas that contributes to lung cancer. Radon-resistant construction techniques in new buildings are very simple and cheap ($350–$500).

If you are constructing or renovating a commercial or institutional building, there is a good way to address all these problems. It's called Leadership in Energy and Environmental Design (LEED), a green building certification program that is taking North America by storm. LEED uses a scoring system that rewards everything from energy efficiency to indoor air quality, green energy, paints, adhesives and recycled products. There will soon be LEED certification for single-family homes and neighborhoods.

The full vision of green building shows great promise for a world with far less cancer.

- *Blue Vinyl* (DVD): www.bluevinyl.org
- Building Green: www.buildinggreen.com
- Canada Green Building Council (LEED): www.cagbc.org
- Citizen's Guide to Radon: www.epa.gov/radon/pubs/citguide.html
- Green Communities: www.epa.gov/greenkit
- Green Building Products, by Alex Wilson, New Society Publishers, 2006
- Healthy Building Network: www.healthybuilding.net
- Indoor Air Pollution (Asbestos): www.epa.gov/iaq/asbestos.html
- Indoor Air Pollution (Formaldehyde): www.epa.gov/iaq/formalde.html
- Indoor Air Pollution (Radon): www.epa.gov/radon
- Indoor Air Pollution (VOCs): www.epa.gov/iaq/voc.html
- Materials to Avoid: www.healthybuilding.net/target_materials.html
- PVC Alternatives Database: http:greenpeace.org/toxics/pvcdatabase
- PVC Facts: www.healthybuilding.net/pvc/facts.html
- PVC-free Materials List: www.healthybuilding.net/pvc/PVCFreeAlts.html
- Radon Resistant Construction: www.epa.gov/radon/construc.html
- Treated Wood Campaign: www.healthybuilding.net/arsenic/arsenic2_newsletter2.htm
- US Green Building Council (LEED): www.usgbc.org
- *Your Green Home*, by Alex Wilson, New Society Publishers, 2006

Zero-energy developments will generate their own power and not need coal-fired or nuclear power. Communities that make walking and cycling easy will encourage us to keep fit. Village centers will allow us to walk to local stores and schools and forgo cars that release benzene and diesel fumes. Local allotments and urban farms will encourage us to grow fresh, local, organic produce.

# 63

# Solutions for Farmers and the Food Industry

## Solutions for Farmers

You, too, can become an organic farmer.

If there is one area of change that is critically important as we work to reduce the record-high cancer rates, it is the movement by farmers to organic agriculture. The food is healthier, the use of chemical pesticides and fertilizers disappears, the phyto-nutrients that protect us against cancer reappear, the soil recovers, wildlife returns, the vet bills fall and farmers feel more at peace with the world, knowing they are contributing something good.

Since the modern farming revolution began with the development of chemical fertilizers in 1843, yields have increased, but everything else has been diminished. The percentage of trace minerals in fruits and vegetables in conventionally grown foods has fallen by up to 76% since the 1940s, as soils have become depleted.[1] Many associations have linked conventional farming to an increased risk of cancer (see p. 41), and evidence grows that parents' exposure to pesticides contributes to their children's cancer risk,[2] as well as to parental infertility.[3, 4]

The public is paying attention. Organic food sales in America are growing by 20% a year, compared to 2% to 4% for food in general. In Britain 50% of all baby food is now organic. Organic shoppers are buying because they think it is better quality food and because they don't want pesticides.

In 2005, 7,700 American farms cultivated 890,000 hectares organically (0.22% of the farmland); in Canada 3,500 farms cultivated 488,000 hectares (0.7%). The leaders are Lichtenstein,

People are applying the precautionary principle to their own lives by purchasing food that has not been produced by industrial methods. From the simple stance of hazard avoidance, organically produced food is the best option that we have.

— Dr. Vyvyan Howard,
toxico-pathologist,
University of Liverpool, UK

where 26% of the farmland is organic, followed by Austria (13.5%), Switzerland (11%) and Finland (7%).[5] By 2013 the Rodale Institute predicts that there will be 100,000 certified organic farmers in the US, representing 5% of its 2 million farmers. For farmers who want to make the change, there is plenty of support available.

## Solutions for the Food Industry

In one year, American fast-food chains spend more than $3 billion on TV advertising. In the US, the typical child will watch 20,000 advertisements for junk food, and the typical adult will drink 240 liters of soft drinks — well over 500 cans — a year. Two thirds of American adolescents drink sodas daily, and even the tots are at it: 20% of children aged 1 and 2 consume soft drinks each day.[6] The resulting accumulation of overweight and obese people is building an enormous problem, laden with diabetes and cancer. A quarter of American children are overweight, and 12% are classed as obese.

What can the food industry do to help us get back to healthy eating?

The World Health Assembly recommends that companies reduce the amount of salt, sugar and fat in their products and the size of servings, and that they create policies for corporate social responsibility and develop staff health programs. It also recommends that nutritional labeling become the standard worldwide.

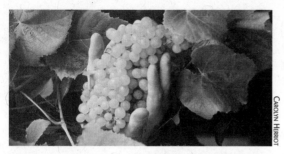

Organic grapes, mouth-watering and healthy.

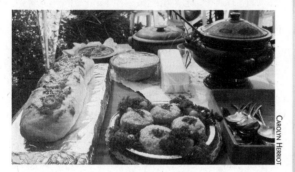

A banquet gathered from local organic farms.

Driven by concerned parents and health professionals, the State of California banned junk food on school campuses, which it may follow with a ban on sodas and other sweetened beverages.

Instead of fighting moves like this, and lobbying in Washington for pre-emptive legislation to stop states from protecting consumers from toxins and other contaminants,[7] the food industry would be wiser to get behind them, and support initiatives such as the demand for nutritional labeling to help people make healthy choices.

The industry can do a lot to promote organic food. On Vancouver Island, BC, Thrifty Foods, a major supermarket chain with many stores, has made a serious commitment to stock organic food, carrying over 70 varieties of organic fruits and vegetables and 400 organic grocery items.

Britain's Marks & Spencer has made commitments called Behind the Label for their food products, including sustainable fish, free-range

- California Project LEAN: www.californiaprojectlean.org
- Canadian Organic Growers: www.cog.ca
- Center for Informed Food Choices: www.informedeating.org
- *Chew on This, Everything You Don't Want to Know About Fast Food*, by Eric Schlosser
- Cyberhelp for Organic Farmers: www.certifiedorganic.bc.ca/rcbtoa
- European Public Health Alliance: www.epha.org
- *Food Politics: How the Food Industry Influences Nutrition and Health*, by Marion Nestle
- International Federation of Organic Agricultural Movements: www.ifoam.org
- National Sustainable Agriculture Information Service: www.attra.org
- The New Farm: www.newfarm.org
- Oregon Tilth: www.tilth.org
- Organic Advocates: www.organicadvocates.org
- Organic Agriculture Centre of Canada: www.organicagcentre.ca
- Organic Monitor: www.organicmonitor.com
- Organic Trade Association: www.ota.com
- Rodale Institute: www.rodaleinstitute.org
- Soil Association (UK): www.soilassociation.org
- Sustainable Agriculture Research & Education: www.sare.org
- Ten Reasons Why Organic Food Is Better: www.earthfuture.com/earth
- *The End of Food*, by Thomas Pawick.
- The New Farm: www.newfarm.org
- Transitioning to Organic Production: www.sare.org/publications/organic/organic.pdf

eggs, no GM food, reduced salt, no hydrogenated fats in ready meals and no artificial colorings, flavorings or flavor enhancers in their chilled ready meals.[8]

Which is smarter — to wait until the juggernaut of liability suits and ignominy hits share prices, or get ahead of the curve and become part of the solution?

# 64

# Solutions for Supermarkets and Retailers

> Consumers want to play an influencing role as active citizens. That's why the Co-op is embarking on the most radical review of a supermarket own-brand range ever undertaken.
> — David Croft, head of Co-op Brand, UK

Retail stores worldwide are overflowing with products,[1] many of which contain dangerous chemicals. The dust in our homes is contaminated with the same chemicals, and traces are showing up in our bodies. Is there a connection? Definitely. Is there anything retailers can do about it? Absolutely.

In a British survey, 9 out of 10 consumers said they wanted tougher monitoring of the retail industry on ethical and environmental issues, and 6 out of 10 said they would be willing to boycott products that are ethically unsound. Some companies are quietly rising to the challenge. Hennes & Mauritz, an international retailer of affordable fashions, has a strict chemical policy that clothing suppliers must meet if they want their business — no azo-dyes, no flame-retardants, no PVC, no formaldehyde and the list of assorted carcinogens and hazardous chemicals goes on.

There is also the question of food. Of American adults 20 years or older, 30% are obese; 16% of those aged 6 to 19 are overweight.[2] Obesity itself is a contributing cause of cancer because many carcinogenic chemicals cling to fat.

Supermarkets could feature fruit and vegetables in their advertising. They could replace candy near the checkout with healthy alternatives and increase their supply of locally grown organic food. They could use bio-based materials for packaging, eliminating plastic and styrofoam that migrates into food.[3, 4] Eggs packed in styrofoam have been found to contain seven times more ethyl benzene and styrene than eggs packed in cardboard.[5]

## Safe Cosmetics

On any given day, a North American consumer may use cosmetics and personal care products containing 200 different chemical compounds, many of them banned in Europe. Popular brands contain acrylamide (linked to mammary tumors), formaldehyde (a probable human carcinogen) and lead acetate (a known carcinogen and reproductive toxin). Many nail polishes and hair sprays contain phthalates that cause birth defects in laboratory animals, particularly males. Underarm cosmetics are being investigated for their possible carcinogenic effects.

The Campaign for Safe Cosmetics has persuaded many companies to sign a Compact for Safe Cosmetics to agree not to use chemicals that are known or strongly suspected of causing

BREAST CANCER FUND ON BEHALF OF THE CAMPAIGN FOR SAFE COSMETICS

**Putting on makeup shouldn't be like playing with matches.**

Which cosmetics company do you trust with your daughter?

When it comes to cosmetics, we shouldn't be forced to choose between health and beauty. Personal care products should be free of chemicals linked to cancer and birth defects.

Read our lips:

No More Toxic Chemicals in Cosmetics.

Paid for by the Safe Cosmetics Coalition          www.SafeCosmetics.org

In *USA Today* by the Safe Cosmetics Coalition. www.safecosmetics.org.

cancer, mutation or birth defects. It has published a Report Card that ranks the progress of the various companies and is pressuring the cosmetics industry to clean up. Some companies, like Avalon Organics, have signed onto the Compact and made major changes in their product formulations to avoid chemicals regarded as suspect.

## Dangerous Chemicals

In Britain Friends of the Earth has a Safer Chemicals Campaign that asks retailers to reduce their use of risky chemicals in a wide range of products. IKEA tops their League Table of good producers.

In the US nine organizations have formed Clean Production Action to run the Safer Products Project, including a Safer Chemicals Pledge in which retailers pledge to inventory the hazardous chemicals in their products and develop plans to eliminate them. Many major retailers have no policies at all to ensure that their suppliers will avoid the use of hazardous chemicals.

- IKEA uses The Natural Step to guide its environmental commitments. It has phased out most high-priority hazardous chemicals and brominated flame-retardants from its mattresses, carpets and furniture. It requires suppliers to follow environmental guidelines and not use anything on a list of forbidden or restricted chemicals, including pesticides, carcinogens and phthalates in children's products. It has set a goal to maximize the use of organic cotton in its furniture.

- Patagonia and the Vancouver-based Mountain Equipment Co-op have both made

- Adverse Health Effects of Plastics: www.ecologycenter.org/erc/fact_sheets/plastichealtheffects.html
- Campaign for Safe Cosmetics: www.safecosmetics.org
- IKEA: www.ikea-group.ikea.com/responsible
- Mountain Equipment Co-op: www.mec.ca
- The Natural Step: www.naturalstep.org
- Obesity: www.cmaj.ca/misc/obesity/usobesity.shtml
- Organic Cotton: www.sustainablecotton.org
- Patagonia: www.patagonia.com/enviro
- Safer Chemicals Campaign: www.foe.co.uk/campaigns/safer_chemicals
- Safer Products Pledge: www.safer-products.org

their sportswear lines 100% organic cotton. In the US 10% of all agricultural chemicals are used to produce cotton.

- Staples Business Depot collects dead cellphones, pagers and rechargeable batteries to prevent mercury, cadmium and lead from contaminating the environment and recycles them through a company called CollectiveGood.

- In Britain the Co-op has developed an "honest labelling" initiative, eliminated GM ingredients from its brand-name products, introduced a comprehensive range of organic products and eliminated 20 pesticides from its produce and many toxic chemicals from its household cleaning products, including fabric conditioners.

- Dell has developed a list of more than 50 banned or restricted materials that won't be used in their computers. It includes all halogenated flame-retardants and all substances that show strong indications of risks to human health. Dell was among the first US electronics manufacturers to publicly adopt a precautionary approach to its choice of materials.

# 65

# Solutions for All Businesses

We contribute to a better world by pursuing sustainability and environmental wisdom. Environmental advocacy is part of our heritage, and a responsibility we gladly bear for future generations.

— Herman Miller's Corporate Values
Statement

Small businesses can be an equally important part of the cancer solution — including the butcher (offer organically raised beef and chicken), the baker (offer whole wheat and organic grains) and the candlestick maker (use beeswax or soy wax; the emissions from petroleum-based wax may include reproductive toxins, neurotoxins, carcinogens and phthalates).[1] The changes are small, but collectively they make a big difference.

Dry cleaners can switch from perchloroethylene (linked to ten kinds of cancer)[2] and silicone-based solvents[3] to citrus and banana juice, wet-cleaning or liquid $CO_2$. Laundries can use biodegradable and non-toxic detergents.

Coffee shops can sell more organic coffee, so that coffee growers are not exposed to pesticides. Hotels can evaluate the cleaners, sanitizers, paints and pesticides they use and substitute safer alternatives.

Golf courses can become organic, as can lawn care companies.

Auto repair shops can change from naphtha-based solvents to water-based washers, minimize the liquids they use, clean up spills immediately using dry clean-up practices and use a squeegee and dustpan or oil mop instead of liquid methods.

Printers can adopt computerized pre-press operations, eliminating the use of photochemicals, use alcohol-free printing and low-VOC inks and recycle their solvents.

Furniture makers can use recycled materials, avoid the use of PVC and seek alternatives to fluorinated fire-retardants.

Every business has a role to play in becoming part of the solution, including hotels, beauty salons, embalmers and restaurants, as well as larger industrial businesses. In San Francisco, the Bay Area Green Business Program has set up a first-class program to help local businesses enjoy the benefits of becoming clean and green that deserves to be copied worldwide. In Halifax, Nova Scotia, the Eco-Efficiency Centre offers small companies advice on good environmental practices.

All businesses have purchasing departments, which provide an opportunity to control what you buy. Many large companies have created a

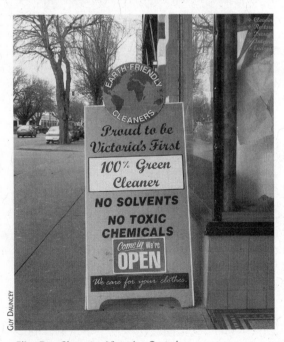

Elite Dry Cleaners, Victoria, Canada.
www.greendrycleaner.com.

demand for less-toxic alternatives through their purchasing policies. Kaiser Permanente, Catholic Healthcare West, Intel, Hewlett-Packard, Bentley Prince Street, IBM and Apple have all developed chemical and material screening programs for their supplies.[4] Other US and EU companies that are working with their suppliers to produce safer products include Herman Miller, Samsung, Sony, Fujitsu, Nike, Marks & Spencer and Boots Group PLC.

**The Big Picture**

As a world, we face enormous problems, from the growing contamination of our bodies to the loss of rainforests. Because of our activities, 60% of all ecosystems are in a state of decline or collapse.[5] Why are we acting as if we had another planet to go to when we have ruined this one? None of us wants to be part of this great ecological destruction, and yet we all are.

In the past, corporations almost single-mindedly pursued profits, with little regard for environmental and health concerns. Many corporate directors act on the assumption that they are required by law to maximize their shareholders' financial interests, regardless of how dubious the means might be. Some directors struggle with this view of the world as a moral wasteland where compassion, integrity and sustainability have no place.

There are solutions. Redefine your company's goals. Choose the corporate path less traveled where higher values guide business success, and carry your customers with you. If IKEA and the Mountain Equipment Co-op can make good

- BE SAFE Precautionary Platform: www.besafenet.com
- Center for Health, Environment and Justice: www.chej.org
- *Mid-Course Correction: Toward a Sustainable Enterprise, The Interface Model*, by Ray Anderson, Peregrinzilla Press, 1999.
- Prevent Cancer *Now*: www.preventcancernow.ca
- *The Natural Step Story: Seeding a Quiet Revolution*, by Karl-Henrik Robert and Ray Anderson, New Society Publishers, 2005.

- Auto Repair Shops: www.greenbiz.ca.gov/BGAuto.html
- Bay Area Green Business Program: www.greenbiz.ca.gov
- Dry Cleaning: www.greendrycleaner.com
- Organic Golf: www.growingsolutions.com/home/gs1/page/123/13
- Organic Lawn Care: www.environmentalfactor.com
- Printers and Publishers: www.ec.gc.ca/nopp/voc/en/secP.cfm
- Small Business Environmental Home Page: www.smallbiz-enviroweb.org

money following this path, so can you. Don't shift your production to countries with lax standards in order to continue polluting. Set your benchmark by countries with the highest standards, not the lowest.

Campaign for good legislation, not against it. Dissociate yourself from industry groups that work to undermine good legislation. Support organizations that are working for solutions to cancer, such as the Center for Health, Environment and Justice and Prevent Cancer Now.

Be open to rethinking how the world works. The cancer epidemic and the ecological collapses are a sign that something is very wrong. So, too, is the global climate crisis. Businesses can play a huge role in making things right again.

# 66

# Build a National Cancer Prevention Strategy

Calling all governments! The following solutions offer a guide to help you build a comprehensive strategy to prevent cancer. Yes, governments already have cancer prevention plans, but we ask you to refocus on stopping cancer before it starts.

### First, Lay the Foundation
Public policy framework is the foundation on which to build a cancer prevention strategy.

The new foundation must be a firm public commitment to achieve a non-toxic society within one generation, as Sweden has done, ensuring that all government departments embrace the goal and work towards its success, with identifiable benchmarks along the way.

By eliminating toxic chemicals to the greatest extent possible, we reduce not only the cancer burden, but also the incidence of birth defects, learning disabilities, asthma and other chronic diseases that come from living with too many toxic exposures.

As part of this foundation, government decision-making must be guided by the precautionary principle and the principle of substitution.

Let's start afresh from this day forward and say that if there is any suspicion that a chemical is harmful, then every decision will be taken with the foremost regard for protecting our health and the environment.

And let's place the substitution principle at the heart of government policy, so that industry begins the task of replacing its most toxic chemicals with safer substitutes.

The Ministry of Sustainable Development is striving to reduce the use of toxic and ecotoxic chemicals. The most hazardous ones must disappear from the market completely.[1]
— Sweden's Environmental Code.

### Next, Set the Cornerstones in Place
The cornerstones are the laws and programs that give strength to the public policy framework. Laws that require the reduction and elimination of toxic chemicals not only result in lower costs for industry, they also promote innovation and clean production. Model your programs after the successful ones we highlight here:

- Sweden's Environmental Code requires all Swedish companies to consider the opportunities for substitution and to replace hazardous chemicals with less hazardous or non-toxic ones by 2020.
- The Massachusetts Toxics Use Reduction Act makes pollution prevention plans mandatory and has led to a reduction in all aspects of toxic chemical use.
- Laws that extend our right to know, like Eugene's Toxics Use Bylaw that proves even a City can force polluters to divulge their secrets, and British Columbia's Workers' Compensation Act that gives workers the right to substitute less hazardous chemicals for carcinogens.
- Laws that ban the use of key toxic chemicals, like the European Union's Cosmetics Directive that bans carcinogens from all cosmetics.
- Chemicals legislation like the REACH regulation in Europe that aims to make companies test and register their chemicals, so that chemicals like carcinogens can be strictly controlled or eliminated.
- Biomonitoring programs and registries that track our body burden and exposure to toxic chemicals.

Austin, Jim and Karen Collier ride for the Breast Cancer Fund's Bike Against the Odds, a cancer prevention event which Jim helped establish in 2003 after his sister Karen was diagnosed with breast cancer. In 2006, he was joined by his son Austin.

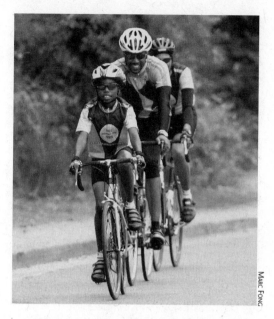

MARC FONG

- Organic action plans that help farmers grow food without harmful pesticides and make organic food, the antidote to cancer, affordable and widely available.

## Now, the Building Blocks that Will Create a Safer Place for Us to Live

- Develop a wholly new framework for chemicals policy and innovation that will simultaneously address the lack of transparent information, the toxicity problems and the need for an industry-wide transition to green chemistry, as the *Green Chemistry in California* report to the California State Senate and Assembly recommended in 2006.[2]

- Green up your government's procurement activities and buy products and services that are carcinogen free.

- Educate the next generation, so that an understanding of nature and a knowledge of green chemistry and clean production will help us to a better future.

- Clean the air, water and land of carcinogens and toxic chemicals that have been flushed and dumped without regard for our health, our children's health or the health of future generations.

- Reward companies that move to clean production with tax breaks, and tax the pollution itself. Prosecute companies that break environmental laws. Name them and shame them so that they become the pariahs of a clean society.

- Pass laws that rein in corporations that hide damning information about chemical hazards from the public or export cancerous products to developing countries.

- Detoxify the military use of our land, and demilitarize.

## Finally, Put up the Roof

The roof is the concluding element of the new structure. Governments must develop their own legislation, but the ultimate solution is for all countries to collectively implement the most effective strategies for cancer prevention and toxics use reduction.

Global treaties such as the Convention on Tobacco Control, the Stockholm Convention and the Basel Convention show how it can be done. We also need nations to sign on to treaties that outlaw asbestos and restrict or eliminate other carcinogens and hazardous chemicals.

These are the responsibilities and opportunities for governments that can move us to a safer and healthier world.

# 67

# Adopt the Precautionary Principle

Adopting the precautionary principle is a way to take out an insurance policy against our own ignorance. We rarely understand environmental risks until after the damage is done.[1]

— Anne Platt McGinn

Instead of asking "How much lead should we allow in paint?" the precautionary principle asks, "What can we use that's safe?" The idea is simple, but it changes the way we decide everything. It says if we have a reasonable suspicion that something will be harmful, even in the face of scientific uncertainty, we should take action to prevent that harm.

For too long, governments have used "risk assessment," investigating one chemical at a time, to decide how many cancers or how much risk we should accept. Although there were early warnings that substances such as benzene, asbestos and radiation could damage our health, governments and other experts used risk assessment data to insist that the dangers were small.

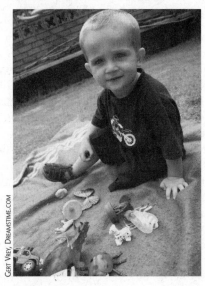

Plastic toys – how safe are they?

Take asbestos, a known cause of lung cancer and the sole cause of mesothelioma. As early as 1906, doctors observed that asbestos workers were dying from serious lung diseases. By the 1960s, the death toll had simply become unacceptable. Exposure levels were lowered, but it was another 30 years before asbestos was banned in Europe. The Dutch calculated if they had banned asbestos in 1965 instead of waiting until 1993, 34,000 victims of mesothelioma would have been spared, and Holland would have saved $24 billion (US) in health costs and building cleanups. Although asbestos is banned in Europe, this deadly mineral is still being mined by countries such as Canada, Russia and China and exported to developing countries.[2] (See Solution 96)

How can governments prevent future tragedies?

## Adopt and Practise the Precautionary Principle

- The 1992 Rio Declaration on Environment and Development, Principle 15, codified the precautionary approach for the first time at the global level: "The lack of full scientific certainty shall not be used as a reason for postponing cost-effective measures to prevent environmental degradation."

- The Cartagena Protocol on Biosafety allows countries to use the precautionary principle to decide whether or not to import genetically modified foods. It is also in the Convention on Biological Diversity, and the Stockholm Convention on Persistent Organic

Pollutants, firmly establishing precaution in international agreements.

- The European Commission has adopted the precautionary principle as the underlying foundation for all environmental laws. When studies linked certain phthalates to reproductive damage, the EU banned them from children's toys and cosmetics.

- Sweden has made the precautionary principle the basis of its chemicals policy, requiring industry to prove that all new chemicals have no carcinogenic, mutagenic or reproductive effects. Sweden banned some flame-retardants, not because they were a proven human health hazard, but because they were accumulating in breast milk.

- San Francisco was the first American city to adopt the precautionary principle. As Article One of its Environmental Code, it guides everything the City does, from environmentally preferable purchasing to its less-toxic pesticide program.

- Invoking the precautionary principle, nearly 200 communities in Canada — from large cities like Toronto and Vancouver to tiny Sainte-Paule, Quebec — have passed municipal bylaws to stop cosmetic pesticide spraying, a position which has been upheld by the Supreme Court of Canada.

**Pass Laws that Protect Children**
Another compelling reason to adopt the precautionary principle is the risk of toxic chemicals to children. Babies in the womb and children are

- Environmental Research Foundation: www.rachel.org
- Our Stolen Future: www.ourstolenfuture.org
- Precautionary Policy Clearinghouse: www.besafenet.com/ppc
- *Precautionary Tools for Reshaping Environmental Policy*, Nancy Myers and Carolyn Raffensberger, Eds., MIT Press, 2006
- *Rachel's Precaution Reporter*: www.precaution.org
- Science and Environmental Health Network: www.sehn.org
- Wingspread Statement on the Precautionary Principle: www.sehn.org/precaution.html

more vulnerable than adults are to contaminants. We now understand that some chemicals can cause damage at levels far lower than previously believed, and mixtures can increase both risk and adverse health effects. With this new understanding, governments need to reconsider legislation that establishes environmental standards in order to protect vulnerable populations. The US Pesticides Act was the first attempt to consider children's health by lowering acceptable levels of pesticide residues on food.

**Create a Fund to Test the Most Suspicious Chemicals**
We are beginning to grasp the risks of chemicals, called endocrine disruptors, that interfere with hormonal activity and affect reproduction. Because of the magnitude of these risks, research scientists worldwide have called for precautionary action in reducing exposures to chemicals like phthalates found in cosmetics and plastic toys and bisphenol A that migrates from clear-plastic baby bottles and can liners. Governments should restrict these chemicals immediately. In addition, they should create a trust fund for testing toxic chemicals financed by those who profit from them, so that manufacturers will not influence the results.

# 68

# Expand Public Health Care

## An Open Letter to Canada's Government

April 18, 2007. Saskatoon, Canada

It's April, which means it is Cancer Awareness Month in Canada, a time when people remember the courage of Terry Fox and his Marathon of Hope. April is also the month my daughter, Tanya, who died of a cancer similar to Terry's, would have turned 25. (See p. 98)

How ironic that you acknowledge Terry's legacy, but you have not acted to prevent other children and youth from suffering the same sad fate.

The Canadian government has very little funding for cancer surveillance programs — none for children's cancer surveillance even though cancer is the number one disease killer of children, and almost no public education campaigns that target carcinogens. We have an unacknowledged epidemic on our hands. Yet, we continue to search for elusive cures that generate a profit, while turning a blind eye to the causes. It's time that we changed our priorities. That's why I am urging you and all national governments to take the following actions:

## Set up Environmental and Occupational Surveillance Programs

National, provincial and state cancer registries track the number of people who are diagnosed with cancer, but they do not ask what they were exposed to. Did they work with pesticides? Did they live beside a chemical plant? Did they drink contaminated water? If you had this information, you could tell us what the risks are, and we could try to protect ourselves and our children. You could see why it matters to clean up contaminated areas. People's work and life histories should be taken every time they are diagnosed with cancer, as the Department of Environmental Health is doing in Cincinnati, creating a breast cancer registry that will collect information on residence, occupation and family history. From this information, they hope to gain a better understanding of the role that chemicals, diet, radiation and genetic factors play in the development of breast cancer.

## Conduct Biomonitoring Studies

We all carry a body burden of chemicals, like brominated flame-retardants that were unknown before World War II. Since 2001 the US Centers for Disease Control has been monitoring the chemicals in our blood and urine, seeking clues to our environmental exposures and looking for signs of abnormal or chronic chemical exposures.

- Best Start: www.beststart.org
- Canadian Partnership for Children's Health and Environment: www.healthyenvironmentforkids.ca
- Canadian Association of Physicians for the Environment: www.cape.ca
- Centers for Disease Control and Prevention: www.cdc.gov/biomonitoring
- Children's Health and Environmental Coalition: www.checnet.org
- Labour Environmental Alliance Society: www.leas.ca
- Terry Fox Foundation: www.terryfoxrun.org
- Trust for America's Health: www.healthyamericans.org

Now Canada will start its own program. Give your federal, state and provincial health departments the mandate and the funding to do extensive biomonitoring studies, to identify chemicals and take action.

### Warn Parents in Pre-natal Classes About Toxics

Effective health promotion programs, like Ontario's Best Start and Early Years, help expecting and new parents develop healthy lifestyles. Ensure that these programs also teach mothers and fathers how to shift to safe products and practices and how to avoid exposing themselves and their children to toxic products.

### Promote Public Education

In Vancouver, BC, the Labour Environmental Alliance Society does audits of toxic chemicals in schools and workplaces. Using material safety data sheets, they help workers to identify carcinogens and endocrine-disrupting ingredients in the workplace and to find safe alternatives. They also teach children how to audit their schools for toxic chemicals in everyday products. What they learn at school, they apply at home with the CancerSmart Consumer Guide. Governments should fund programs like this that help people recognize the carcinogens in everyday products and reduce their risk by avoiding them.

### Establish a National Carcinogen Registry

The Finnish government's ASA[1] registry requires companies that use carcinogens to report the type of chemical and the exposure of their workers to

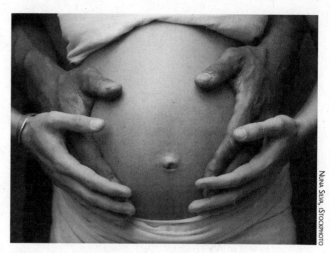

NUNA SILVA, ISTOCKPHOTO

This should be the safest place in the world.

the government every year. If workers develop cancer later, it can be linked with their exposure, and if too many people are getting cancer from one chemical, its use can be stopped. The registry gives employers an incentive to avoid cancer-causing chemicals in the workplace. Canada has a carcinogen registry but only for radiation — the National Radiation Dose Registry.[2] Dosimeters measure the exposures of hospital workers, uranium miners, nuclear plant workers — anyone who works with cancer-causing radioactive materials. If they have had too much radiation, they must be transferred to a safer job. This too can help prevent cancer. The "war" on cancer will never be won with money and a military mentality. We need a change of strategy. We need political will in Canada, the United States and in every country to locate and legislate the carcinogens out of our environment. We hope you will demonstrate this political will.

Yours sincerely, Donna Ell,
Tanya's mother.

# 69

# Control the Chemicals

No ecosystem has been left untouched. No human has been born since the middle of the 20ᵗʰ century without some exposure, in the womb, to hormonally active synthetic compounds.

— Theo Colborn, *Our Stolen Future*

Teflon and flame-retardants are modern miracles, but the darker side of the miracles is the discovery that these chemicals are pervasive and their health effects unknown. The breast milk of new mothers contains brominated flame-retardants. Perfluorooctanoic acid (PFOA), a key ingredient in Teflon, has been found in virtually every human blood sample taken worldwide. Over 100,000 chemicals are on the market, but only 7% have had full safety tests. For decades governments let companies develop and produce these chemicals, with "innocent until proven guilty" being the fatal rule.

Alarmed by the consequences of these free-floating, untested chemicals, countries are now trying to deal with the chemical data gap. Under the Canadian Environmental Protection Act, Canada categorized 23,000 chemicals, and those deemed most likely to be toxic based on persistence, bioaccumulation and inherent toxicity as well as exposure will be subjected to risk assessments. The problem is that it may take decades to finish this task. In the US the Toxic Substances Control Act has failed totally in its attempt to screen toxic chemicals and protect us from their nasty effects.

It is time for a new strategy to treat the sea of chemicals around us. Sweden has set a national objective of achieving a Non-Toxic Environment within one generation (by 2020), by eliminating the man-made and extracted chemicals that threaten human health.

## Ban or Phase Out Hazardous Chemicals
Bans are effective. In 1975, after scientists showed that lead damaged children's brains,

California ordered the lead out of gasoline. As a result, from 1976 to 1980, lead levels dropped by 40% in gasoline, air and the blood of everyone tracked by the US Centers for Disease Control.

Since 2006 cadmium, lead, mercury and hexavalent chromium have not been allowed in any electric or electronic goods sold in the European Union. Companies like Panasonic and Sony developed lead-free solder for their products well ahead of the deadline.

## Require Safer Substitutes
The substitution of hazardous chemicals with less hazardous or non-toxic ones is another effective strategy. At present, when regulations target a chemical for control, there are no specific guidelines to achieve green chemistry, clean production or sustainable product design. The replacement chemicals are often just as hazardous, or simply a less concentrated version of the same toxic substance.

By making the substitution principle the heart of new chemical policies and regulations, hazardous chemicals would be replaced with less hazardous or preferably non-toxic alternatives. This would hasten the uptake of green chemistry. A German law requiring the development of lists of "safer substitutes" has led to a wave of safer chemistries and changes in production.

To meet its goal of a toxic-free future by 2020, Sweden has made the substitution principle the core of its chemicals policy. Successful companies like Skanska, the construction giant, or H & M, an international clothes retailer, have replaced

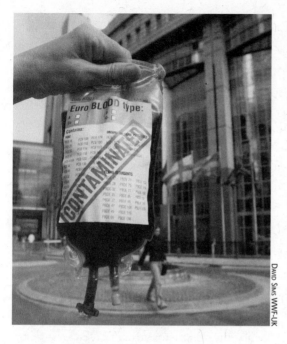

DAVID SIMS WWF-UK

- Green Chemistry Institute:
  www.greenchemistryinstitute.org
- Green Chemistry Network:
  www.chemsoc.org
- Louisville Charter Chemicals Policy:
  www.louisvillecharter.org
- Lowell Center for Sustainable Production:
  www.sustainableproduction.org
- Greenpeace on REACH:
  www.greenpeace.eu/issues/chem.html
- REACH White Paper:
  www.ec.europa.eu/enterprise/reach/whitepaper/
  index_en.htm
- Sweden's Environmental Objectives:
  www.sweden.gov.se/sb/d/5400/a/43592
- What Is REACH?
  http://detox.panda.org/the_solution/what_is_reach.cfm

toxic chemicals with safer ones, proving that companies can substitute and prosper.

Incentives also work. The Danish government operates a Cleaner Products Support Program that gives subsidies to companies that are developing safer products and processes. The US EPA's Green Chemistry Program also promotes green chemistry through grants to industries and universities.

## Adopt the Goals of REACH

The European Union has introduced a new approach to chemicals regulation known as REACH — the Registration, Evaluation and Authorisation of Chemicals. Under REACH, industry must take responsibility for testing the chemicals it uses and for passing on information about their effects.

Over 11 years, starting in 2007, chemical producers will phase in the registration of their chemicals and provide safety-testing data, starting with the highest volume and most hazardous ones. After that, chemicals that have not been registered cannot be used. In the second phase, chemicals that are suspected of being hazardous must undergo more intensive evaluation. If they are found to be a danger to human health or the environment, they may either be restricted or listed as chemicals of "very high concern."

If a company wishes to use a chemical of very high concern, authorization will be granted only if the risks can be adequately controlled. If it can't be, it can still be authorized if there are strong socio-economic reasons for its use, and no suitable alternatives exist. REACH's goal is to provide comprehensive information on all chemicals and to use that information to reduce the risk to human health and the environment.

REACH, as it was proposed originally, has been considerably weakened by industry lobbying. The goal for all governments must be to adopt the principles and ideas for REACH that were first set out in the European Union's White Paper.[1]

# 70

# Strengthen Your Regulatory Arm

> Industry proved much more clever and creative at exploiting the loopholes than Congress expected.
>
> — Donald Kettl, Clean Air Act New Source Review Panel, 2003

Toxic air has always been a problem in Texas. In counties like Galveston, El Paso and Harris, the only thing that separates some communities from the chemical plants and oil refineries are the chain-link fences. More than 142,000 children go to school in the shadow of these plants, exposed to chemicals wafting into their schoolyards that are known to cause cancer, birth defects and learning disabilities.

During the 1970s governments passed laws designed to clean the air and water and protect the environment, but like many of us, the citizens of Texas have found that their laws contain loopholes big enough to push a smokestack through. In Texas there is no consistent air monitoring at schools or on the fencelines of neighboring plants, and the thresholds for

chemicals have been set so high that they do not protect human health. When cancer-causing chemicals such as butadiene are found over the standards, no action is taken. Not surprisingly, cancer rates are unacceptably high.

What can governments learn from Texas? Close the loopholes and enforce the existing legislation.

## Learn from the PFOA Disaster

Perfluorooctanoic acid (PFOA) is used to make Teflon and protective finishes like Scotchgard and Gore-Tex and is recognized as a probable carcinogen by the US Environmental Protection Agency. In Parkersburg, West Virginia, the DuPont Corporation has been dumping PFOA into the town's drinking water for years. In 2005 DuPont finally agreed to pay more than $100 million to compensate the people of Parkersburg.

When they were passed, laws like the US Toxic Substances Control Act and the Canadian Environmental Protection Act did not require safety data for chemicals that were already being used, like PFOA. Companies were, however, required to submit information to the government if they discovered problems with their chemicals. DuPont knew that PFOA was linked to serious health problems, but it took years before they made the government or the community aware of it. Now we know that PFOA is a persistent, bioaccumulative health risk.

What can governments learn from PFOA? Strengthen and enforce your toxic chemicals legislation. Require companies to thoroughly test all new chemicals before they are approved, and to fill in the data gaps on those already in use.

© GREENPEACE/PIERRE VIROT

Greenpeace activists with e-waste outside Hewlett Packard, Geneva, Switzerland.

## Learn from Citizen Suits

In 1970 US environmental laws gave citizens the right to bring legal action against polluters, or against the EPA to force them to apply the laws. Armed with Discharge Monitoring Reports that exposed permit violations, US citizens have used their rights under the Clean Water Act to force polluters to clean up. What can governments learn from these citizen suits? Give citizens more enforcement powers.

## Learn from Canada

It used to be that sentences for environmental crimes paled in comparison to sentences for drug trafficking or street crimes. In Canada the courts are now treating environmental crimes more seriously and giving prison terms to managers and company directors, levying high fines, requiring public apologies, ordering remediation and directing fines into environmentally oriented projects and programs. In Ontario a pulp and paper company, Provincial Papers of Thunder Bay, was found guilty of polluting fish-bearing waters and fined $200,000.[1] The judge ordered that $160,000 be paid to the local community for the enhancement of fish habitat and to local colleges for environmental studies programs.

What can governments learn from Canada to discourage environmental crimes? Promote stiffer penalties and creative sentencing.

## Learn from New Jersey

New Jersey has collected more than $42 million in 10 years through its Natural Resource Restoration

- Canadian Environmental Law Association: www.cela.ca
- Environment Canada: www.atl.ec.gc.ca/enforcement
- Environmental Compliance Consortium: www.complianceconsortium.org
- Environmental Damages Fund: http://atlantic-web1.ns.ec.gc.ca/edf
- Environmental Working Group: www.ewg.org
- Massachusetts Environmental Strike Force: www.mass.gov/dep/about/organization/aboutesf.htm
- New Jersey Natural Resource Restoration: www.nj.gov/dep/nrr
- Refinery Reform: www.refineryreform.org
- Sierra Legal Defence Fund: www.sierralegal.org

Program by demanding compensation from companies that have damaged the environment through oil spills or discharges. They have used the money to restore aquifers and wetlands and save valuable wildlife habitat. In 1999 one of New Jersey's notorious Superfund sites, Chemical Leaman, gave the State $3.7 million in damages and paid for the preservation of a bald eagle habitat.[2] What can governments learn from New Jersey? Create a Natural Resources Damage program. Use money from settlements and fines to fund environmental restoration.

## Learn from Massachusetts

Massachusetts is fighting polluters with an Environmental Crimes Strike Force. Its Department of Environmental Protection is working with the state police to share their technical, investigative and legal talents. Together they've set state records for enforcement, including the longest prison term ever handed out for an environmental crime and the largest fine ever imposed in the state. What can governments learn from Massachusetts? Set up a special Environmental Strike Force to investigate and prosecute environmental crimes.

# 71

# Tax Pollution, Instead of People

We tax the wrong things. Mostly, we tax things we want more of, such as paychecks and enterprise, not things we want less of, such as pollution and resource depletion.
— Alan Thein Durning, *Tax Shift*

Everyone complains about taxes, except perhaps the Swedes. That's because in Sweden income taxes have been going down while pollution taxes go up.

The Swedes know it as a green tax shift, and it pays a double dividend. Higher taxes on environmentally harmful activities make it more expensive to pollute, while people's work is rewarded with lower taxes. Since Sweden committed itself to a green tax shift in 2000, it has reduced income taxes every year. At the same time, it balances its budget with higher taxes on carbon dioxide, diesel fuel, electricity, pesticides and chemical fertilizers.

Although the tax system can't replace regulation, it's one more tool in the government kit. It can be used on activities that governments want to discourage, or even encourage. If governments want to discourage the use of toxic chemicals that damage human health, they tax toxic chemicals. It is a strategy that's already proven itself.

Massachusetts charges fees on companies that use large volumes of toxic chemicals, which help the state pay for its successful Toxics Use Reduction Program (see Solution 72). Even Eugene, Oregon, with its municipal Toxics Right to Know law, funds its toxics use reporting program with fees paid by polluters.

Several states impose taxes on dry cleaners that use perchloroethylene, a known carcinogen. Not only is perchloroethylene a hazard to workers, but it has found its way into many drinking water supplies. Connecticut imposes a 1% surcharge on all dry-cleaning services to help clean up the contamination from dry-cleaning solvents and organize prevention programs. Texas has a similar fund in which the distributors collect fees on the sales of dry-cleaning solvents. These taxes promote reduced solvent use and a shift to effective, non-toxic alternatives such as citrus-based or wet cleaning.

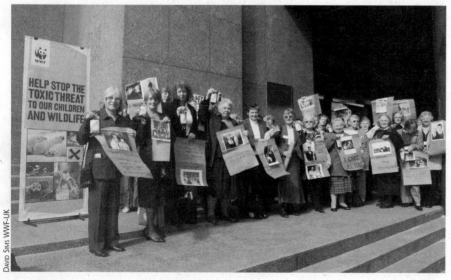

Grannies in Brussels campaigning for strong REACH legislation.

DAVID SIMS WWF-UK

Denmark uses taxes to target specific undesirable chemicals such as chlorinated solvents, phthalates and soft-plastic polyvinyl chloride, popular ingredients in many products, making these chemicals expensive enough that companies seek out safe substitutes. Danish taxes on three chlorinated solvents resulted in a 70% drop in their use over three years.

Sweden and Denmark have also used taxes as one of several strategies to cut their countries' use of pesticides and fertilizers in half. In 1996 Denmark raised its pesticide taxes from 3% of the retail price to as high as 37%. They calculated that for every 15% increase in the price of pesticides, there would be an 8% reduction in use.

France, one of the largest pesticide users in the world, announced in June 2006 that it aims to cut the country's use of the most harmful pesticides and biocides by 50%, in part by imposing new taxes on them.

Just as governments can tax "bad" things, they can also support the good alternatives. A large part of the money that Denmark collects from pesticide taxes goes to fund research and support for organic farming. At the same time, the Danish government has reduced taxes on farmland.

Tax breaks are another way of gently directing people towards positive choices. Currently, though, most governments send the wrong signals. Instead of the polluter paying, our governments often pay polluters with ill-advised tax breaks and subsidies. In Canada and the United States, sales tax exemptions handed out by governments encourage the use of fertilizers and pesticides.

The Canadian government also gives the swimming-in-profits oil and gas sector an estimated annual $1.4 billion tax subsidy[1], according to the Green Budget Coalition. Most of the subsidy is in the form of tax breaks, including accelerated capital cost allowances for tar sands development[2]; yet, the oil and gas companies are among the largest air polluters in the country.[3]

The US Green Scissors campaign targets environmentally wasteful subsidies that could be eliminated by governments and save both money and the environment. It has also identified some of the worst abuses of the American tax system, such as subsidizing the mining of mercury and asbestos through depletion allowance costs.[4] The Green Scissors Campaign also recommends green taxes that will transfer some of the government's burden back to industry.

The message? Green taxes and tax shifts are another tool we can use to prevent cancer.

- Connecticut Dry Cleaning Remediation Fund: www.ct.gov/ecd/cwp/view.asp?a=1101&q=249814
- Environmental Taxation Worldwide: www.greentaxes.org
- Fiscal Ecological Reform: www.fiscallygreen.ca
- Green Budget Coalition: www.greenbudget.ca
- Green Scissors Campaign: www.greenscissors.org
- Green Tax Shift: www.progress.org/banneker/shift.html#new
- Tax Shift: www.sightline.org/research/taxes

# 72

# Reduce the Toxics

> We need to set the agenda and push for what we want — not just for what we don't want.
>
> — Beverley Thorpe

Imagine a day when every company in your community drastically reduced its carcinogens and other damaging chemicals. For a lesson in how-to, governments can look to Massachusetts, which provides a sterling example of what political will and an ambitious strategy can achieve.

The Toxics Use Reduction Act was introduced in 1990, and by 2000, Massachusetts' largest industries had reduced their:

- toxic chemical use by 40%,
- toxic transfers offsite by 36%,
- toxics shipped in products by 47%,
- toxic by-products by 58%, and
- toxic releases to the environment by 90%.

And they saved money doing it. An evaluation showed that more than two-thirds of the firms collectively saved $14 million, while increasing production by one third. They also reduced releases of carcinogens to the environment by 76%.

A typical success story is LePage's, an adhesive tape manufacturer. After hundreds of tests with different solvents and adhesives, it created adhesive formulations that were free of cyclohexane and vinyl acetate. As a result, it was able to develop new and better products, while significantly reducing its toxic chemical use.

How did Massachusetts get so far so fast? And how can other governments do the same?

*Step 1*: Pass a Toxics Use Reduction Act with the goal of promoting safer and cleaner production, while enhancing the economic viability of your companies. Change from controlling end-of-the-pipe pollutants to controlling the chemicals themselves, and how they are used.

*Step 2*: Set targets such as reducing the amount of chemicals used, and toxic waste released, in your province, state or nation by 50% within seven years.

*Step 3*: Require companies to produce pollution prevention plans that describe how they can reduce their use and release of toxic chemicals over a prescribed period of time, with updates every two years. Require them to do detailed accounting of the amounts used, generated as waste and shipped in or used as product (known as materials use accounting). Charge them a fee, and use it to provide technical support. (See Steps 4 and 5)

In Massachusetts the planning process begins when the company solicits ideas from its employees. This recognition — that employees have valuable knowledge — can translate into using chemicals more efficiently. Poly-Plating, one company that produces nickel-plated parts for other industries, involved its employees in redesigning its nickel-plating methods. The redesign reduced the company's use of acid by 96%, its acid waste disposal costs by 91% and its water and sewage fees by 98%. The company had a total annual savings of $107,000 and a 25-month payback period for its investment.

Initially about 1,000 companies were required to report their chemical use and emissions. However, by 2005, 450 of these companies no longer produced enough chemicals to meet the reporting thresholds. The Robbins Company that does metal finishing

- Massachusetts Toxic Use Reduction Act: www.mass.gov/dep/toxics/toxicsus.htm
- Office of Technical Assistance Case Studies: www.mass.gov/ota/cases
- Toxics Use Reduction Institute: www.turi.org

slowly changed its processes to reduce or eliminate all of its reportable toxic substances. By 1994 it had re-engineered the annealing process to get rid of ammonia, its last reportable substance under the Toxics Use Reduction Act.

The Massachusetts experience shows that simply requiring companies to write pollution prevention plans pays off. Although companies are not legally bound to implement them, 80% of them do. The plans help companies understand why they are using toxic chemicals, how they are using them and how they can reduce them. To ensure consistency and an appropriate level of detail, the plans must be signed by certified trained planners.

**Step 4**: Set up an Office of Technical Assistance, funded by the toxics fees, to help businesses with confidential onsite engineering and technical advice on how to replace and reduce their toxic chemicals.

**Step 5**: Establish a Toxics Use Reduction Institute, financed by the same fees, to test and promote alternatives to toxic chemicals, and to provide training, information and a laboratory service.

The Institute also works with small businesses and community groups in Massachusetts to extend the reach of the program. Grants are awarded to groups such as the Healthy Boston

Schools Janitorial Project to cut down their use of toxic cleaners.

**Step 6**: Require companies to make progress reports every year and to publish them on the Internet.

With these reports, everyone knows what has been accomplished. They know that pollution has been reduced inside and outside the plants, that companies have saved money buying and disposing of chemicals with less paperwork and fewer permitting problems, and that industries in their communities can export their products to places like Europe that have higher standards.

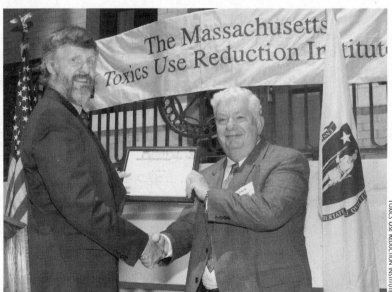

Michael Ellenbecker, Director of TURI, presenting an award to Jack Bailey of Bose Corporation.

# 73

# Let the People Know

Mandatory disclosure has done more
than all other legislation put
together in getting companies to
voluntarily reduce emissions.
— Dow Chemical Executive

Although the old adage tells us that what we don't know won't hurt us, today it's the exact opposite. In this jet age of modern products and pollution, one line of defense is to know what's in the drinking water, the air, the shampoo and the cleaning products we use every day.

This information, held in government and company files, was considered privileged until the 1980s when workers and citizen groups convinced governments to pass right to know laws. New Jersey's law gives people "the inherent right to know the full range of the risks they face, so that they can make reasoned decisions and take informed actions concerning their employment and their health."[1]

These laws oblige polluters to publicly report what they are putting into the air, the water and the toxic dump site out back. Using just a zip code, US citizens can find out how much pollution is in their neighborhood by consulting the Toxics Release Inventory (www.scorecard.org). Canadians can look it up on their National Pollutant Release Inventory (www.pollutionwatch.org).

Being in the spotlight has driven many companies to clean up. When Novopharm in Scarborough, Ontario, topped the list as Canada's largest emitter of methylene chloride, a suspected carcinogen, the company changed to using water in its pill-coating process, and its releases dropped from almost 500 tonnes a year to nothing.[2] Ohio Citizen Action, using toxics reports, negotiates "good neighbor agreements" with companies like Brush Wellman in Elmore, Ohio, that reduced its beryllium releases to the air by 96%.

Under California's Proposition 65, citizens must be warned through labels, in-store signs and toll-free

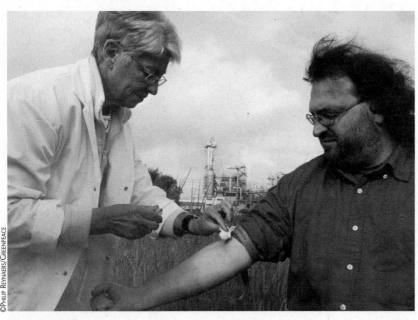

Wendel Trio from Greenpeace Belgium gives a blood sample in a protest at a Bayer plant inviting the chemical industry to substitute for safer substances.

©PHILIP REYNAERS/GREENPEACE

information services when businesses knowingly expose them to chemicals that cause cancer or reproductive harm. To avoid warnings, companies often choose to remove the carcinogens from products such as nail polish removers and ceramic faucets.

As good as these laws are, however, there is a need to know more. *An estimated 95% of all toxic releases do not have to be reported.* If we want to get rid of carcinogens, governments need to strengthen existing laws to give people the right to know not only about emissions but also the use and fate of all toxic chemicals.

The citizens of Eugene, Oregon, did just that, voting for a unique municipal Toxics Right-to-Know law. They recognized that the Toxics Release Inventory reported only a fraction of the chemicals used in their community. Now Eugene manufacturers give an exact accounting of all their chemicals. Every year they have to file a sheet, like an income and expenses ledger, that balances the toxic chemicals they buy and use with the ones that leave the plants in products or as emissions. This balancing of the chemical accounts has helped companies improve controls and find safer chemicals. The citizens of Eugene also voted to have industry pay for the program's costs (see also Solution 29). State laws in Massachusetts and New Jersey also require this kind of materials-use accounting for toxic chemicals (see Solution 72).

The Eugene Toxics Board, which oversees the program, wants it extended to smaller businesses like gas stations and paint shops, because of evidence that even small sources can pose a risk.

- *Hooked on Poison,* Pesticide Action Network: www.panna.org
- Eugene Toxics Right-to-Know Law: www.ci.eugene.or.us/toxics
- New Jersey Right to Know Act: www.state.nj.us/health/eoh/rtkweb/rtkact.pdf
- Ohio Citizen Action: www.ohiocitizen.org
- Oregon's Pesticide Right-to-Know Law: www.pesticide.org/
- Oregon Toxics Alliance: www.oregontoxics.org
- Toronto Environmental Alliance: www.torontoenvironment.org

Full reporting of pesticide use is also left out of the current national laws, so both California and New York have set up their own pesticide use reporting laws. California was the first state to require monthly pesticide reports, making it possible to track all pesticide use. Since the start of the program in 1990, it has become evident that the use of the most hazardous pesticides, including those that cause cancer, has been on the rise.

In Canada and the US, successful campaigns have won workers the basic right to know about chemical hazards such as carcinogens in the workplace through training, labeling and data sheets. Now workers need the right to find *substitutes* for carcinogens. Where a carcinogen has been identified by a safety data sheet, workers should have the right to a safer alternative. The Canadian Auto Workers successfully worked with the large automakers in Ontario to replace widely used metalworking fluids, linked to skin and other cancers, with canola oil.

British Columbia[3] and Quebec laws require employers to look for safer chemicals or products and substitute them for ones that may cause cancer. European directives also promote substitution for carcinogens. It is time for all governments to extend the right to replace workplace carcinogens to all workers.

# 74

# Control the Corporations

*There was a growing gap between the efforts to reduce the impact of business and industry on nature and the worsening state of the planet.[1]*
— United Nations

Corporations are, by definition, obliged to make money for their shareholders and prohibited from activities that would reduce their profits. Money can only be spent to protect the environment and public health if it contributes to the bottom line. This corporate imperative has led to a rush on destructive projects worldwide that have severely damaged the environment and put our health at risk.

The only restraint on companies is their obligation to comply with public laws, which means that governments play a crucial role in curbing corporate practices through laws, regulations and policies. With globalization upon us, however, many corporations wield a power greater than any national government. Of the top 500 economies in the world, 51 are countries and 49 are corporations.

Some multinational companies skirt their environmental responsibilities by operating in countries where regulations are not as strict or not enforced. Some push governments for political favors that benefit them, while destroying the environment.

What can governments do to make corporations accountable?

**Rewrite Corporate Charters**
National governments need to rewrite the corporate charters that determine how companies operate.

Under a new charter, companies should be compelled to report on the social and environmental impacts of their activities and products as part of their legally required annual reporting. Many companies *voluntarily* adopt guidelines, promising to reduce their impacts, but there's no way to hold them legally accountable or to impose sanctions when they don't live up to them. In some cases, companies pay lip service to environmental principles as a form of marketing and then blithely damage communities where they operate — a practice known as greenwashing. Shell, the world's second-largest oil and gas company, while committing itself to sustainable development, continues to flare gas in the Niger delta, ignoring a 1969 ban on gas flaring by the Nigerian government.[2]

Under corporate law, directors are required to consider company profit in all their business decisions. Governments should expand their legal duties by adding a simple 28-word amendment, as proposed by the activist corporate lawyer, Robert Hinkley: "The duty of directors henceforth shall be to make money for shareholders *but not at the expense of the environment, human rights, public health and safety, dignity of*

- Aurora Institute: www.aurora.ca
- Corporate Responsibility Coalition: www.corporate-responsibility.org
- Friends of the Earth: www.foe.co.uk/campaigns/corporates
- Program on Corporations, Law and Democracy: www.poclad.org
- Robert Hinkley: www.thesunmagazine.org/345Hinkley.pdf and www.commondreams.org/views02/0322-07.htm

*employees and the welfare of the communities in which the company operates"* (italics in original).

Corporations should also be required to follow the same rules and regulations wherever they operate. In 2005 Britain introduced a Company Law Reform Bill that (among other things) would require company directors to "have regard to" communities and the environment. It falls short of Friends of the Earth's calls for a "duty of care" that would require directors to minimize their company's damage to local communities and the environment, and that allow citizens and communities abroad who are harmed by the activities of a British company to take action against them in a British court.

### Require Companies to Report Pollutants

Whether it is emissions, operating permits or legal violations, transparency increases corporate accountability.

Most developed countries now require large companies to publicly report their air, water and waste emissions. This reporting has been more effective in reducing toxics than any other regulatory scheme. After 11 years of reporting to the US Toxics Release Inventory, emissions were reduced by 46%,[3] and companies that emitted carcinogens were more likely to reduce them.[4] All countries need to expand their pollutant registries by adding more companies, longer chemical lists and lower reporting thresholds.

For developing countries, the Indonesian environment agency has pioneered an innovative reporting scheme.[5] With weak enforcement capacity and a limited budget, the agency decided to

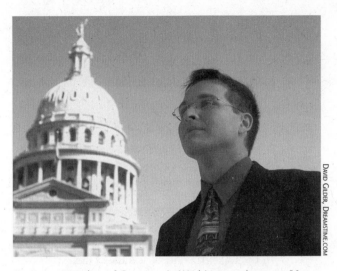

For every Member of Congress in Washington, there are 20 paid lobbyists. Whose interest are they lobbying for?

rank polluting companies on a scale of black to gold and publicize the results. Within one year, the number of plants complying with Indonesia's regulations leapt from one-third to one-half, and pollution was reduced by 40% as companies scrambled to upgrade the color of their performance.

### Shame the Bad Companies

In England and Wales, companies operating illegally or with a poor environmental record are named and shamed in the Environment Agency's annual *Spotlight on Business* report. The report highlights companies that have been convicted each year and the fines meted out to their directors. It includes the stock market listed parent companies, so that shareholders, investors and the public can identify the bad actors.

Two more ways to force improvements are to establish a government blacklist of companies with a poor environmental record when procuring services, and to ask the courts for restoration orders that force companies to repair the environmental damage they cause.

# 75

# Revive Democracy

**Democracy is a device that ensures we shall be governed no better than we deserve.**

— George Bernard Shaw

Political electroshock therapy — that's what is needed to revive our rusting democracies and give health concerns a chance against corporate self-interest. Here's what forward-thinking governments are doing.

## Reform Campaign Financing

In the wake of political scandals, three state governments have been nudged by public pressure towards voter-owned elections. Connecticut, Maine and Arizona have become the first to embrace what is known as "clean money, clean elections." Corporations and wealthy individuals who influence politicians with their checkbooks will now find it harder in these states.

The new legislation allows candidates the option to refuse private money and have their campaigns publicly financed. A candidate has only to raise a small amount of seed money from supporters to qualify. During the election, they are freed from fundraising to address the issues and the voters. If elected, they are answerable only to their constituents. In Maine, where the movement began, more than 80% of the candidates in the last election ran publicly financed campaigns.

With the Political Financing Act of 2003, Canada also created public financing of federal elections. Government money goes to all political parties that win 2% or more of the vote, and parties are paid an amount based on the number of votes garnered in the last election. The 2006 Accountability Act bans contributions from corporations and unions to parties and leadership contests, and caps individual donations at $1,000. Even that's not enough, says Democracy Watch, which wants legislation that makes secret donations to party leadership campaigns illegal.

## Control the Lobbyists

But corporate influence doesn't begin and end with elections. Everywhere in the world, lobbyists work against health regulations by exaggerating the costs and downplaying the benefits — aided and abetted by company-financed scientists, lawyers and public relations firms.

When the adverse health effects of exposures to substances such as beryllium, vinyl chloride, benzene or other carcinogens are raised, scientists are paid by industry to do studies that challenge the legitimate evidence incriminating these chemicals. By manufacturing doubt, companies successfully stall or block public health

DREAMSTIME.COM

Trustworthy – or not?

protection measures. This ensures that cancer-causing products such as tobacco and asbestos remain on the market.[1]

Canada's Accountability Act prevents all ministers, political aides and senior public servants from becoming lobbyists for at least five years from the time they leave office. Laws should also require anyone with decision-making powers to disclose all those who communicate with them to influence their decisions in a Lobbyist Registry, and make this information publicly accessible on an easily searchable website. Nor should decision-makers be allowed to dine, travel or receive gifts on the expense accounts of professional lobbyists.

### Adopt Proportional Voting

Democracy works when we all have a voice, but our "first past the post" electoral systems in Canada and the US leave large blocks of people unrepresented. Governments need a system of proportional representation that rewards voters with the representation they choose. Holland, Germany, Denmark and New Zealand have opted for a system that mixes proportional representation with representation from local constituencies.

Under this mixed-member proportional system, each voter has two votes — one for the local representative, chosen by the "first past the post" system, and one for the party of their choice. If a party's seats do not reflect the overall number of people who voted for it, representatives are added from the party's list to balance the representation. Other systems such as the Single Transferable Vote are also more democratic.

- Consumer Protection for Elections: www.blackboxvoting.org
- Corporate Accountability International: www.stopcorporateabuse.org
- Corporate Corruption of Science, International Journal of Occupational and Democracy Watch Canada: www.dwatch.ca
- Environmental Health, Vol. 11(4), Oct/Dec. 2005: www.ijoeh.com
- Fair Vote Canada: www.fairvotecanada.org
- Public Campaign: www.publicampaign.org
- Working for Change: www.workingforchange.com

### Reform Electronic Balloting

The introduction of electronic voting machines in the US and in some Canadian cities, marketed by private companies with links to political parties, has created new possibilities for destroying democracy through vote tampering and computer "error."

According to Black Box Voting, a computer programmer can create an invisible backdoor for millions of votes and rig elections without having to stuff or steal a ballot box. Incorrect programming has been identified in over 100 elections, often flipping the election to the wrong candidate, even when the election was not close. Worst of all, electronic voting machines that produce no paper ballots to recount or check for machine error or tampering lend themselves to enormous abuse.[2]

Some states are now trying to guarantee their constituents that their votes will not disappear. Legislation in New Mexico would establish a uniform system where voters fill out paper ballots and feed them into an optical-scan voting machine. In Wisconsin, legislation requires that electronic voting machines produce a verifiable paper trail.

# 76

# Green Up Your Government

The elite of our nation have failed to internalize the ecological principle that every poison we put out into the environment comes right back to us in our air, water and food.

— Anil Agarwal

Ten million sheets of copy paper an hour. That's how much paper the US government uses every working day of the year. If you decide that all this paper must be 30% post-consumer waste, you've created a huge market for recycled paper. That's exactly what the US government did.

Governments are big spenders. With $8 to $12 billion to spend every year, the Canadian government is the largest single buyer in the country. Add all the provincial governments and agencies, and you can have a powerful influence on what products and services are available, and how toxic they are. The US government spends more than $200 billion a year, while state and local governments together spend more than $1 trillion annually.

From copy paper to computers, pesticides to printing, federal governments, states, provinces and several ambitious cities are adopting laws or policies that require buying environmentally preferable goods and services. "Environmentally preferable" means goods and services that don't waste energy and water and don't persist in the environment, harm children's health or generally pollute. It can also mean products without cancer-causing chemicals.

## Adopt Environmentally Preferable Purchasing Policies

Santa Monica pioneered green purchasing in the early 1990s with recycled content and less-toxic chemical products. In 1994 it developed a Sustainable City Plan that established environmentally preferable purchasing as one of the city's eight guiding principles. It was also the first government to demand cleaning products without carcinogens, reproductive toxins or ozone-depleting chemicals, under its Toxics Use Reduction Program. By doing this, Santa Monica spares the environment 3,200 pounds of hazardous materials every year and saves 5% on safer products.

Since 2001 they have been purchasing flat-screen computers because of their energy efficiency and because they contain fewer heavy metals. All requests for outside printing specify the use of recycled or tree-free paper and vegetable-based inks. The City also assists its businesses, agencies and residents to adopt sustainable purchasing practices.

In 2006 the governor of Maine issued "An Order Promoting Safer Chemicals in Consumer Products and Services," with action plans to replace toxic chemicals like mercury, lead, brominated flame-retardants and pesticides with safer alternatives. It directs the government to avoid purchasing products with chemicals that cause cancer or are toxic, persistent and bioaccumulative. A task force will look at ways to expand university research into green chemistry, focusing on non-toxic bio-based plastics from Maine potatoes and wood waste.

Washington State has developed a program to phase out its use of persistent toxic chemicals such as mercury, dioxins and PCBs. To achieve this goal, the City of Seattle is eliminating chlorine-bleached paper, PVC building materials and office supplies, utility poles treated with pentachlorophenol and mercury auto switches.

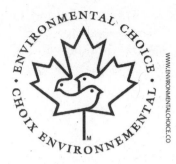

The EcoLogo™ is used to certify environmental leaders in 300+ categories of products.

Minnesota's Central Stores, which supplies government agencies, promotes plant-based cleaning products that contain no toxic or cancer-causing agents, no phosphates and nothing that would irritate the skin or cause allergic reactions.

It's not always easy to know what makes a product green. Richmond, British Columbia, is the first Canadian municipality to develop an Environmental Purchasing Guide to help its staff choose the best environmental products. The guide explains why products like printing inks without heavy metals are environmentally preferable, and gives tips on how to avoid paints or carpeting that emit volatile organic compounds.

One shortcut to finding the least damaging products is a trustworthy labeling system:

- Green Seal, a nonprofit US organization, awards the Green Seal of Approval and works with governments to assist with green purchasing and operations.

- Canada's EcoLogo identifies products that meet environmental criteria, such as being free of known carcinogens.

- The Nordic Swan in Scandinavia and the well-known Eco-Label in Europe are used for many green products and services, from household cleaners to hotels.

## Make Environmental Product Declarations Mandatory

Sweden has introduced "environmental product declarations" so that consumers can understand

- City of Richmond Environmental Purchasing Guide: www.richmond.ca/services/environment/policies/purchasing.htm
- EcoLogo: www.environmentalchoice.com
- EPA Environmentally Preferable Purchasing: www.epa.gov/opptintr/epp
- European Eco-Label: www.europa.eu.int/comm/environment/ecolabel
- Government Purchasing Project: www.gpp.org
- Green Seal: www.greenseal.org/greeninggov.htm
- Green Suppliers Network: www.greensuppliers.gov
- Minnesota Environmentally Preferable Purchasing: www.moea.state.mn.us/lc/purchasing
- Natural Resources Council of Maine: www.maineenvironment.org
- Procurement Resources: www.newdream.org/procure/stateres.php
- Purchasing for Pollution Prevention: www.informinc.org/p3_00.php
- Santa Monica Sustainable City Program: www.santa-monica.org/epd

the life cycle of products and make informed choices. Although it is voluntary, Volvo and Electrolux have made their product declarations public, posting them on the Internet.[1] Electrolux, for instance, declares that the plastics used in its refrigerators contain no lead, mercury or cadmium.[2]

Sweden and Denmark have also created lists of harmful chemicals to help purchasers, manufacturers and product developers avoid high-risk chemicals. In Denmark, the List of Undesirable Substances targets 7,000 chemicals that are known to cause serious and long-term damage. These lists also serve as a warning that certain chemicals will eventually be phased out.

> We should no longer accept the counsel of those who tell us that we must fill our world with poisonous chemicals; we should look around and see what other course is open to us.
>
> — Rachel Carson, *Silent Spring*

# 77

## Encourage Education for a Sustainable World

H.G. Wells had it right, when he said we are in a race between education and catastrophe.

— David W. Orr

You have just been appointed Minister or Secretary of State for Education, and you want schools to join the national effort to stop cancer. You have also decided that your nation needs schools that connect students with the natural environment, and graduates who can tackle the planet's most daunting environmental and health problems. So you draw up plans to make health and sustainability fundamental parts of the educational experience, from kindergarten to college.

### Detoxify the Schools

No school should expose its students to carcinogens like asbestos, lead paint and pesticides and to toxic cleaning products. In 2005 New York State required all schools to use safe carcinogen-free cleaning products, joining Massachusetts, Vermont, Minnesota, Pennsylvania and Washington in adopting an environmentally preferable cleaning products program. You pass a Schools Environmental Protection Act that bans the use of pesticides in schools, and requires the use of integrated pest management.

### Build Healthy Schools

Halifax West High School in Nova Scotia has become the model for public buildings provincewide. Thanks to persistent parent involvement, the school burns no fossil fuels, the gym floor used less-toxic finishes and the indoor air is cleaner than outdoor air, to name a few of the school's green features, now enshrined in Nova Scotia's Design Requirements Manual. Studies have shown that students with the most daylight perform better at math and reading tests than students in classrooms with less natural light.[1]

### Infuse Nature into the Entire Curriculum

You pass an Education and Environmental Initiative, as California did in 2005, integrating environmental principles and concepts into every subject from history to mathematics. In this way, children will learn about the environment in a comprehensive way from kindergarten through high school.

### Encourage Hands-on Natural Learning

Experiences with the natural world teach skills and improve academic performance, especially

- Association for Experiential Education: www.aee.org
- Center for Ecoliteracy: www.ecoliteracy.org
- Citizens for a Safe Learning Environment: www.chebucto.ns.ca/Education/CASLE
- Eco-Schools: www.fee-international.org
- The Edible Schoolyard: www.edibleschoolyard.org
- EPA Tools for Schools: www.epa.gov/iaq/schools
- Green Street: www.green-street.ca
- Green Teacher Diploma: www.greenteacher.org
- *Green Teacher Magazine*: www.greenteacher.com
- *Last Child in the Woods*, by Richard Louv
- *Planet U: Sustaining the World, Reinventing the University* by Michael M'Gonigle and Justine Stark
- Teacher's Garden: www.kidsgardening.com/teachers.asp
- *Teaching Green*, by Tim Grant and Gail Littlejohn
- University of Massachusetts Green Chemistry Program: www.greenchemistry.uml.edu

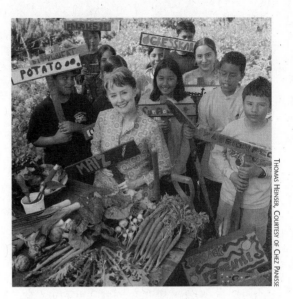

Alice Waters and Berkeley students in the Edible Schoolyard.

THOMAS HEINSER, COURTESY OF CHEZ PANISSE

for children in cities. From pond and watershed projects, children can learn about the chemistry of aquatic ecosystems, as well as reading and writing. Across Quebec, students in the Adopt a River Program sample water quality for pH and bacteria, and monitor insects, mollusks and worms that live in the rivers. In California, Grade 4 students at Brookside School in San Anselmo successfully re-established freshwater shrimp by creating new habitat for them in creek beds near their school.[2]

Even lunch programs can teach sustainability and improve nutrition. In Berkeley, California, the Edible School Yard Program at Martin Luther King Jr. Middle School combines garden work and cooking classes, serving up the fruits of the students' labors in the cafeteria (see Solution 19). The children practice Spanish while cooking Spanish food and learn math by costing the meal's ingredients. A study by Harvard Medical School showed that students in the program had better ecological understanding and academic performance.[3] In Richmond, BC, the community gardens of the Edible School Yard teach students farming for social studies, measurements for math and plants for science.[4] And of course, you ban the sale of junk food in schools across the nation.

**Get the Kids Moving!**
The lack of exercise in today's schools is a terrible teacher of bad habits, so you announce that schoolchildren must exercise for two hours a week if their schools want government funding, as the Prime Minister of Australia did in 2004. But is that enough? France requires three hours;

in Britain, all students are to be offered five hours a week.

**Educate Green Chemists**
The toxic aspect of chemicals should be taught in chemistry, and green chemistry should become an integral part of chemistry courses from grade school to university, because it will be the chemists of the future who decide whether a new product will release hazardous substances or be designed in harmony with the environment. The University of Massachusetts offers the only green chemistry doctoral program in the US, but having seen the trend, many universities are working to set up similar programs.

**Make Sustainability Part of Higher Education**
Colleges and universities should incorporate sustainability into the curricula for disciplines such as economics, business, architecture and engineering. Medical schools must spend more than the average 18 hours teaching nutrition so that our future doctors know how to counsel patients about the importance of healthy foods, preferably organic, for cancer prevention.[5]

# 78

# Clean Up the Toxic Sites

> **Four out of every five toxic-waste dumps in America is in a black neighborhood. The largest toxic-waste dump in America is in a community in Alabama that is 85% black.**[1]
>
> — Robert F. Kennedy Jr.

Toxic waste sites are poisoned pieces of real estate, and the people who live near them are more likely to have cancer. Take Clinton County, Pennsylvania, home of the Drake Chemical Superfund site, where scores of carcinogens including benzidene and benzene were manufactured and stored for years. Many types of cancer found here — lymphomas, leukemias in women, bone cancer in men, cancers of the salivary glands and others — are much higher than normal.[2]

## Clean up the Toxic Waste Sites

This is why governments simply have to clean up these sites. Consider it cancer prevention. Fixing them will reduce the amount of toxic chemicals that we are exposed to, and protect our health. It will give us cleaner air and water and the possibility of using the land again.

Currently there are 77,000 hazardous waste sites in the US, and 200,000 more are expected to be added by 2033.[3] Including 3 to 4 million children, 11 million people live within one mile of a hazardous waste site.

In Canada there are 3,600 contaminated sites on federal land alone, and countless others that haven't been catalogued.

The Stringfellow Acid Pits in Riverside, California, is a notorious Superfund site. From 1956 to 1972, millions of gallons of chemicals were dumped into this old quarry. In 1978 exceptionally heavy rains caused the lagoons to flood, carrying the chemicals down the hill into people's homes and into a school. When mothers saw their children coming home with asthma, rashes and headaches they formed Concerned Neighbors in Action, and picketed, protested and sued until site cleanup finally got underway.

Yet governments are backing away from these cleanups. In both the US and Canada, the money for remediation has almost vanished. In the US, before 2001 when the new administration withdrew its support, 85 Superfund sites were being cleaned up every year. Since then, the number has been cut in half. Scheduled cleanups have been slowed down or postponed.

## Restore the Superfund

For 25 years, the US Superfund provided funds to clean up hazardous waste sites. The legislation was passed in response to public outcry over the chemical contamination of the Love Canal

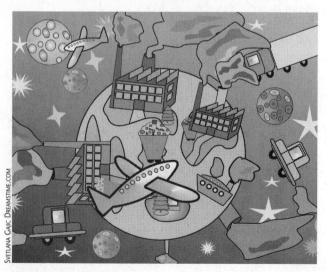

One Earth, many toxic polluters.

neighborhood in upstate New York and the Valley of the Drums in Kentucky. It embraced the "polluter-pays" principle by making the responsible parties pay for cleanup. If an owner couldn't be found, the cost was covered by a trust fund, financed by a tax on the chemical and petroleum industries.

Superfund cleanups brought annual benefits of $3.6 billion on an investment of less than $1.5 billion. It also inspired states to set up their own funds and to clean up more than 2,000 hazardous sites.

But in 1995, the tax provisions of the fund expired. To save companies the price of a pizza — $12 on every $10,000 of corporate profit,[4] Congress refused to renew it. Since 2000, when the remaining Superfund money was exhausted, tax revenues have had to cover the high costs of cleanups.

## Create a Polluter-Pays Cleanup Fund

Canadian provincial governments need their own Superfund legislation so that they too can collect money from known past polluters and create a fund for abandoned sites. Unlike most developed countries, Canada has no legislation or national program to deal with its contaminated sites, which include airports, harbours, military bases, abandoned mines and native reserves.

In her 2002 report, the Federal Commissioner for the Environment and Sustainable Development found that the government did "not have a complete picture of its contaminated sites, or a timetable for assembling one." In 1989 Canada's Green Plan made $250 million available for five years to clean up a number of high-risk contaminated sites and to develop an inventory, but when the money ran out in 1995, so did the government's interest.

Since then, local communities have been left on their own to cope with the contamination. The people living on Frederick Street in Sydney, Nova Scotia, want the government to relocate them away from the yellow toxic mud that oozes into their backyards. Their neighbor, the Sydney Tar Ponds, is one of North America's largest toxic waste dumps, abandoned after 100 years of steel-making. It contains more than 700,000 tonnes of chemically contaminated sediments, enough to fill 60 storeys in a building the size of a football field.[5] The people of Sydney have a 16% greater chance of dying of cancer than people in other parts of Canada, which they blame in part on the Tar Ponds.

- BE SAFE: www.besafenet.com/superfund.html
- EPA Superfund: www.epa.gov/superfund
- Mining Watch Canada: www.miningwatch.ca
- Safe from Toxics: www.safefromtoxics.org
- Scorecard Superfund Locator: www.scorecard.org/env-releases/land
- Sierra Club: www.sierraclub.org/toxics/superfund
- Superfund costs by state: www.sierraclub.org/toxics/factsheets
- US PIRG: www.safefromtoxics.org

# 79

## End the Use of Tobacco

The best thing to do with cigars is give them to your enemy.

— Fidel Castro

In Shangri-La it is illegal to smoke in public or sell tobacco. The tiny Himalayan country of Bhutan, also known as the Last Shangri-La, made headlines in December 2004 when it became the first nation to force its citizens to butt out. Any Bhutan citizen caught smoking in public will be fined.

Tobacco is the world's most famous and preventable cause of cancer. This has put it in the forefront of cancer prevention programs and made it a global concern.

More than 190 countries signed the Framework Convention on Tobacco Control, an international agreement coordinated by the World Health Organization that came into force in February 2005. The countries that have ratified it have agreed to ban advertising of tobacco products, post clear and visible health warnings on cigarette packages, protect people from exposure to tobacco smoke in workplaces and indoor public places, and curb cigarette smuggling.

Worldwide the pressure to phase out tobacco has been steadily growing. Organizations such as the American Society of Clinical Oncology have called for its total elimination, but most countries are slow to go as far as Bhutan or France, Scotland and Ireland, which have all now banned public smoking. Still, they are moving at varying paces towards benchmarks that once were unimaginable. According to the US Centers for Disease Control, the most effective way for governments to control tobacco is through the synergistic effect of different programs.

### Increase Tobacco Taxes

Higher taxes are the key to cutting cigarette consumption, especially for the young, the poor and the less educated.[1] The British medical journal, *The Lancet*, has recommended that governments increase cigarette prices by 50% every year to stem the global rise in lung cancer. In Canada cigarette consumption fell by 50% when prices were increased significantly starting in the late 1980s. At 20%, Canada now has one of the lowest smoking rates in the world.[2]

California has also used taxes effectively. In 1988 California voters approved a 25-cent tax on every package of cigarettes, with 5 cents earmarked for prevention programs, and by 2004, California's adult smoking rate had dropped to a historic low of 15%.[3] At the same time, lung and bronchial cancer rates for men and women

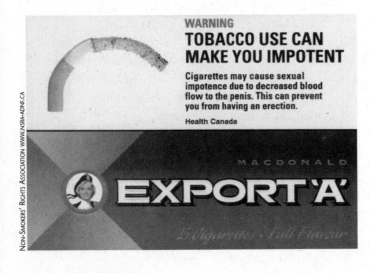

**WARNING**

## TOBACCO USE CAN MAKE YOU IMPOTENT

Cigarettes may cause sexual impotence due to decreased blood flow to the penis. This can prevent you from having an erection.

Health Canada

MACDONALD

EXPORT 'A'

25 Cigarettes · Full Flavour

Non-Smokers' Rights Association www.nsra-adnf.ca

- Americans for Non-Smokers Rights: www.no-smoke.org
- Non-Smokers' Rights Association: www.nsra-adnf.ca
- Ontario Campaign for Action on Tobacco: www.ocat.org
- Physicians for a Smoke-Free Canada: www.smoke-free.ca
- Tobacco Free Kids: www.tobaccofreekids.org
- WHO Tobacco Free Initiative: www.who.int/tobacco/en

in California declined significantly compared to other US states.

### Advertise Against Tobacco

Studies show that well-funded mass-media campaigns against tobacco, along with control programs, bring down smoking rates, but it is a David and Goliath battle between the government and the tobacco industry.

In the US, tobacco companies spend more than $30 million on advertising every day, 23 times as much as state governments spend to prevent smoking. A survey by the US Centers for Disease Control found that the increase in tobacco marketing, discounted cigarette prices and scaled-back prevention programs had stalled the reduction in youth smoking between 2002 and 2004.[4]

This is why it is essential for governments to counter the industry's messages. Many countries run media campaigns encouraging smokers to quit and warning people about second-hand smoke. Sweden, Lithuania and Thailand have instituted outright bans on tobacco advertising and sponsorships. Canada and Brazil require explicit health warnings on cigarette packages. In Canada half of every package carries a graphic illustration of the damage, with 16 different messages such as Cigarettes Leave You Breathless, or Children See, Children Do. For those who disregard the warnings, the Canadian and Thai governments have another caution, Tobacco Use Can Make You Impotent.

In addition to issuing warnings, governments can use Tobacco Industry Denormalization campaigns that expose the industry's manipulative marketing and unethical behavior. Both California and Massachusetts have run successful denormalization campaigns, countering the industry's attempts to make smoking acceptable.

### Ban Smoking in Workplaces and Public Places

Smoke-free laws not only protect people from the deadly effects of second-hand smoke — they also lead many people to quit. The World Bank found that total bans on smoking in the workplace and public places led to an 8% decline in smoking.

Norway was one of the first countries to ban smoking in restaurants and bars. Many governments are going further, making it illegal to smoke in workplaces and many public places. In 2004 Ireland made it illegal to smoke in any enclosed workplace, including pubs and restaurants. Italy has banned smoking in all indoor spaces unless there is a separate ventilated smoking area.

### Help Farmers Exit Tobacco Farming

As governments phase out tobacco, they must help the farmers who will lose their livelihoods. Ontario has set up a $50 million tobacco transition fund for farmers, while the US has legislated a tobacco quota buyout. Physicians for a Smoke-Free Canada, however, say that tobacco companies, not governments, should pay farmers to quit tobacco farming.

# 80

## Promote Clean Production

Sustainability takes forever. And that's the point.
— Bill McDonough

Think durable, not disposable. Think clean, not dirty. Think life cycle, not instant obsolescence. Clean production is the ideal way in which all products and processes should be designed.

Instead of re-engineering to use fewer toxic chemicals and waste less, clean production is free of any and all carcinogens. It looks at everything that goes into making a product — where the raw materials come from, how and where they are processed, what wastes are generated and what happens to the product at the end of its useful life. It aims to work in harmony with natural systems.

Clean production might be a technical innovation in material such as a ramie-wool blend, a furniture fabric made with non-toxic dyes that decomposes harmlessly.

It might be a new product line, such as the Sony televisions that have been designed for disassembly and recycling, with more snap-together parts and fewer screws, and Sony's vegetable-based plastic packages made from plant starch that provide casings for Walkmans.

It might be an industrial plant like Interface's, the world's largest carpet manufacturer, whose most popular floor covering, the Entropy, consists of individual tiles that can be replaced as they wear out.

Clean production is a win-win for governments. Industries become more efficient and save money, while protecting the environment, workers and consumers. The United Nations is promoting the idea, setting up more than 20 Cleaner Production Centers from Brazil to Sri Lanka.

**Pass Extended Producer Responsibility Laws**
These laws make those who create a product responsible for choosing safe materials and taking it back at the end of its useful life. Europe is the leader in this kind of legislation. In 2000 the European Union (EU) made automakers fund the recycling of vehicles that were headed for the junkyard. Hot on the heels of this initiative, they tackled electronic wastes, the most hazardous and fastest-growing waste stream in the world, which contributes 70% of the heavy metals that leach from landfills.

The EU's electronics legislation — the Waste from Electrical and Electronic Equipment Directive (WEEE) and the Restriction on Hazardous Substances Directive (ROHS) — have had a global impact. WEEE makes manufacturers responsible for the recovery of used electric and electronic equipment, from computers to televisions, refrigerators and hair dryers. ROHS phased out the use of carcinogens like lead, mercury, cadmium and hexavalent chromium in these products by 2006.

The laws have already spurred ecological design changes, as companies such as Panasonic developed lead-free solder for their products. Producer responsibility laws promote cleaner production by making companies rethink their product design, creating an incentive to make them less hazardous and more recyclable.

Although North America lags behind, some states and provinces are following Europe's lead. California and Alberta have passed legislation that charges consumers a fee on the purchase of new televisions, computer monitors and other

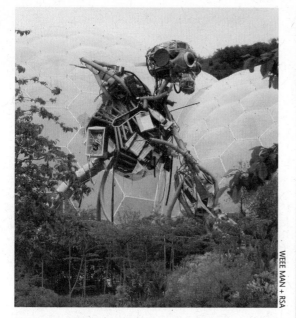

The WEEE MAN, made from waste electrical and electronic products. www.weeeman.org.

- Bay Area Green Business Association: www.greenbiz.abag.ca.gov
- Clean Car Campaign: www.cleancarcampaign.org
- Clean Production Action: www.cleanproduction.org
- Computer Take Back Campaign: www.computertakeback.com
- Eco-Efficiency Centre (Dartmouth): www.eco-efficiency.management.dal.ca
- Extended Producer Responsibility: www.informinc.org/epr_00.php
- Extended Producer Responsibility (Canada): www.ec.gc.ca/epr/en
- Hannover Principles: www.mcdonough.com/principles.pdf
- The Next Industrial Revolution (video): www.thenextindustrialrevolution.org
- Silicon Valley Toxics Coalition: www.svtc.org
- Sony Environmentally Conscious Products: www.sony.net/SonyInfo/Environment
- UNEP Clean Production: www.unepie.org/pc/cp
- Zero Emissions Research Initiative: www.zeri.org

products containing cathode-ray tubes, which pays for their recycling, since every cathode-ray tube currently contains eight pounds of lead. The California law also prohibits the sale of electronic products with heavy metals that cannot be sold in Europe. Although several states and provinces have introduced legislation aimed at recovering used electronic equipment, Washington is the only state that has made producers responsible.

### Help Small Businesses Make the Change
Large corporations like Panasonic or Interface can do this themselves, but smaller businesses need support. Governments can extend clean production practices to small and medium-sized businesses with programs that lend an expert helping hand such as the Eco-Efficiency Centre in Dartmouth, Nova Scotia, and the Bay Area Green Business Program in California. With their own specialists, they can offer companies advice on how to improve their energy efficiency, reduce their use of toxic chemicals and, in some cases, develop new green businesses. Governments can also support small businesses by giving extra points for good environmental practices when awarding contracts for supplies and services.

### Adopt Zero Waste as a Goal
In New Zealand, the first country in the world to set a target of zero waste by 2015, every city that adopts the target receives $25,000 to find the best ways to reduce their garbage. Zero waste encourages us to think of everything we throw away as a resource in disguise. The Ciba Geigy textile mill that produces the ramie-wool fabric, for instance, gives local strawberry growers the scrap material to use as mulch.

# 81

# Promote Organic Food

> Our dream is to make organic the only way farming is done, because it is the only true way farming should be done.
>
> — Vandana Shiva

Around the world, the market for organic food is growing by 20% a year as consumers view organic food as a way to avoid pesticides and protect themselves against cancer.

There is growing evidence that food that has been grown organically protects us. Research at the University of Leicester in England shows that compounds in food called salvestrols trigger an enzyme to attack cancer cells, while leaving healthy cells unharmed. The salvestrols are generated when a plant is exposed to fungus, so they are either missing or significantly diminished in food that has been sprayed with fungicides. To meet the growing consumer demand, governments are coming up with policies to promote organic farming, especially in Europe.

### Create an Organic Action Plan
In 2002 Britain launched an Organic Action Plan to increase organic farmland in order to meet the consumer demand. The government is paying farmers to convert to organic, and in two years the share of organic produce provided by British farmers (as opposed to imported) increased from 30% to 44%. The goal is to reach 70% by 2010. The European Union has developed an Action Plan to promote organic agriculture, including marketing campaigns and support programs for farmers, and is encouraging member countries to develop their own targets and action plans.

### Set Targets for Organic Farming
In the 1990s Sweden set a target of 10% of farmland to be organic by 2000. They achieved this in 1999 by funding pilot projects, helping develop markets and rewarding organic farmers for converting their land and contributing to the environment. The new target is 15% by 2010. Sweden and Denmark help finance their organic farming initiatives through a tax on pesticides and with support from the European Union. France, Britain, Denmark, the Netherlands, Ireland, Austria, Germany and Finland have all set targets for organic farming.

### Support Organic Farmers
Since 2003 Britain has been providing organic maintenance payments for farmers, promoting

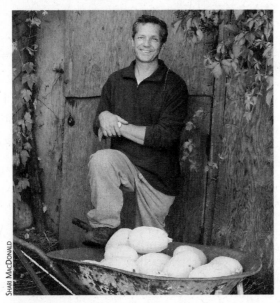

SHARI MACDONALD

Peter Briner, a leukemia survivor, with a barrow of spaghetti squash at his organic farm in Surrey, BC, Canada.

- Canadian Organic Growers: www.cog.ca
- International Federation of Organic Agriculture Movements: www.ifoam.org
- Organic Consumers Association: www.organicconsumers.org
- Organic Europe: www.organic-europe.net
- Soil Association: www.soilassociation.org
- Sustainable Farming: www.farmingsolutions.org

public procurement and encouraging schools and hospitals to buy organic. The Darlington Hospital in northern England serves 5,000 pints of organic milk a day to patients, staff and visitors. The government is also planning to strengthen local supply networks and eliminate the obstacles to marketing organic food. Germany provides funding for advisory groups to help farmers through the transition out of chemical farming.

### Aim for All Baby Food to Be Organic

Researchers at Liverpool University have found that low levels of pesticides, previously thought to be harmless, could cause cancer in babies and young children, and they recommend that parents consider switching to organic foods to avoid contamination.[1] European regulations that severely limit chemical residues in baby food have prompted some baby food companies in Europe to go organic. In Germany, where the leading baby food manufacturer, Hipp, began using organic ingredients 20 years ago, almost all baby food is now organic.

### Require Schools and Hospitals to Provide Organic Food

Concern about the quality of food and children's health has led to the introduction of organic food in schools. A 2006 study found that when organic food was substituted for conventional food in school children's diets, the pesticide levels in their bodies dramatically decreased. When they switched back to a conventional diet, their pesticide levels went up again.[2]

Italy has boosted its organic food production with a law that requires school cafeterias and hospitals to serve some organic food every day. In Modena province, 22 of the 47 towns serve organic foods in their schools. In 2004 the Seattle School District adopted a policy banning junk food in cafeterias and encouraging organic food, following the lead of school districts in Berkeley, Santa Monica and Palo Alto, California. In Sweden more than 25% of the cities serve some organic food in their schools and hospitals.

### Protect Organic Farmers against GM Contamination

In Canada and the US, agriculture departments have chosen to promote genetically modified food and chemical farming, rather than organic, even though genetically modified crops are a major threat to the viability of organic farming. In Saskatchewan, where organic farming is growing fast, farmers have been fighting Monsanto and Bayer Crop Science to get compensation for losing their canola crops to genetic contamination. Since zero contamination is the only standard that is acceptable to organic farmers and consumers, the International Federation of Organic Agriculture Movements wants governments to adopt coexistence and economic liability schemes to protect organic farms.

# 82

## Clear the Air: Promote Sustainable Energy

> I'd put my money on the sun and solar energy. What a source of power! I hope we don't have to wait 'til oil and coal run out before we tackle that.
>
> — Thomas Edison (1847-1931)

Governments around the world are facing critical choices about their future energy supplies. Of all the energy we use, 85% comes from fossil fuels, which are the primary cause of global climate change, creating an urgent need to find sustainable substitutes.

Benzene and diesel fumes from cars, trucks and transport such as cruise liners, and chemical leachates from coal-fired power plants[1] are all contributing causes of cancer. Radiation from nuclear power plants is also a cancer hazard, with the potential for disastrous impacts if another Chernobyl-style accident were to happen. (see p. 52)

Where does that leave us? With fossil fuels and nuclear energy off the table, what are we to do? As well as being a cause of cancer, oil is going to become more and more expensive as the remaining global supply shrinks. Future historians will talk about 1850 to 2050 as the Age of Fossil Fuels and explain how humanity made a transition to energy from the sun, wind, biofuels and other kinds of safe, sustainable energy.

The purpose of this Solution is not to solve the whole problem, but to show that there are many options to achieve what is needed.

### Can We Heat Buildings Without Fossil Fuels?

- Most buildings could be twice as efficient as they are today.
- Homes that use passive solar design need 50% less energy.
- Buildings with heat-recovery ventilators recycle their heat so that little is lost.
- Buildings can be heated with solar walls, solar thermal systems, heat from the ground, heat from a lake or the sea, air-source heat pumps or biodiesel and wood pellet furnaces.
- In Dockside Green, Victoria, BC, homes are heated with gasified wood wastes that also generate electricity. In Sweden homes are heated using gasified compost wastes.
- In Zurich, Switzerland, homes are warmed with heat from the sewer pipes.
- In Okotoks, outside Calgary, Alberta, homes are heated with solar hot water that is gathered in summer and stored underground for use in winter.
- In China 50 million homes use solar hot water systems.
- In Spain all new homes must be fitted with solar hot water systems.

- Association for the Study of Peak Oil: www.peakoil.net
- BC Sustainable Energy Association: www.bcsea.org
- Plug-In Hybrid Cars: www.pluginamerica.com
- *Plug-in Hybrids: The Cars that Will Recharge America* by Sherry Boschert, New Society Publishers, 2006
- Post-Carbon Institute: www.postcarbon.org
- Rocky Mountain Institute: www.rmi.org
- *Stormy Weather: 101 Solutions to Global Climate Change* by Guy Dauncey with Patrick Mazza, New Society Publishers, 2001

## Can We Travel Without Fossil Fuels?

This is the next big challenge. We can redesign our communities to make them more pedestrian friendly and install bicycle facilities to make cycling safe and easy, as did Odense, Denmark. We can encourage car-sharing and make public transit more user-friendly and accessible as Curitiba, Brazil, and Boulder, Colorado, have done. In Calgary, Alberta, the C-train light-rail transit is powered by energy from the wind.

Then there's the "Plug-In Hybrid." By adding extra batteries to a gas-electric hybrid vehicle such as the Toyota Prius, it can become an electric vehicle for all local trips, costing only $20 a month to run. Biodiesel and ethanol from crop wastes can provide liquid fuel. Trucks and buses can use similar technology. Only airplanes remain a difficult problem. Flying is a big contributor to global climate change, and we really need to question how easily we jump on and off planes.

## Can We Generate Electricity Without Fossil Fuels?

Almost every appliance, light bulb and piece of factory equipment could use half the power it does today. We can generate electricity from the sun, wind, microhydro, geothermal, tides, waves, biomass and biogas, and we can store it using hydro dams and other systems.[2]

If we adopt policies that really encourage sustainable energy systems, such as Germany's Advanced Renewables Tariff, we will be astonished at how quick the energy transition can be. North Dakota has enough wind energy potential for two-thirds of the entire US grid if everything was twice as efficient. Every south-facing roof could have a solar system on it. All household and farm compost and sewage could generate energy from biogas.

Governments should not be afraid of planning a complete switch away from fossil fuels. Sweden has announced that it will end its dependency on oil by 2020. There are many energy solutions that contribute to neither cancer nor climate change. There is an urgency about this that calls for immediate action.

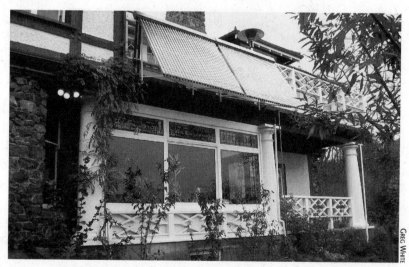

Solar hot water evacuated tubes on a house in Victoria, BC, Canada.

# 83

## Let the Waters Flow Clearly

**Filthy water cannot be washed.**
— **African Proverb**

What's in the water? In 300 California communities, every glass is tainted with tiny bits of rocket fuel called perchlorate; in Massachusetts, traces of a gasoline additive known as MtBE; and almost everywhere, the solvent trichloroethylene, now considered up to 40 times more carcinogenic than previously thought.[1] These contaminants are just the toxic tip of the drinking water "iceberg."

The US Safe Drinking Water Act requires testing for 40 known or suspected carcinogens, out of over 80 regulated drinking water contaminants. In Canada standards vary from province to province. The carcinogens generally looked for include arsenic and trihalomethanes, created in the treatment process when chlorine is added. Both have been linked to a higher incidence of bladder cancer. For bottled water, there are almost no government standards and infrequent testing.

Although drinking water generally meets the standards, many potential contaminants in drinking water, surface water and groundwater go unmonitored and unregulated. Take drugs, for example. Pharmaceutical drugs, given to both humans and animals, are finding their way into the environment through flushed toilets, manure and sewage sludge spread onto the land. Tested properly, a typical water sample may contain a cocktail of 30 to 60 pesticides, antibiotics, painkillers, tranquillizers and chemotherapy agents. No one knows what the long-term effects might be.

This disregard for our water can have serious consequences. In Toms River, New Jersey, children have suffered from unexpectedly high rates of many different cancers.[2] The prime suspect is groundwater, poisoned by two highly contaminated toxic waste sites that have infiltrated the community's drinking water supplies.

### Protect Drinking Water Sources

To reduce cancer, it is critical that we pass laws to keep our drinking water clean and protect drinking water sources.

In the US the Safe Drinking Water Act requires cities to identify where contaminants in drinking water are coming from, and protect drinking water from contamination. Similarly, Ontario has passed a Clean Water Act that will require every community to protect the source of its drinking water.

So tempting — but do you trust your children to play in it?

RAYNA CANEDY, DREAMSTIME.COM

The province of New Brunswick's Watershed Protection Program has established buffer zones around all lakes and rivers that supply drinking water. Because the province relies heavily on groundwater, there is also a Wellfield Protection Program. To protect the wells, municipalities identify the recharge areas and establish ground rules for what can be done around them. In the recharge areas, potentially harmful activities such as dry cleaning or auto repair shops are not allowed.

New York City, in cooperation with the State and the US EPA, has developed an ambitious plan to protect the reservoirs that supply the drinking water for its nine million residents. The Watershed Protection Agreement prioritizes the acquisition of sensitive lands and voluntary farm plans that protect key waterways, thereby avoiding the billions of dollars needed for filtering out contaminants.

### Support Local Clean Water Initiatives

Governments can also support local initiatives such as local Watershed Stewardship Councils. Working with local, state and provincial governments, these independent councils involve people in developing programs that improve local rivers and streams.

Minnesotans want their state government to pass the Clean Water Legacy bill — a citizens' initiative to test, protect and restore all contaminated waters in Minnesota within 10 years. A coalition of 40 groups has proposed a long-term funding plan that will generate $80 million through user fees on sewers and septic systems. Only 8% of Minnesota's rivers and 14% of its

- Campaign for Safe and Affordable Drinking Water: www.safe-drinking-water.org
- Canadian Environmental Law Association: www.cela.ca
- Clean Water Fund: www.cleanwaterfund.org
- Minnesota Clean Water Legacy Project: www.cleanwateraction.org/mn/cwl.html
- Natural Resources Defense Council: www.nrdc.org/water/drinking
- Safe Drinking Water Foundation: www.safewater.org
- *The Water You Drink: Safe or Suspect?* by Julie Stauffer

lakes have been fully tested. In 2004 testing identified almost 2,000 water pollution violations.

### Reform Sewage Treatment Systems

Governments can also clean up our water by reducing pollution from sewer systems and investing in environmental treatments. Because industrial and domestic waste is mixed in the sewage system, sludge disposal poses a challenge for most governments.

The City of Toronto has used its Sewage Treatment Bylaw to reduce industrial wastes flowing into the sewer system.[3] Borrowing from the Massachusetts Toxic Use Reduction Act, businesses such as metal finishers, commercial laundries and dental offices now have to develop pollution prevention plans. Within eight months, mercury discharges to the sewers dropped by 40% to 68%.

Constructed wetlands and wastewater gardens that treat sewage have been used in some urban areas, where they also enhance the landscape and increase biological diversity. The sewage from Estevan, Saskatchewan, is processed through a wetland created by SaskPower. The sewage is cleaned up naturally and provides 40% of the annual cooling water to a local power plant.

The water we drink flows through every part of our bodies. Let it flow clearly.

# 84

# Stop Military Abuse of the Environment

The preparations for war and war itself are responsible for thousands of cancers. Take the workers who contracted cancer making nuclear bombs for the Cold War, or the Vietnam veterans exposed to Agent Orange, now eligible for compensation for 23 different cancers.

These are the obvious casualties, but we give little thought to the cancer risk in the communities that host the military establishment — like the people downwind of the Nevada Test Site with thyroid cancer from nuclear fallout, or the women in Cape Cod with lung cancer from the burning of excess artillery propellant at the Massachusetts Military Reservation.[2] The military enjoys a special but unwarranted status that immunizes it from many legal responsibilities related to health and the environment.

## Stop the Military Contamination of Air, Water and Land

The US Defense Department, the country's largest toxics polluter and a major source of contamination in communities where it trains and tests,[3] generates more toxic chemicals annually than the top-five chemical companies combined. It is the largest user of trichloroethylene, a carcinogen that contaminates almost every US military installation.[4]

What makes the military's activities so insidious is not just the magnitude, but the nature of its pollution. In addition to familiar toxics like pesticides and solvents, the military produces unique wastes, including unexploded ordnance, depleted uranium and chemical weapons. They threaten communities with contaminated

There is a lot of talk these days about sustainability, and very little sense of what it means. It is impossible to imagine that our society will ever move to anything remotely resembling "sustainable" until we demilitarize and detoxify.

— Center for Community Action and Environmental Justice[1]

plumes of groundwater, uranium exposure from weapons production and testing, and poisonous air emissions from burning solid rocket fuel.

One of the gravest problems is munitions contamination. According to the US Government Accounting Office, more than 15 million acres of military land are contaminated with used or dumped munitions. A recently closed US Navy firing range on Vieques Island, Puerto Rico, is contaminated by unexploded ordnance and depleted uranium weapons.[5] In Tooele, Utah, concerned citizens have been trying to stop the incineration of 30,000 tons of expired sarin, VX and mustard gas at the Deseret Chemical Depot.

Military sites are also a major source of water contamination. At the Hanford Nuclear Reservation in Washington State, 450 billion gallons of waste from making weapons-grade plutonium were dumped onto the desert soil of eastern Washington State and into the groundwater. Despite multimillion-dollar cleanup attempts, it is moving inexorably to the Columbia River.[6]

## Test People Who Have Been Exposed, and Keep Records

Military families at Camp Lejeune, North Carolina, drank water laced with trichloroethylene and volatile organic compounds for almost 20 years. In 1985, after 50,000 to 200,000 people had been exposed, it shut down the last contaminated well.[7] Preliminary work by the Agency for Toxic Substances and Disease Registry showed childhood

- Arc Ecology: www.arcecology.org
- Chemical Weapons Working Group: www.cwwg.org
- *Enough Blood Shed: 101 Solutions to Violence, Terror and War,* by Mary-Wynne Ashford with Guy Dauncey
- Military Toxics Project: www.miltoxproj.org

cancers and birth defects in Camp Lejeune families high enough to warrant further study.[8]

Around such military sites, families want to understand their risk. Governments must provide free screening, treatment and compensation for disabilities resulting from exposures. They should also create a comprehensive database of people's exposure to the military's toxic chemicals and radioactive pollutants, and make it available for research.

### Require Government Military Agencies to Meet Legal Cleanup Obligations

Many active or former military sites are notorious hazardous waste sites. The US Defense Department is responsible for 11,000 "hot spots," 100 of which have been proposed for, or are on, the Superfund list.[9] Instead of tackling these cleanups estimated at billions of dollars, though, the Department has proposed exemptions from major air and toxics legislation.

Canada has also neglected its responsibility for military cleanup. The Royal Canadian Air Force Base at Winisk on Hudson's Bay, a relic of the Cold War effort to detect Soviet air attacks, is one of dozens that were closed in the mid-1960s.[10] Left behind at these bases are asbestos, PCBs and buried fuel drums, but because they are in remote areas, the Department of National Defence has been able to stall the remedial work. George Hunter, former chief of the Winisk First Nation, observed, "It seems the military has all the engineers it wants when it comes to putting something up, but none for cleaning up the mess they leave behind."

Countries from the Philippines to Panama are also struggling to remediate closed US bases.

### Redirect the Military Budget to Restoration

The answer for governments is to clean up the military bases and the contaminated lands around them. Yet, despite huge increases in military spending, the funding for cleanup has decreased. The money that governments allocate to train soldiers and build weapons should be used to detoxify the existing sites.

And demilitarize. Governments should direct all their efforts at peace, and relegate the industry of war to the scrap heap of history.

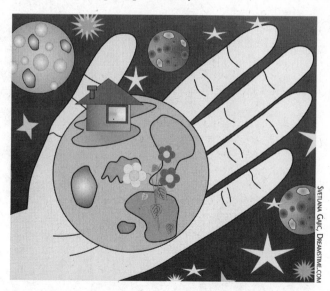

*From a distance there is harmony, and it echoes through the land. And it's the hope of hopes, it's the love of loves, it's the heart of every man.* — Julie Gold

# 85

# Support the Global Movement

**Primary prevention is far too low down on the political agenda, and for patients that's unacceptable. For us it is not just gaining access to the best treatments available. It is about not getting cancer in the first place.**

**— UK Breast Cancer Coalition**

By allowing carcinogens into everyday products, the British government has exposed millions of women to risky chemicals and let breast cancer run rampant, charges the UK Working Group on the Primary Prevention of Breast Cancer.[1] Their answer: control the chemicals.

It is hard for any one government to ban or restrict certain chemicals. International trade rules and powerful corporate interests have made health protection a tricky business. A determined government must prove that the chemical is a hazard and then stand up to the corporate scientists and lawyers who will challenge the process. But there are ways for countries to make progress on the international front.

### Ratify and Implement the International Environmental Agreements

One very important achievement has been the agreement on the Stockholm Convention on Persistent Pollutants (POPs) (see Solution 93) banning 12 groups of chemicals that are known to harm the environment and human health. Ratified by the requisite 50 countries, it became international law in May 2004.

Similarly, the Basel Convention (see Solution 95) has been instrumental in halting the export of hazardous wastes from industrialized to developing countries. The Basel Action Network, a watchdog on the international trade in hazardous wastes, campaigned successfully against the export to India of the *Clemenceau*, a French aircraft carrier containing tons of asbestos and PCBs, for decommissioning.[2] They argued that the ship was a hazardous waste subject to the Basel Convention, and in February 2006,

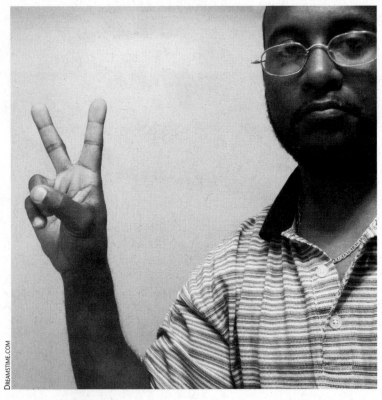

DREAMSTIME.COM

- Basel Action Network: www.ban.org
- Countries signing the POPs agreement: www.pops.int/documents/signature/signstatus.htm
- UK Working Group on the Primary Prevention of Breast Cancer: www.nomorebreastcancer.org.uk

the French President announced that the *Clemenceau* would not be sent to India.

The task now is to persuade all governments, especially the United States which has not ratified any of them, to ratify and implement these agreements without weakening them.

### Cooperate Internationally to Improve Chemical Control

The most ambitious attempt to redress the worldwide chemicals problem is the European Union's REACH legislation (see Solution 69). REACH's original intention — a job that is still outstanding — was to test the 100,000 chemicals that are in daily use about which we know little or nothing, and to protect the environment and our health from the most hazardous ones. The EPA found that of the 3,000 most heavily used chemicals in the US, 93% do not have a full set of basic safety data, and 43% have none at all.[3]

REACH will require companies to register chemicals and provide information on their hazards. In the US companies are generating basic safety data through a voluntary program called the High Production Volume Challenge Program, in which industry "adopts" and tests chemicals that are used in large quantities. In Canada, the government has categorized thousands of chemicals according to their toxicity. They have identified many chemicals that are damaging to our our health and the environment, and should be eliminated.

All countries should cooperate in order to fill in the gaps of our chemical knowledge, and all countries should pass legislation that requires the substitution of less-hazardous chemicals for carcinogens and other toxic chemicals. A binding international agreement to implement the original goals of REACH should be undertaken by the United Nations.

### Implement the International Chemicals Agreement

The UN has already taken a step in this direction. With chemical production shifting from industrialized to developing countries, the UN Environment Program has developed a policy framework for international action that would help all countries, especially developing countries, to produce, transport and dispose of chemicals safely. In February 2006, 100 health and environment ministers adopted a voluntary framework, the Strategic Approach to International Chemicals Management (SAICM) (See Solution 94). One of its accomplishments was to provide funding from European countries for programs to help developing countries handle chemicals safely.

### Establish National Cancer Prevention Plans

In addition to international cooperation to control chemicals, governments must establish national cancer plans that focus on primary cancer prevention. This means national legislation and international agreements that focus on the elimination or reduction of environmental and occupational carcinogens. The ultimate responsibility for the primary prevention of cancer lies with governments.

# 86

# Make Prevention Your #1 Strategy

So what do we do in India? We have to take the preventive route, especially because we have far too many poor people who cannot afford treatment.
— Anil Agarwal, Centre for Science and Environment, Delhi

*As authors from the "developed" world, we note that the same toxic practices that are causing cancer here are being exported to the "developing" world by Western interests. Our food chains have landed in droves to serve up empty junk food; agribusiness corporations promote chemical farming and GMO seeds; heavily polluting industries abandon Canada and the US to set up shop wherever labor is cheapest; and electronics companies dump huge amounts of toxic waste anywhere they can. At the same time, Western-dominated financial agencies such as the World Bank and the International Monetary Fund impose structural adjustments that demand that developing nations spend less on public health care, to speed the repayment of debts to Western banks. In many ways, it is the West's way of life itself that is toxic. We need to reject the direction that Western civilization is taking, and steer our world instead towards a green, sustainable future.*

Public health care providers in most developing nations face enormous challenges. Among other demands, they have to provide clean water and healthy sanitation, overcome hunger and malnutrition, and prevent the spread of infectious diseases in huge and growing populations.

They also have to confront rapidly increasing rates of cancer, as cancers of the developed world that are being caused by modern carcinogens, intensive farming and Western diets (breast, prostate, colorectal) join the infectious cancers that are more prevalent in the developing world (stomach, liver, cervix).[1]

Already, 60% of the world's burden of cancer and 84% of new childhood cancer cases occur in the developing world. By 2020, when cancer occurrences are due to rise by 50%, 75% of the deaths will be in the developing world.[2]

What are countries like India, China, Egypt and Brazil to do? By the time the cancer sufferers come to a hospital, it is usually too late for treatment, even if they could afford it. By the time they are diagnosed, 80% to 90% have advanced or incurable cancer.

Some cancers call out for public health interventions, including vaccination and the prevention of infections and infestations. Infectious agents are responsible for 22% of the cancer deaths in the developing world, compared to only 6% in the industrialized countries:

- Cancer of the cervix, caused by the human papilloma virus, spread through sex. When caught early with Pap smear screening, it is treatable and curable.

- Cancer of the liver, caused by viral hepatitis B and C, and by aflatoxins from moldy peanuts and maize.

- Stomach cancer, for which the risk is increased by the bacterium Helicobacter pylori.

- Oral cancers in south Asia and Taiwan, caused by chewing betel and Areca nuts, mixed with tobacco. India has banned the manufacture and sale of some betel products; community education programs have also led to a decline in use.[3]

- Bladder cancer, for which the risk is increased in some countries by the parasitic infection schistosomiasis, transmitted by the liver fluke.

- Alliance for Cervical Cancer Prevention: www.alliance-cxca.org
- Centre for Science and Environment: www.cseindia.org
- Toxics Alert, India: www.toxicslink.org

For these types of cancer, it is essential to integrate cancer prevention into family planning, pregnancy and dietary advice, involving traditional healers as well as trained professionals; to strengthen public health programs; and to train public health care activists, professionals and barefoot workers. "Pouring money into national health systems is not cost effective, because 70% of it gets siphoned into big hospitals," says Dr Hakan Sandbladh, Senior Health Officer with the International Federation of the Red Cross.

The reality for most developing nations is blunt: most will never be able to afford the cost of treatment and drugs for new cancer cases. Prevention *must* become the number one strategy.

Prevention means tackling the fundamental causes of cancers:

- Stop the market-hungry expansion of the global tobacco, junk food, agro-chemical, and asbestos industries. (See Solutions 87 and 96)

- Support a rapid transition to organic, GM-free agriculture. (See Solution 88)

- End air pollution from diesel vehicles, industry and other sources. (See Solution 89)

- End toxic water pollution and the spread of carcinogens into our bodies from toxic wastes, incineration and the chemical and plastics industries. (See Solution 90)

- Pass legislation that prohibits carcinogens in products and gives workers the right to substitute non-toxic chemicals for carcinogens.

- Generate strong citizens' lobby groups that can pressure politicians for the legislation and regulations that are needed to achieve these goals.

Because developing nations have such limited resources, the best place to invest is with citizen-based public health advocacy groups such as India's Toxics Alert, based in Delhi, that can push for the best legislation, and open the doors of democracy.

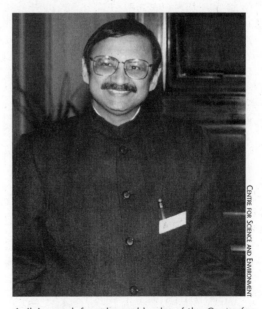

Anil Agarwal, founder and leader of the Centre for Science and Environment, who died on January 2, 2002 after a seven-year battle against cancer. Anil was a rare thinker and advocate, and a staunch supporter of the rights of the poor.

# 87
# Stop the Tobacco Industry

If you look at why Thailand has been successful [in curbing tobacco], you can't ignore the role of civil society in pushing governments to take action and mobilizing public opinion.
— Bungon Rittipakdee, Southeast Asia Tobacco Control Alliance

As public awareness increases and anti-smoking measures succeed in the developed world, the global tobacco industry is desperate to replace the smokers it is losing.

Their prime focus is the developing world, especially Asia, where companies such as Philip Morris/Altria and British American Tobacco are increasingly targeting all youth, including young women, "the largest untapped market," by sponsoring beauty pageants, sports, arts and music events.

In Malaysia they organize free discos with a light show on the buses and pay scantily clad girls to sell cigarettes to male teenagers and young adults.

In China more than 60% of the men and 7% of the women smoke, totaling 300 million adults who either smoke or are exposed to second-hand smoke at home.[1] As a result, China is heading towards the worst tobacco-related health crisis in the world. Already, a third of young Chinese men are afflicted with tobacco-related diseases.

- Advocacy Tools: www.tobaccofreeasia.net/advocacy.htm
- Economics of Tobacco Control (World Bank): www1.worldbank.org/tobacco
- Southeast Asia Tobacco Control Alliance: www.tobaccofreeasia.net
- *Tobacco Control in Developing Countries*, Edited by Prabhat Jha and Frank Chaloupka, Oxford University Press, 2000
- Tobacco News: www.tobacco.org

Of global tobacco sales, 65% are in developing nations. Every day of the year, 50,000 new Asian teenagers take up smoking.[2] By 2020, unless the tobacco industry is stopped, annual deaths from lung cancer worldwide will grow to over 9 million, with 7 million in developing nations.

The personal and family cost is enormous. Every dollar spent on smoking is a dollar not used to build a family's resources. In Vietnam cigarettes consume 8 billion Vietnamese dollars a year, enough to build 20,000 health stations, while causing 1.3 million people to fall below the poverty threshold. If the money spent on cigarettes was used to buy food, 11% of Vietnam's most needy families could escape hunger and malnutrition.[3]

*Step 1*: **Ratify the WHO's Framework Convention on Tobacco Control.** This lays the foundation for strong legislation and practices. It is important to understand the tobacco industry's attempts to derail the Convention, and know how to fight them.

*Step 2*: **Increase the Tax on Tobacco Sales.** A price rise of 10% will decrease consumption by 8%. In Malaysia a percentage of the tobacco tax is earmarked to fund the Malaysian Health Promotion Foundation.

*Step 3*: **Ban Smoking in Public Places.** The small Himalayan kingdom of Bhutan has banned the sale of tobacco and smoking in all public places, punishable by a fine equivalent to two months' wages. Vietnam also has a ban on smoking in public places, but it is widely ignored because it is not enforced, since the Ministry of

Health has no budget for the job. Saudi Arabia has an anti-smoking campaign in Mecca, where anyone caught smoking is handed the sugi plant, used by Prophet Muhammad to clean his teeth, and a pamphlet on the bad effects of smoking. There is a Muslim *fatwah* against smoking, defining it as *Haram*, "unclean, forbidden."[4]

**Step 4: Ban Tobacco Advertising, Promotion and Sponsorship.** In 1992 Thailand banned all tobacco advertising, promotion and sponsorship. By 2001 this had contributed to a 20% decline in smoking, even though enforcement has been weak. Philip Morris/Altria tried to undermine the legislation but met determined resistance from Thai NGOs and the Thai Health Promotion Institute.

**Step 5: Place Large Pictorial Warnings on the Packages.** In Singapore and Brazil, cigarette packets bear grim graphic pictures that warn smokers about the dangers of their habit, as they do in Canada, where it has proven to be an effective deterrent.

**Step 6: Support Quit-Smoking Efforts and Anti-Smoking Groups.** In Brazil organized campaigns have reduced the number of smokers from 32% in 1989 to 18.8% in 2004. Among other measures, the Ministry of Health provides assured treatment in public hospitals for addicted smokers.

**Step 7: Stop Public Displays of Cigarettes by Vendors.** In Thailand vendors have had to remove all cigarettes from display or face a $50,000 fine. Thailand has also increased the price of cigarettes and banned their sale to youths under 18.

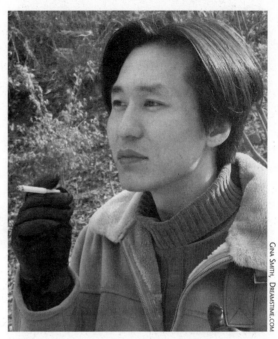

The new cool in South Korea. Short-lived and painful, for those who succumb.

**Step 8: Ban Smoking in Films.** When the film stars smoke, they send a powerful message. In India films made there are no longer allowed to display characters smoking, which is still a common practice in the US.

**Step 9: Clamp Down on Tobacco Smuggling.** In Brazil 32% of the cigarettes are contraband or counterfeit, which may explain why the government cannot increase the price. (They are among the cheapest in the world.)

**Step 10: Support Anti-Smoking NGOs.** A government needs a strong civil society campaign to support its programs. The International Union Against Cancer gives $10,000 grants to anti-smoking campaigners in developing countries to educate people about the dangers of tobacco and to lobby their governments to sign, ratify and comply with the Framework Convention on Tobacco Control.

# 88

# Clean the Air

Where is your concern? The power? The city? What will you choose? So choose one thing: the city, your citizens, your kids. Politics has to make a difference.
— Enrique Peñalosa, Mayor of Bogota, 1998-2001

In India, if you live in Bangalore, Mumbai, Chennai or Delhi, your chance of getting cancer is 7% to 11%. That is much lower than in North America, but it is twice as high as in a rural area such as Barsi, Maharashtra.[1]

In many big cities of the developing world, the air is disastrously polluted, day after day.[2] It comes from vehicles, power plants and industry.

Between 1975 and 1995, when India's economy grew by 250%, the pollutants released by vehicles increased by 800%. From Durban to Dhaka and from Surabaya to Shanghai, it's the same filthy story. Every day, millions of motorcycles, auto-rickshaws, poorly maintained cars, ancient buses and inefficient trucks spew pollution into the air. Uncontrolled industry adds to the stew. In Calcutta 56% of the population suffers from lung trouble, and 40% suffer from upper respiratory tract infections. In Delhi 40% of the population suffers from lung, liver or genetic disorders.[3]

Diesel exhaust contains over 450 different compounds, many of which are known to cause cancer, respiratory ailments and reproductive problems. Benzene is a carcinogen, and ultrafine particles from air pollution reach deep into the body's tissues, where they are associated with diseases of the heart, lung and brain, including lung cancers.

We also know that children who live close to high-traffic streets have a significantly greater risk of developing cancer, including childhood leukemia.[4] The death rate from lung cancer increases by 8% for every increase of 10 micrograms of fine particulate matter per cubic meter.[5, 6]

The end of affordable oil and gas is looming, so it makes sense to plan now for a world without fossil fuels. There are many solutions, and all are needed to make our cities healthy, green and sustainable.

## Convert to Cleaner Vehicles

Calcutta has ordered all of its pre-1990 vehicles off the streets unless they convert to liquefied petroleum gas or natural gas; Shanghai has done likewise. Jakarta requires all of its four million vehicles to pass emissions tests. China has adopted fuel efficiency

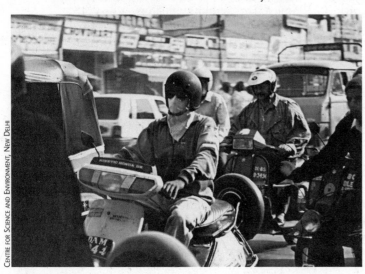

CENTRE FOR SCIENCE AND ENVIRONMENT, NEW DELHI

A trip to work in New Delhi before the city-wide shift to compressed natural gas.

standards that are far tougher than those in the US. Progress is possible, but unless there is a simultaneous investment in public transport, the benefits will be offset by the yearly increase in diesel vehicles. If diesel is necessary, at least make sure it is ultra-low-sulfur diesel, not low-sulfur diesel.

In China and India's rural areas, the widespread use of inefficient three-wheeled "Chinese rural vehicles" is an enormous source of diesel pollution. With re-engineering, they could be twice as efficient and cleaner.[7]

### Expand Public Transit

Curitiba, Brazil, is designing its future around a superb system of public transit. Bogota, Colombia, has created a bus rapid transit system that carries half a million people a day, reclaimed the sidewalks from motorists, established 300 kilometers of cycleways, created the world's longest pedestrian street (17 km), reduced the traffic by 40%, and inaugurated an annual car-free day. A city where people can breathe clean air and get around easily by foot, bicycle and transit is indeed a civilized city.

### Clean Up Rural Air Pollution

In rural areas, kerosene lamps and inefficient cookers (chulhas, in India) are a major air pollutant. Two thirds of the female lung cancer victims in the developing world are non-smokers, and the impact of kerosene smoke and indoor coal-burning is very high.[8] Nationwide solar village programs are needed to encourage

- Centre for Science and Environment: www.cseindia.org
- Clean Air Initiative: www.cleanairnet.org
- Improved Cookstoves: www.mnes.nic.in/ichulha.html
- *The Leapfrog Factor: Clearing the Air in Asian Cities*, 2006: www.cseindia.org
- Light Up the World: www.lutw.org
- Solar Electric Light Fund: www.self.org
- UN Habitat Urban Transport: www.unhabitat.org/programmes/urbantransport

solar lighting and alternative cookers, supported by groups such as the Solar Electric Light Fund and Light Up the World.

### Support Non-Governmental Organizations

After years of dilly-dallying, Delhi finally converted its entire public transport fleet of 80,000 vehicles to natural gas; banned taxis, buses and auto-rickshaws that are more than 15 years old; eliminated leaded gas; brought in tough new penalties for vehicles emitting visible pollution; increased enforcement; and launched its first underground trains.

Left to the politicians, these changes would never have happened. It was a citizens' group, the Centre for Science and Environment, that made things happen by launching a public interest lawsuit. As a result the Supreme Court set up an independent committee — the Environment Protection Control Authority — that advised the Supreme Court about the technical aspects, which then issued the legal orders. There was huge opposition and a strike by the bus company owners, but in the end, the Supreme Court prevailed. The best lever for this kind of change is strong, independent, nonprofit organizations. Support them. Finance them. Join them.

# 89

# Support Organic Farming

There is no other way out. How much can a person run? Punjab is very tired now, with no stamina left. Organic is the only way out.[1]
— Harjant Singh, Punjabi organic farmer since 2002

For millions of farmers across the developing world, the Green Revolution no longer brings higher yields and good fortunes. It has become instead a source of pesticide poisoning, depleted soils, falling yields, crippling debt and suicide.

Over the years, the use of chemical fertilizers and pesticides has undermined soil fertility and its ability to retain water. It has also destroyed the natural biodiversity of the land. As pest damage increases and yields fall, farmers' costs increase and their incomes shrink, while powerful agro-food corporations make good profits from food distribution and sales.

- "Can Organic Farming Feed Us All?" *World Watch Magazine,* May 2006
- Farming Solutions: www.farmingsolutions.org
- Morarka Foundation, India: www.morarkango.com
- Navdanya, India: www.navdanya.org
- Nayakrishi Centers, Bangladesh: www.membres.lycos.fr/ubinig/naya/centers.html
- Organic Food and Farming, Myth and Reality: www.soilassociation.org
- Pesticide Action Network International: www.pan-international.org
- The Real Green Revolution: www.greenpeace.org
- Sekem, Egypt: www.sekem.com
- *Stolen Harvest: The Hijacking of the Global Food Supply* by Vandana Shiva, South Island Press, 2000
- Vandana Shiva: www.en.wikipedia.org/wiki/Vandana_Shiva

For some the only way out of the crushing burden of debt has been suicide, hanging from a tree or swallowing pesticides. Since 1997, in India more than 25,000 farmers in Andhra Pradesh, Karnataka, Maharashtra and Punjab have taken their own lives.

The suicides are just one sign of the failure of the Green Revolution. The evidence of links between pesticides and cancer is a second sign. The argument that chemical farming prevents plants from being exposed to pests and fungi, causing them not to develop the very phytonutrients and anti-oxidants that protect us against cancer, is a third very persuasive sign.

These facts create a powerful argument for developing nations to make a rapid transition back to fully organic farming.

### Can Organic Farming Feed the World?

There is a belief among some that organic farming simply cannot feed the world. This is not true.

In 2006 the Worldwatch Institute reported on a survey of 200 studies that examined the yields when farmers went organic. The news is very encouraging: in the developing world, yields almost doubled (a 93% improvement), with increases being the highest and most consistent in the poor, remote areas where hunger is the most severe.[2]

When a team from the University of Michigan asked what would happen if the whole world were to go organic, they found that the available calories increased by 75% to 4,381 calories per person a day, 90% more than we need to be healthy.

In Brazil the use of green manure and cover crops has increased yields of maize by between 20% and 250%.[3] In Peru the restoration of traditional Inca terracing has seen increases of up to 150% for a range of upland crops.[4]

Farmers in China doubled their rice yields by planting a mixed crop of rice, rather than just one variety.[5] In Nepal farmers who are using local seed to plant their rice earlier without flooding the fields are increasing their yields by 28% to 100% with much less use of chemicals.[6]

In Ethiopia, when 12,500 farm households adopted sustainable farming methods, yields rose by 60%, and nutrition levels by 70%.[7] In Cuba, where 65% of the rice and 50% of the fresh produce is grown organically, thousands of organic farms and urban gardens flourish, and a complete system of organic support, research and development has been established.[8]

In Chiapas, Mexico, where the Mayan peasants produce 2 tonnes of corn per acre, when the women and small farmers grow beans, squashes, vegetables and fruit trees on the same patch of land, their overall yields increase to 20 tonnes per acre.[9]

And in Egypt where the Sekem group of companies employs 2,000 people to grow organic rice, cotton, vegetables and herbs, the use of pesticides in cotton fields has fallen by 90%, while yields have increased by 30%.[10]

## What Should Governments Do?

- Establish organic training programs, extension agencies, R & D centers and integrated

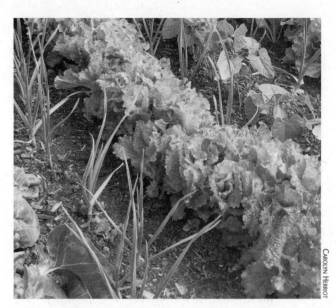

CAROLYN HERRIOT

Organic salad greens provide excellent nutrition around the world.

pest management training, as Jamaica, Cambodia and Ethiopia are doing.

- Require organic training for all agricultural extension agency workers and withdraw support from chemical training.

- Using a selective tax on chemical pesticides and fertilizers, establish transition financing for organic farmers in the early years when yields are lower.

- Control the large agro-trading companies that use packaging standards and pseudo hygiene standards to push small farmers out of the market.

- Ban the use of pesticides that are banned elsewhere.

- Defend the farmers' rights to say no to GM food and to protect local seed varieties.

- Support community seed banks, such as the Nayakrishi centers in Bangladesh.

- Fight the false claims on patents and intellectual property rights for native plants.

# 90

# Leapfrog over the Western Path

It has become crucial that we also talk about — and implement — an alternative urban development strategy. Because if we don't, nothing will survive in the villages of the Third World.

— Anil Agarwal, Centre for Science and Environment, India, who died January 2, 2002, after a seven-year battle with cancer, aged 54.

Villages along the Huaihe River in Henan Province, China, are known as "the cancer villages," since so many people are falling sick from the filthy polluted water from hundreds of unregulated industries.

In Bhopal, India, tens of thousands still live with pain and deep scarring from that night in December 1984 when 40 tonnes of methyl isocynate leaked silently from Union Carbide's pesticide plant, killing 3,000 people outright and 15,000 in the aftermath and injuring up to 600,000.

At Map Ta Phut, Thailand, oil refineries and petrochemical industries have turned a small rural fishing and farming community into a notorious industrial estate, poisoning the local residents with a shocking mix of toxic wastes.

Out of the pollution and the toxic spills, however, a new wisdom is emerging, built around the principles of harmony with nature. The Indian Supreme Court has ruled that "the right to life" includes the right to clean air and clean water: how simple is this self-evident truth.

The West has pioneered a path of development that is causing cancer, global climate change and environmental destruction. Progressive leaders in the developing world are taking a more sustainable path that leapfrogs over the polluting technologies and achieves a healthier, more sustainable form of economic development.

In Taiyuan, a highly polluted Chinese city that has been designated by the United Nations to experiment with clean production, the City has invested $200 million in 15 clean production projects, and 20% of its backbone enterprises are engaged in clean production.

In Kovalam, a scenic tourist spot in Kerala, India, that was becoming notorious for its beaches covered with garbage, a government proposal to build a garbage incinerator met with loud protests from the local community because of fears about cancer from the resulting dioxins and other pollutants. A project called Zero Waste Kovalam was formed, with help from Greenpeace and the Global Alliance for Incinerator Alternatives; since 2001 the community has moved ahead with

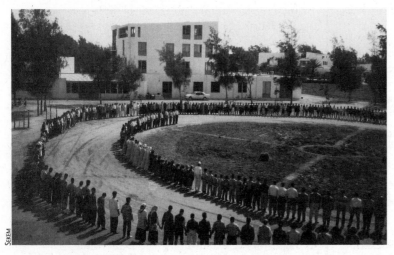

Sekem employees at the start of the working day.

source separation, biogas plants, resource recovery parks and vocational training for women to make eco-friendly products from local waste materials. A hundred women have changed to growing organic vegetables and bananas, ending their use of chemical fertilizers and pesticides. Kovalam is not alone in its goal. Buenos Aires, Argentina, has set its own goal of Zero Waste by 2020.

In Belbes, 60km northeast of Cairo, Egypt, 2,000 people in the Sekem Initiative are practicing a successful version of social capitalism, growing, processing and packaging herbs, spices, medicines, cotton, vegetables, fruit, oils, teas and jams for sale in specialty shops throughout Europe, all grown organically. They are doing this on land reclaimed from the desert, combining their work with educational initiatives from kindergarten to college level, a vocational training center, an educational program for handicapped children, an illiterate children's program and a medical center that serves the whole local community of 30,000 people. *Sekem* means "vitality from the sun," and their motto is "Healing the earth for sustainable development."[1]

In 2005 Greenpeace India produced *Clean Production: A Strategy for a Toxics Free Asia*, a paper that called for governments to embrace legislation including:

- Extended producer responsibility — requiring producers to take responsibility for their products' entire life cycle.
- Ecological tax reform — taxing pollutants, instead of income.

- Bhopal: www.en.wikipedia.org/wiki/Bhopal_disaster
- Cleaner Production in China: www.chinacp.com/eng
- Global Alliance of Incinerator Alternatives: www.no-burn.org
- Global Community Monitor: www.gcmonitor.org
- Greenpeace India: www.greenpeaceindia.org
- The Next Industrial Revolution: www.thenextindustrialrevolution.org
- Sekem: www.sekem.com
- Sipcot Area Community Environmental Monitors: www.sipcotcuddalore.com
- South Durban Community Environmental Alliance: www.h-net.org/~esati/sdcea
- Thailand Toxics: www.gcmonitor.org/thailand.html
- Zero Waste International Alliance: www.zwia.org
- Zero Waste Kovalam: www.zerowastekovalam.org

- Public access to information — guaranteeing that people have the right to know about local pollutants.
- Toxics use reduction legislation — charging a fee on chemical use and using the income to assist companies to reduce their toxic emissions, as Massachusetts has done (see Solution 72).

The vision of a developing nation leapfrogging right over the dirty, polluting phase of industrial development into a world of healthy, sustainable communities is exciting. It may seem an impossible vision, since poverty and pollution are still so widespread, but the other choice — the Western path of development — is so wasteful of resources and bent on consumerism that it is leading to cancer, global warming and ecological collapse.

There is no future for humanity on this path, so it makes good sense to choose a better way. As many people around the globe are saying, another world is possible.

# 91

# Fulfill the Dream of Sustainable Global Governance

> Unless someone like you cares a whole lot, nothing is going to get better. It's not.
>
> — Dr. Seuss's *The Lorax*

We now come to the final section of the book, where we consider the global solutions that are needed to end the epidemic of cancer that is sweeping the world.

Some global measures are obvious, such as applying more resources to close down the tobacco industry (see Solution 79) and tighten the implementation of the Montreal Protocol on ozone depletion, eliminating the loopholes and dawdling that will cause millions to suffer and many to die from skin cancer (see Solution 97). We must also accelerate the implementation of the Stockholm Convention on persistent organic pollutants (POPs) and add more chemicals to the list for future phase-out (see Solution 93).

There is also a much wider perspective that needs our attention.

A hundred years ago, the world consisted of nation-states, the many colonies of imperial powers such as Britain and France, and areas that still had tribal self-governance. There was no concept of global law or governance.

In 1919, following the misery and death of World War I, 44 countries formed the League of Nations, but they failed to stop the advance of fascism. In 1948, after the misery and death of World War II, they tried again and formed the United Nations.

Since then there has been a steady advance in global governance. We now accept that in order to tackle such immense challenges as the spread of nuclear weapons, poverty and disease, pollution of the oceans and climate change, we must work together, however imperfect the results.

The process is incomplete, however. The Earth Charter declares that we must "prevent pollution of any part of the environment and allow no build-up of radioactive, toxic, or other hazardous substances," but the reality is otherwise. Where global treaties do not apply, rogue nations, rogue companies and many corporations that are fully legal are treating the world and its ecosystems as something they can use, exploit and contaminate with toxic emissions and trash. It is no surprise that there is a growing accumulation of poisonous substances in the world, fuelling the record high rates of cancer.

We must end the corporate piracy and contamination of the world that is occurring in the absence of coherent global governance.

We must reframe the way our world operates, so that ecological sustainability, precaution and intergenerational equity become fundamental principles of all human conduct.

We must write a Universal Declaration of Ecological Rights, establishing a legal foundation for environmental sustainability in all global conventions and instruments of international law, following the precedent established by the Earth Charter.

We must find a way to end the destructive influence of the global corporations and to include them as participants, not as lobbyists for a selfish agenda focused solely on profit and market share.

We must write a new Global Charter for Corporate Sustainability, adding 28 new words to the legal duties of corporate directors, so that they are entitled to make money for their

- Earth Charter: www.earthcharter.org
- Redefining Progress: www.rprogress.org

shareholders, *but not at the expense of the environment, human rights, public health and safety, dignity of employees and the welfare of the communities in which the company operates* (see Solution 69). We must agree that, by a certain date, corporations that have not signed the Charter will lose the right to trade across national borders.

We must establish a World Environment Organization with the power to negotiate global agreements on air quality, water quality, ionizing radiation and chemical contamination and establish producer responsibility for the health, safety and disposal of their products, without these goals being trumped and undermined by the lesser goals of the World Trade Organization.

We must change the way the World Trade Organization works, so that its decisions reflect the new principles and not the bad old ways.

We must change the way in which the IMF and the World Bank work, so that they too serve these new principles, instead of acting on behalf of the global corporations as if they were the world.

We must reframe the way we keep our national accounts, so that we include social, health and environmental indicators in our calculations, as well as simple financial wealth.

We must also ensure that these global efforts are properly funded through a global tax either on national GDP, aviation or currency transactions. We must have global governance, which requires global taxation, so we should welcome it.

All of these changes must be part of the worldwide effort to stop cancer. It is not an isolated disease that can be cured with some quick-fix drugs or regulations. It is a consequence of many decisions that have become embedded in the way we run our world, and that need to be changed.

The global epidemic of cancer is one of the most pervasive failures of public health care in human history, which we are called upon to correct.

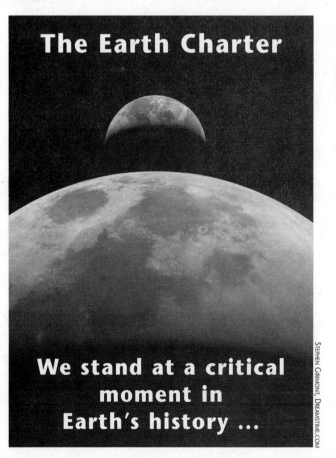

**The Earth Charter**

**We stand at a critical moment in Earth's history ...**

Stephen Cirimont, Dreamstime.com

# 92

# Show Global Leadership on Cancer Prevention

> Our food is contaminated, our air is contaminated and our bodies are contaminated. Something is desperately wrong here and we need to resolve the problem.
> — Elizabeth Salter Green, WWF-UK

There are three organizations that work to fight the colossal challenge of cancer on a global scale, two governmental and one non-governmental.

**World Health Organization (WHO)**
The WHO, based in Geneva, Switzerland, operates under the World Health Assembly of the United Nations. In 2005 its Director General approved a major new Global Cancer Control Strategy to help countries implement comprehensive cancer prevention and control programs, and accelerate their progress.

When you dig into the details, however, it is "more of the same," based on the outdated Doll and Peto premise that only 5% of cancers result from occupational or environmental causes (see

p. 8). As a result, the WHO's Global Strategy is still focused on early detection, treatment and palliative care. There is a small mention of "avoiding exposure to carcinogens" in the Global Strategy, but nothing that would cause a cancer agency to rethink its standard approach.

**International Agency for Research on Cancer (IARC)**
IARC is part of the WHO, based in Lyon, France. It carries out scientific research with the goal of identifying the causes of cancer, so that preventive measures may be adopted against it. That sounds good, and IARC acknowledges that 80% of cancers are directly or indirectly linked to environmental factors, and are thus preventable. IARC has 20 scientific research programs, but only 4 focus on causes that lend themselves to prevention, addressing radiation, tobacco, infections, and nutrition and hormones. There's nothing on toxic chemicals and not much on primary prevention.

Like that of many WHO agencies, IARC's work is heavily influenced by corporations and "business as usual" agendas. IARC programs are being pushed to find their own funding, inviting further corporate influence and pressure to produce business-friendly results.

In 1998 IARC's Evaluation Task Group voted 17 to 13 to classify butadiene, widely used in the rubber industry, as a known human

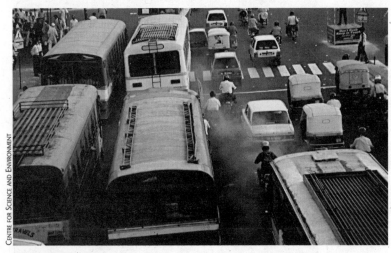

A New Delhi street before the shift to natural gas. People are being exposed to multiple carcinogens in cities throughout the world, due to air pollution.

CENTRE FOR SCIENCE AND ENVIRONMENT

- IARC Research Programs: www.iarc.fr/ENG/Structure/organigramA.html
- International Agency for Research on Cancer: www.iarc.fr
- International Union Against Cancer: www.uicc.org
- World Health Organization: www.who.int/cancer

carcinogen. But then something strange happened. One of the scientists who had voted in favour of the decision left the meeting immediately to return home. The next morning there was an unprecedented revote and the decision was overturned by 15-14, downgrading butadiene from a *known* to a *probable* human carcinogen. Lorenzo Tomatis, founding director of the IARC group, wrote of the decision: "One may question whether interests other than purely scientific were possibly involved," which is a polite way of crying foul.[1]

**International Union Against Cancer (UICC)**
The UICC, a nonprofit, non-governmental association with 270 member organizations in 80 countries, is also based in Geneva. The Union works as a catalyst, sharing knowledge about best practices among its members, which include voluntary cancer leagues and societies, cancer research and treatment centers and some ministries of health. Although the UICC is well set up to transmit new ideas or approaches to its members, it is wedded to the old paradigm, like the WHO. It has a vision of "a world where cancer is eliminated as a major life-threatening disease for future generations," but with little commitment to prevention, it is limited to the same old approaches that have used up vast amounts of money but have failed to stop the worldwide cancer epidemic.

The WHO, IARC and the UICC need to abandon the old paradigm and eliminate corporate influence from their committees, that encourages the old model and feeds it money. This means that the WHO and IARC must receive secure funding from the UN via national governments, so that they can serve the public interest and not the corporate sector. This in turn means that all governments (including the US) must pay their annual dues to the UN. All three organizations should publish details of their finances, so that they are publicly transparent.

Once free of the old influence, the WHO should establish a whole new area of work, with multiple programs designed to tackle the primary prevention of cancer. It should establish a program, for instance, to promote the use of organic food during pregnancy and infant feeding, including exclusive breast-feeding to six months. It should establish a program to support new public health initiatives in the developing nations, so that community health workers, barefoot workers and native healers can be trained in the early detection and prevention of infectious cancers.

IARC should be tasked to lead a global research effort focused on primary prevention and the elimination of carcinogens, with an independent global scientific panel.

The UICC should use its network to share information about the best community cancer-prevention programs, the best practices in labor unions and businesses and the best legislation to reduce and eliminate toxics. It should create new international networks, linking schools, cities and businesses to work together to end the cancer epidemic.

All three organizations could make an enormous difference if they abandoned the flawed paradigm of cancer causation and worked together to prevent cancer at its source.

# 93
# Build Stronger Global Treaties

> We cannot solve the problems that we have today by thinking in the same way that we did when we created them.
>
> — Albert Einstein

Because thousands of tonnes of hazardous products are manufactured and shipped around the world every day, we need the best possible global standards to rid the Earth of the toxic influences that are contributing to record high cancer rates.

We need strong and relevant global treaties that are respected and adhered to by all nations. The chemical industry, which employs more than ten million people and accounts for 7% of the world's international trade,[1] works hard to avoid regulation, so this is not an easy process.

The chemical industry started in Europe in the early 1800s, with the Industrial Revolution's need for chemicals to make things like soap, glass and cotton. Rachel Carson's book *Silent Spring*, which laid out the profusion of harms done by chemical pesticides and ionizing radiation and effectively launched the global environmental movement, was not published till 160 years later in 1962. The first global treaty, the London Convention to stop the dumping of chemical wastes at sea, was signed in 1972.[2] Since then there have been three additional global conventions, seven voluntary International Labour Organization (ILO) conventions and various regional agreements. But this is nowhere near enough.

The ILO conventions, for instance, are non-binding. They set commitments that countries promise to adopt. One convention aims to prohibit worker exposure to carcinogenic substances and agents.[3] Others seek to protect workers from asbestos,[4] ensure the safe management of chemicals in the workplace[5] and guarantee workers' right to know about the chemicals they use.[6]

The US has ratified none of these, and Canada has ratified only one, ironically, on the safe use of asbestos, a carcinogenic substance that Canada profits handsomely from and that is the target of a worldwide ban. To see the list of countries that have ratified these conventions, search Google.com for APPLIS.

The other binding global conventions are the Basel Convention on the shipment and disposal of Hazardous Wastes (see Solution 95), the Rotterdam Convention on Prior Informed Consent and the Stockholm Convention on Persistent Organic Pollutants.

*The Rotterdam Convention* addresses the problem of dangerous chemicals being shipped around the world. It lists 28 pesticides and 11 industrial chemicals that have been banned or severely restricted by countries signing the convention, and allows importing countries to exclude them if they think they cannot manage them safely. The convention came into force in 2004, but in many ways, it gives implicit approval to the trade in toxic chemicals.

*The Stockholm Convention* on persistent organic pollutants (POPs), which came into force in 2004, was designed to end the global production and use of 12 of the world's most poisonous chemicals associated with cancer and other severe health effects. It targets the chemicals for reduction and eventual elimination and sets up a system to tackle other hazardous chemicals that can be added over time. It provides financial resources to clean up the stockpiles and dumps of POPs that litter the world and uses the precautionary principle as its guide.

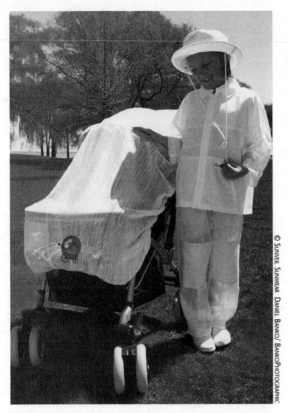

Child wearing Sunveil clothing. By 2065 or later, the ozone layer will hopefully have healed, thanks to the Montreal Protocol (see Solution 97). We urgently need global treaties to address the other hazards that face us.

© SUNVEIL SUNWEAR. DANIEL BANKO/ BANKOPHOTOGRAPHIC

- ILO Conventions:
  www.ilo.org/ilolex/english/convdisp1.htm
- International POPs Elimination Network:
  www.ipen.ecn.cz
- International POPs Elimination Project (IPEP):
  www.oztoxics.org/ipepweb
- Basel, Stockholm and Rotterdam Conventions:
  www.pops.int/documents/background/hcwc.pdf
- Rotterdam Convention: www.pic.int
- Stockholm Convention: www.pops.int
- Toxics Treaties Country Report Cards:
  www.ban.org/country_status/report_card.html

These global conventions are very important, but only eight of the world's nations have ratified all four: Denmark, France, Germany, Norway, Spain, Sweden, Switzerland and the United Kingdom. Forty-four nations have not ratified a single one, including the US, Russia, Israel, and most of the world's smaller, dysfunctional or impoverished nations. Every government should sign and ratify the global and the ILO conventions and encourage others to get on board. The chemicals that trigger cancer do not need passports to cross national borders. We are all in this together, and we must work to eliminate the danger together.

The flame of determination is carried by the International POPs Elimination Network, representing public interest organizations in 65 countries whose members attend all the relevant conferences, where they work to achieve stronger, mandatory, properly financed agreements. They also run the International POPs Elimination Project, helping NGOs in developing nations create awareness about the danger of these chemicals and build protective capacity. The Network's goal is the elimination of all hazardous chemicals by 2020 so that the world can enjoy a toxics-free future.

What is next? Europe has developed its REACH legislation (see Solution 69), which would be a good start for the world as a whole. In 2006 most of the world's governments signed onto an agreement known as SAICM (see Solution 94), but it is voluntary and nowhere near strong enough to achieve what is needed.

We need all government leaders, cancer societies and other nonprofit societies to stick their necks out for strong, binding regulations that will stop the flow of carcinogens into the world.

# 94

## Eliminate All Hazardous Chemicals by 2020

> **It is not enough that governments decide that protecting the health of their population and the environment is voluntary.**
>
> — **Karen Suassuna, Associaco de Combate aos POPs, Brazil**

In 2002 the world's nations signed onto a broad commitment that, by 2020, the global community would ensure that all chemicals would be "used and produced in ways that lead to the minimization of adverse effects on human health and the environment." This was one successful outcome of the World Summit on Sustainable Development in Johannesburg.

How can we achieve such a goal? One approach is to trust industry to make a voluntary commitment to clean up its act. Since the chemical industry has been kicking and screaming against most kinds of regulation, and doing its utmost to sabotage the existing global agreements, its conduct does not give much confidence that it is up to the task. With the US refusing to ratify the global conventions, and US delegations being little more than the voice of the chemical industry, the chances of this happening are next to nil.

Alongside the global conventions, the United Nations Environment Program has worked with the world's nations to craft a very broad, all-encompassing voluntary agreement known as the Strategic Approach to International Chemicals Management (SAICM). This stems from a desire by many to pull together a complicated jigsaw of regional and global voluntary agreements on different aspects of safe chemical management into one coherent approach.

The SAICM Declaration and Global Plan of Action were finally agreed on at Dubai in 2006, after "teetering on the brink of disaster as the Bush Administration demanded sweeping concessions, rebuffed all efforts to find common ground and stood alone against over 140 countries to resist the agreement." The US was determined that "the environment and public health protection would always take a back seat to trade."[1]

The Plan lists 271 activities that governments, industry and others have agreed to undertake. Among them:

- Assess national chemicals management.
- Identify gaps and prioritize actions.
- Promote the use of safe and effective alternatives.

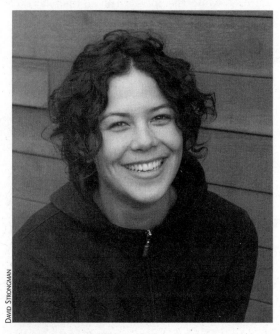

Severn Suzuki in 2007.

DAVID STRONGMAN

- Provide training in clean production techniques.

It is encouraging that the world has agreed to such a plan, since global chemical production is set to climb by as much as 80% by 2020. Throughout the negotiations, however, the United States fought the idea that the plan would ever be anything more than voluntary and balked, unsuccessfully, at the inclusion of the precautionary principle. Both Canada and the US fought the idea that there should be liability and compensation. The European Union wanted an agreement regarding all chemical products, but the US refused to include the chemicals in food and medicines.

We have a long way to go. For the next few years, the world needs to develop a dual-track approach. On one track, we need to ensure that the commitments of the Dubai Declaration are implemented, and press our governments to act on each of the Global Action Plan's 271 components.

On the other track, we need to push for zero emissions, toxics use reduction, mandatory phase-outs and clean production. We need to support the International POPs Elimination Network (IPEN) and its small band of committed staff as they work for a truly meaningful global commitment to eliminate the most persistent organic pollutants (see Solution 93). During the Dubai Conference, IPEN launched a Declaration for a Toxic Free Future with 25 points that describe what is needed with clarity and purpose. When the Dubai Declaration was adopted,

however, the world's media ignored it completely. We need to elevate this decree to the global importance that it deserves.

Imagine if people from cancer agencies, support groups and action groups all over the world were to attend such conferences and inform their members about progress on an hour-by-hour basis. Imagine if we were to besiege our politicians with letters, demanding that they sign mandatory agreements, not voluntary ones. Imagine if a child could be invited to speak at the next such conference, as the 12-year-old Severn Suzuki did at the 1992 Rio Earth Summit, giving voice to her hopes and fears for the future.

"What you do makes me cry at night," she said. "You grown-ups say you love us. I challenge you, please make your actions reflect your words."

- International Forum on Chemical Safety: www.who.int/ifcs
- International POPs Elimination Network (IPEN): www.ipen.ecn.cz
- International Program on Chemical Safety: www.who.int/ipcs
- Inter-Organizational Program for the Sound Management of Chemicals: www.who.int/iomc
- Severn Suzuki's Speech at Rio: www.thespeechsite.com/famous/SevernSuzuki-1.htm
- Strategic Approach to International Chemicals Management: www.chem.unep.ch/saicm
- UNEP's Chemicals Program: www.chem.unep.ch

# 95

# Stop the Global Trade in Hazardous Wastes

I n the 1980s the word "globalization" was just beginning to appear. With it came the discovery of barrels of mixed industrial poisons dumped on tropical beaches and "vessels laden with toxic trash plying the coastlines of developing countries searching for a port-of-call."[1]

The developed world had consumer fever, but it was running out of places to dump its wastes, especially those labeled "hazardous." Thanks to the West's environmental movement, far fewer of the most flagrant wastes could be taken to the local landfill or poured into a river (although this still occurs). Where better, the toxic companies thought, than a poor nation needing the cash? If they needed any further encouragement, the chief economist of the World Bank, Laurence Summers, had this to say in 1991: "I think the economic logic behind dumping a load of toxic waste in the lowest-wage country is impeccable, and we should face up to that. I've always thought that under-populated countries in Africa are vastly under-polluted."[2]

In 1987, prompted by growing anger over the trade in hazardous wastes, the United Nations began negotiations for a convention to control the trade. In 1989, 118 nations met in Switzerland and signed the Basel Convention on the Control of Transboundary Movements of Hazardous Waste and their Disposal.

The vast majority of the world's nations wanted a complete ban on the trade, but a few developed countries, led by the United States, insisted that the treaty should only monitor the trade, not attempt to stop it. The delegates from the developing nations were infuriated and

> You industrialized countries have been asking us to do many things for the global good — to stop cutting down our forests, to stop using your CFCs. Now we are asking you to do something for the global good — to keep your own wastes.
> — A Bhattacharjya, head of India's delegation to the Basel Convention talks

walked out of the meeting. A group of African nations went ahead with their own treaty banning the import of wastes to Africa, and they were followed by others, so that by 1992, when the Basel Convention came into force, 88 countries had banned the trade through local and regional initiatives.

This tidal wave of legislation persuaded the delegates from Switzerland, Norway, Sweden and Denmark that they should join the developing world and countries from Eastern Europe to push again for a global ban, in spite of opposition from Germany, Holland, Britain, the US, Canada, Australia and Japan. The developing nations stood together, refusing to back down, and in March 1994 the parties to the Basel Convention adopted a full ban on the trade in toxic wastes. The ban needs 62 nations to ratify it. At the time of writing (December 2006), it needed just one more nation for it to come into force. Every major nation and almost every smaller nation has ratified it,[3] but not the United States. The other holdouts include Afghanistan, Haiti, Iraq, North Korea, Myanmar, Somalia and Sudan.

The story does not end here. After the ban was proposed, the same nations that opposed it, led by the US, started working to undermine it, arguing over the definition of "waste" and claiming that it was "recycled." This destructive effort continues to this day.

The latest chapters in the saga focus on two areas: electronic wastes and shipbreaking.

With the electronics revolution in full swing, the manufacturers of computers, monitors and

- Basel Action Network: www.ban.org
- Basel Convention: www.basel.int
- *Exporting Harm: The High-Tech Trashing of Asia*: www.ban.org/E-waste/technotrashfinalcomp.pdf
- Shipbreaking: www.greenpeaceweb.org/shipbreak

other high-tech devices forgot to ask what happens to the components when their products die or need to be replaced. Every attractively designed computer is full of toxic chemicals, heavy metals and plastic compounds that can cause cancer, kidney failure, endocrine disruption, neurological failure and birth defects. Many are shipped to China, where children pull them apart for "recycling," exposing themselves to the toxins. The US allows it because it has not signed the Basel Convention. Canada allows it *in spite of* having signed the Convention.[4]

The same loopholes apply to the trade in shipbreaking, which avoided the Basel Convention and is now established as a major trade in India, Pakistan, Bangladesh, China and Turkey, with no safeguards for the workers against the toxins (including asbestos) that many ships contain.

In spite of these formidable problems, the Basel Convention has been a huge success for the world, notwithstanding the serious attempts to derail it. The Basel Action Network, the Seattle-based NGO that has persistently and doggedly tracked the issue, has served as a champion for the health of future generations. This work must continue. The world is not yet safe from the toxic trade.

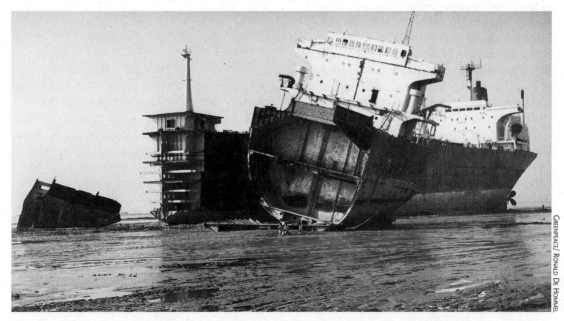

GREENPEACE/ RONALD DE HOMMEL

A partly scrapped tanker hulk on the beach at the shipbreaking yard in Chittagong, Bangladesh.

# 96

# Ban Asbestos

There is only one useful thing you can do with asbestos. Ban it.
— International Metalworkers' Federation

Every five minutes someone dies from asbestos. A worker who made brake linings. A son who sat on his father's lap when he came home from work. A wife who washed her husband's asbestos-covered overalls. All breathed the deadly dust that lodged in their lungs and became cancerous.

We have long known that asbestos causes asbestosis, lung cancer and mesothelioma, a cancer of the lining of the lungs and digestive tract that is usually fatal within one year of being diagnosed. Although its use has been dropping in North America and Europe, the number of deaths continues to climb because of the long period between exposure and the appearance of disease, and Europe expects that there will be 250,000 cases within the next 35 years. Although asbestos is the number one carcinogen in the world of work, anyone who lives or works near an asbestos-contaminated building that is being renovated or demolished is also at risk.

The first miners began to dig out asbestos in 1879 at Thetford, Quebec. By 1920 Canadian, South African and Russian mines were supplying fiber to Europe and North America to manufacture asbestos products. Because of its resistance to high temperatures, it was regarded as a "miracle" mineral. The evidence that it could also be a killer showed up shortly after its first use, when inspectors in British factories noticed high rates of lung disease. For years, however, Canadian companies and the doctors on their payrolls refused to acknowledge the sick and dying miners. One Thetford doctor admitted that he advised workers not to quit and seek compensation because it would do nothing to stop the progress of their disease: "I figured it was in their best interest to stay at their jobs."[1]

Because of its extreme carcinogenicity, unions and anti-asbestos campaigners have been working for the last three decades to ban it. By 1996 nine European countries, including France, had stopped using asbestos. Canada and its industry allies were shaken by the loss of France, since it was Europe's leading consumer of asbestos, taking 6% of Canada's exports. Canada sought to overturn the ban by appealing to the World Trade Organization (WTO), but in 2001 the WTO found in France's favour and pronounced that:

- All forms of asbestos are carcinogenic.
- There is no known threshold of safety for asbestos.
- Building and brake-lining workers and others who handle asbestos products are at risk.
- The efficiency of the "controlled use" of asbestos had not been demonstrated, and the residual risk to workers would still be significant.[2]

A Europe-wide ban quickly followed, outlawing activities such as the extraction or manufacturing of products by 2006 that would expose workers to asbestos.

As a result of the tightening restrictions, by the mid-90s the worldwide production was finally going down. But, like the tobacco industry, the asbestos corporations launched an international campaign targeted at developing

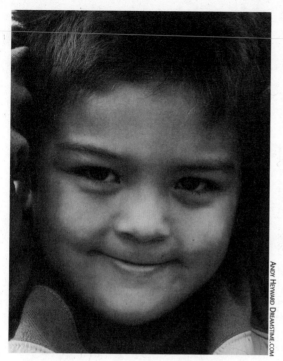

- Asbestos Disease Awareness Organization: www.asbestosdiseaseawareness.org
- Asbestos Epidemic in America: www.ewg.org:16080/reports/asbestos
- *Asbestos: Medical and Legal Aspects* by Barry Castleman, Aspen, 2005
- Ban Asbestos Canada: www.bacanada.org
- European Trade Union Institute: http://hesa.etui-rehs.org/uk/dossiers/dossier.asp
- *Hazards Magazine*: www.hazards.org/asbestos
- International Metalworkers' Federation: www.imfmetal.org
- *Libby, Montana* (DVD): www.highplainsfilms.org/fp_libby.html
- White Lung Association: www.whitelung.org

Will he grow up in a world still threatened by exposure to asbestos? We need to eliminate its use worldwide.

Andy Heyward Dreamstime.com

countries that sent sales back up again. Canada's asbestos industry is the third largest in the world, and Canada has cultivated new markets in China, South Korea, Pakistan, Indonesia, Thailand and Malaysia. Russia and China, the two largest producers, also continue to mine tonnes every year, much of it for use in their own countries.[3]

Canada has been described as an "international pariah" for the way it has marketed asbestos to developing countries and blocked international agreements to control it. Canada refused to allow asbestos to be listed under the Rotterdam Convention on hazardous wastes (see Solution 93).

Even in countries where there is little or no education or protection for workers, Canada perpetrates the fiction that asbestos can be safely used under controlled conditions. In response, Dr. Philip Landrigan, President of the Collegium Ramazzini, has said, "The argument that workers can be protected against asbestos in nations that have no legal infrastructure in occupational health is a cruel joke."[4]

The global campaign to ban asbestos is gaining momentum. The Collegium Ramazzini, set up to translate scientific research into public policy in the environmental and occupational health fields, has called for an international ban. The International Labour Organization is calling for a partial ban, and in 2006 a campaign supported by other Global Union Federations introduced a resolution supporting a complete global ban. These efforts should be supported, along with just transition programs to help asbestos workers find new employment or compensation.

Because there is no safe level of asbestos, the only way to prevent needless cancer deaths is a global convention to ban all mining and use of asbestos. Every country in the world must sign on.

# 97

# Stop Ozone Depletion

The incidence of non-melanoma skin cancer is expected to increase by approximately 2% for every persistent 1% loss in average ozone concentration.
— Dr. Frank R. de Gruijl, Dermatology Dept., University of Utrecht, Holland

High in the atmosphere, 6 to 30 miles above our heads, there is a super-thin scattering of ozone molecules. It was created two billion years ago when oxygen from early bacteria in the oceans rose into the atmosphere and reformed as ozone molecules, creating the shield that protects life on Earth against the sun's deadly ultraviolet radiation.

Now, fast-forward to humans and a chemist called Thomas Midgley who in 1930 was asked by General Motors to develop a refrigerant less dangerous than sulfur dioxide and ammonia. Within three days, he had developed Freon, which led to a family of chemicals called chlorinated fluorocarbons (CFCs) that were soon used as refrigerants in cars and freezers and as propellants in spray cans.

No-one knew that the chlorine in CFCs would attack the ozone layer and begin to blast it apart. It was not until 1974 that scientists suggested this might be happening, and not until the 1980s that they realized it was a certainty.

By this time, it was too late. A massive hole had formed over Antarctica, and the sun's UVB rays were pouring through. Doctors were seeing a growing number of people with skin cancer, both the dangerous malignant (invasive) melanoma and the more easily treated basal cell and squamous cell carcinomas. They also saw evidence of cataracts and immune system damage caused by exposure to the UVB rays.

Today over half of all new cancers are skin cancers. The process of cause and effect is complex because the most vulnerable pale-skinned people have been doing more sunbathing and wearing fewer summer clothes, but there is strong evidence that ozone depletion is associated with non-melanoma skin cancers, and that UVB radiation enhances the development of invasive melanomas.[1]

Each year over a million new cases of skin cancer are diagnosed in North America, and 11,000 people die from them. Globally, continuing ozone depletion contributes to 53,000 deaths a year.[2]

In 1987 most of the world's nations signed the

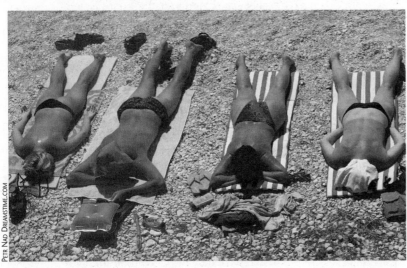

Caution: this is not a recommended activity!

PETR NAD DREAMSTIME.COM

Montreal Protocol, phasing out CFCs, halons and brominated chemicals. The CFCs were to be gone from the developed world by 1995 and elsewhere by 2010. Their replacement, the HCFCs, which cause 95% less damage, are being phased out from the developed world by 2010 and elsewhere by 2040. Methyl bromide, used as a pesticide on strawberries and melons, is being phased out in the developed world by 2005 and elsewhere by 2015.

Many people point to the Montreal Protocol as a successful treaty. The trouble is, they are wrong. The ozone holes are not improving. CFCs are leaking from carelessly discarded fridges and illegally stockpiled CFCs. Illegal substances are still being used in North America, particularly CFC-113, used as a flux remover and solvent in the electronics industry.[3] US farmers have lobbied hard to continue using methyl bromide on their strawberries.

There is also a big illegal trade in CFCs in the developing world. In 2005 staff from the non-profit Environmental Investigation Agency posing as purchasers were offered 122 tonnes of illegal CFCs for car air conditioning and refrigeration by Chinese companies cashing in on China's planned phase-out of CFCs by 2007.

There is also concern that the Space Shuttle, Ariane and Air Force Titan IV rockets are damaging the ozone layer by injecting chlorine from ammonium perchlorate fuel directly into the upper stratosphere, where the chlorine does far more damage than in the lower stratosphere because the atmosphere is so thin. The entire US aerospace plan and ballistic missile-shield program are

- Environmental Investigation Agency: www.eia-international.org
- Greenfreeze: http://archive.greenpeace.org/ozone/greenfreeze
- Health Effects of UV Radiation: www.epa.gov/sunwise/uvandhealth.html
- Montreal Protocol: www.theozonehole.com/montreal.htm
- Ozone Crisis: http://archive.greenpeace.org/ozone
- Ozone Depletion: www.epa.gov/ozone
- Ozone Hole: www.theozonehole.com
- Ozone Hole Tour: www.atm.ch.cam.ac.uk/tour
- Stratospheric Ozone: www.ozonelayer.noaa.gov
- Sunsmart: www.sunsmart.org.uk

premised on using this fuel, which received an unlimited exemption under the Montreal Protocol. Since the damage may be far greater than is commonly understood, especially at the 43km level, the exemption should be re-examined.[4]

We are paying dearly for our abuse of the ozone layer through increased skin cancers. Because of these loopholes and abuses, it is now unlikely to repair itself before 2065 *or later.*

The Montreal Protocol nations must speed up the phase-out dates for all ozone-depleting substances. They must enforce the rules more toughly to prevent smuggling, and they must ensure that developing nations have the resources needed to enforce the bans.

There is no need for any of the ozone-depleting substances, as there are alternatives for all of them. The Greenfreeze refrigerator, developed by Greenpeace, is an award-winning technology that damages neither the ozone layer nor the global climate. There are 100 models available in different parts of the world, and by 2006 over 12 million fridges had been produced. They are not being allowed into North America, however, due to industry resistance. They need to become the new global standard, everywhere.

# 98

# Ban Depleted Uranium

> I hope God slam-dunks their butts,
> because this is absolutely criminal.
>
> — Dr. Doug Rokke, former Director of the
> US Army Depleted Uranium Project

In addition to the cancer risks posed by nuclear power and nuclear weapons, there is another alarming nuclear danger we must address.

Depleted uranium (DU) is a waste product that is created during the enrichment of uranium for nuclear reactors and weapons. It is a very hard metal, and when used on the tip of a bullet or missile, it slices through the armor like a knife through butter.

When a DU bullet or missile strikes its target, the DU oxidizes, scattering radioactive uranium oxide particles much smaller than a face mask can protect against. Penetrating deep within the lungs, they emit alpha radiation, which has been classified as carcinogenic by all the nuclear regulatory and environment health agencies. Studies show that when a particle under 5 microns enters the lungs, the surrounding tissue is exposed to 270 times the radiation permitted for workers in the radiation industry.

The US military has used DU munitions in Bosnia, Kosovo, Afghanistan, Iraq, Kuwait and Saudi Arabia. It used as much as 800 tons in the first Gulf War, and 1500 tons in the 2003 invasion of Iraq, including in the guided missiles and bunker-buster bombs that were used to attack buildings.[1]

The immediate danger is to military personnel who inspect the tanks after they have been hit, children who play in the dust of the destroyed tanks and buildings, and pregnant women who live nearby (as well as the soldiers who were in the tank).

In Basra, southern Iraq, doctors have been treating people with double and triple cancers. One hospital there reported treating upwards of 600 children per day with symptoms of radiation sickness.[2] Doctors in Iraq have estimated that birth defects have increased 2 to 6 times since 1991, and childhood cancers 3 to 12 times.[3] A 1998 report in *The Lancet* reported that cases of lymphoblastic leukemia in Iraq had quadrupled since 1991.[4]

Soldiers returning home are also getting sick. From 1991 to 2004, 7,000 US troops were wounded in the two Gulf wars, but by 2004 the Pentagon was paying disability pensions to 518,000 Gulf War veterans. Although the causes of Gulf War Syndrome are disputed, many sick soldiers remember being exposed to the black soot of DU, and DU accumulations have been found in the bones and lungs of veterans who died after long illnesses.[5] In studies of soldiers who had normal babies before the war, 67% of their infants born after the war had blood diseases and severe birth defects, missing brains, eyes, organs, legs and arms.[6]

The Uranium Medical Research Centre (UMRC) is a nonprofit organization that offers

- Campaign Against Depleted Uranium: www.cadu.org.uk
- *Depleted Uranium Is WMD*, by Leuren Moret: www.commondreams.org/views05/0809-33.htm
- International Action Center: www.iacenter.org/depleted
- International Coalition to Ban Depleted Uranium Weapons: www.bandepleteduranium.org
- Uranium Medical Research Centre: www.umrc.net

veterans and others at risk medical assessment and clinical treatment. Its Research Director, Dr. Asaf Durakovic, Professor of Radiology and Nuclear Medicine at Georgetown University in Washington, was a US Army colonel who left the military because he was so distressed at what he saw. In October 2003, when a UMRC research team conducted a field trip to Iraq, they collected air, soil and water samples that contained "hundreds to thousands of times" the normal levels of radiation. There are also reports of DU weapons being recycled as scrap in Iraq.[7]

The larger danger is to all of us. As DU contamination builds up in the atmosphere, it is spread around the world by wind currents and dust storms. The dust has a radioactive half-life of 4.5 billion years, which is as long as the Earth has existed.[8]

"Since 1991, the US has released the radioactive atomicity equivalent of at least 400,000 Nagasaki bombs into the global atmosphere ... 10 times the amount released during atmospheric testing, which was the equivalent of 40,000 Hiroshima bombs." [9]

At least 16 countries keep uranium weapons in their arsenals, including France, Israel, Pakistan, Russia, Saudi Arabia, UK and the US. Only Britain and the US are known to have used DU weapons in conflict and during peacekeeping operations in the former Yugoslavia.

In October 2003 the International Coalition to Ban Depleted Uranium Weapons was formed after a conference in Belgium. It called for a ban on the military use of uranium and drafted a global convention that would prohibit the use of uranium weapons and require parties to the treaty to destroy their arsenals.

The use of depleted uranium is a global disgrace. As individuals, we can sign the petition on the Coalition's website. As organizations, we can add our voices to the call for a global ban by becoming Friends of the Coalition. As governments, we must pass national legislation banning the use of DU and mobilize other nations to achieve a global ban.

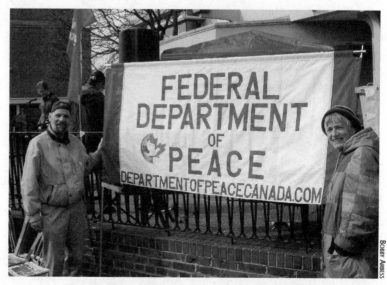

Saul Arbess and Penny Joy campaign for a Canadian Department of Peace. With persistent citizen involvement, we can make a better world.

# 99

## A Solution for the World's Religions

Preaching for me is not behind the wooden desk, or the glass desk, or the gold desk. Preaching for me is rolling up your sleeves as a minister of the gospel of Jesus Christ, and getting busy.
— Charlotte Keys, Jesus People Against Pollution, Columbia, Mississippi

Around the globe, spiritual and religious beliefs form the core of many people's worlds and shape the principles they live by. Many aboriginal groups practice what they preach when they believe that nature is inseparable from the Great Spirit. An Arapaho proverb says, "When we show our respect for other living things, they respond with respect for us."

If you are not a religious believer, and prefer to be guided by your own innate sense of the value of life, and by scientific reason, please move right on to Solution 100.

The world's religions have many differences, but at their core they all agree that we should

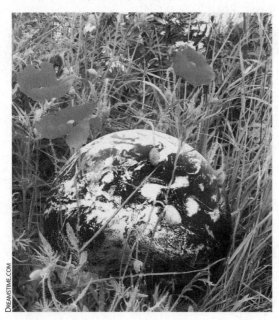

Beauty discarded, or beauty found?

DREAMSTIME.COM

strive to love and support each other, that we do unto others as we would have them do to us. God does not want us to argue, fight or kill.

The world's religions also agree on a second point: that we should love God's creation, and take care of it as we would our own garden. As Shehe Mlekwa Lissani Bambi, a Muslim religious leader in Tanzania has said, "We are the guardians of God's creation. He asks us to protect what he created."[1]

"Greater indeed than the creation of man is the creation of the heavens and the earth," says the Koran.[2]

In the Hebrew Bible, the words "adam" (man) and "adamah" (earth) are closely related.

The Jewish and Christian religions share this belief. "The Earth is the Lord's and the fullness thereof, the world, and they that dwell therein," says Psalm 24:1.

In the Jewish faith, when God created Adam, he showed him all the trees of the Garden of Eden and said:

> See my works, how lovely they are, how fine they are. All I have created, I created for you. Take care not to corrupt and destroy my universe, for if you destroy it, no-one will come after you to put it right.[3]

This is a mitzvah, a divine commandment.

Right now we are abusing and polluting the trust that has been given to us. We are overharvesting the fish of the oceans and the forests of the world. By spreading pollution, we are creating distress and loss throughout God's creation. The pollution is arriving in our bodies, creating the conditions where cancer, asthma and many other diseases take hold. Our children are suffering. Our families and friends are suffering.

As we come to the end of this book, we appeal to all who find comfort in God, however you worship. We need your help to tackle this scourge of cancer, so that the world can be made safe for ourselves, for our children and for future generations. We encourage you to meet in your congregations and ask what you can do to help.

In Columbia, Mississippi, the Jesus People Against Pollution work to obtain justice for people affected by toxic poisoning through the misuse of hazardous chemicals.

In the Bronx, New York, the Sisters of Mercy bought stock in Synagro, a fertilizer pellet-maker, and used activist shareholder resolutions to pressure them to clean up the emissions they were causing by burning New York City sewage.

The American Baptist Churches have called on their members to learn about the environmental crisis and become involved in organizations and actions to restore the environment.[4]

The United Methodist Women are forming Green Teams in their environmental justice program.

Among Catholics, the Coalition for Children and a Safe Environment is working to educate the larger community.

**Our task must be to widen our circle of compassion to embrace all living creatures, and the whole of nature in its beauty.**

**— Albert Einstein (1879 – 1955)**

- Catholic Coalition for Children and a Safe Environment: www.usccb.org/sdwp/ejp/case
- Coalition on the Environment and Jewish Life: www.coejl.org
- Earth Sangha: www.earthsangha.org
- Evangelical Environment Network: www.creationcare.org
- Faith and the Common Good: www.faith-commongood.net
- Greening Congregations: www.earthministry.org/Congregations/handbook.htm
- Guardians of the Natural Order (Muslim): www.amse.net/News_2003_Guardians.html
- Indigenous Environmental Network: www.ienearth.org
- Interfaith Center on Corporate Responsibility: www.iccr.org
- National Council of Churches: www.nccecojustice.org
- National Religious Partnership for the Environment: www.nrpe.org
- United Church of Canada: www.united-church.ca/ecology
- United Methodist Women: http://gbgm-umc.org/umw/green_team.cfm
- Web of Creation: www.webofcreation.org

Many churches and congregations are learning how to save money and reduce air pollution by making their churches more energy efficient, carpooling and avoiding the use of chlorine-bleached paper.

Equally important, we need you to speak out against the toxic pollution that is causing cancer. The beauty of God's creation is being corrupted in the cells of our bodies and the bodies of our children, and we need your help to stop it.

**Glance at the sun. See the moon and the stars. Gaze at the beauty of the Earth's greenings.**

**— Hildegard von Bingen (1089 – 1179)**

# 100

# Heal the Earth's Cancer

> The ecological crisis is doing what no other crisis in history has ever done — challenging us to a realization of a new humanity.
>
> — Jean Houston

Throughout this book, we have shown that many of the actions that are needed to stop the global epidemic of cancer are the same as those that are needed to build a healthy, green, sustainable world. We need to:

- Restore the purity of air and water that existed before the industrial age.
- Replace industrial junk food with wholesome, organic food.
- Replace toxic production with clean production.
- Rebuild our cities, towns and suburbs with traditional communities where people enjoy moving around on foot.
- Replace fossil fuels and nuclear power with clean, sustainable energy.
- Replace corporate influence over science with authentic, independent science, and end corporate influence over democracy.

This may seem utopian, but if we work together, we can meet the challenges and make the dream a reality.

There is another perspective, however, which places a far greater urgency on our choice whether or not to get engaged.

Think of the Earth as a living body. The ecosystems are her limbs and organs; the species are the cells of her body. For millions of years, clean air and water, nutrients and warmth have flowed through her body, keeping her cells and organs healthy.

For millions of years, the emerging species known as *homo sapiens* co-existed with Earth's ecosystems. Our early tools were fairly harmless; without them, we might not have survived. During the last few hundred years, however, our tools have become much more powerful.

We started burning coal — with no awareness that the emissions would cause global climate change, mercury pollution and cancer, or that coal's sulfur dioxide emissions would cause acid rain, locking up the selenium in the soil, depriving us of one of nature's defenses against cancer. Even when we knew this, we continued burning coal because those who profited from it were more powerful than those who wanted it to stop.

We started using fossil fuels to make synthetic chemicals — with no awareness that some would cause cancer, birth defects and other suffering. Even when we learned this, we continued to make them because those who were profiting were more powerful than those who wanted it to stop.

We started on the path of industrial agriculture — with no awareness that pesticides and fungicides would cause plants not to defend themselves against pests and fungus, depriving us of the cancer-fighting compounds that plants have always possessed. When we learn this — will we stop?

Our tools are now all-powerful. We can drive around the world, empty the oceans of fish and fell the world's rainforests. As a result, we have global warming, the oceans are dying and the rainforests are falling. And yet when it profits those who are doing it, they will move heaven and Earth to continue rather than consider the cost to the greater whole.

This is how a cancer cell behaves. It follows the blind instinct of "more!" until it has destroyed the cells and organs it feeds on. It is not "development" that is the problem: it is blind, selfish, unsustainable development based on how much someone can profit, not how they can profit the whole. This is what makes it like a cancer — it acts in willful disregard for the health of the whole, the ecosystems our lives depend on. The larger cancer of unsustainable development is a direct cause of the individual cancers that grow in our bodies.

If we are going to overcome the personal cancers, we must also overcome the larger cancer that feeds toxic substances into our bodies and deprives us of healing food.

We must ourselves become the Earth's immune system, engaging with the cancer cells — the forces within ourselves and within our corporations and governments that continue to pursue blind, cancerous growth.

We must defeat the cancer cells, forming a global movement in the body of the Earth to bring healing to every corner of the Earth.

We must link up with those who are working to stop global climate change and with those who are working for more organic farming.

We must link up with those who are working to make our towns and cities green and healthy and with those who are working to stop chemical contamination.

We must link up with those who are working to restore democracy and with those who are working to change our laws so that corporations serve the greater good of the Earth, not just their selfish desires.

There are millions who have walked, run and climbed mountains to raise money to find a cure for cancer. Think what we could do if we directed some of this effort to heal the Earth as a whole, and remove the causes of cancer.

Just think what we could do.

**Think big. One dollar for the search for a cure, one dollar for prevention. One for one.**

**— Dr. Ross Hume Hall, Professor Emeritus of Biochemistry, McMaster University Health Sciences Faculty**

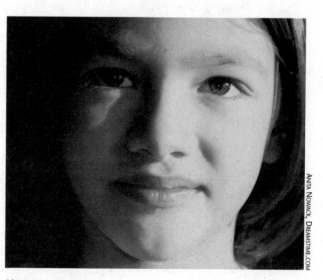

ANITA NOWACK, DREAMSTIME.COM

Hope.

# 101

# Don't Sit This One Out

**Anything else you're interested in is not going to happen if you can't breathe the air and drink the water. Don't sit this one out. Do something.**
— Carl Sagan, astronomer (1934–1996)

*Do something.* Such practical, down to earth advice from Carl Sagan, the brilliant American astronomer and educator. Sagan's own life was cut tragically short at 62 by bone marrow disease, a precursor to cancer.

Who have *you* loved and lost to this heartbreaking disease? In whose memory will you do something to stop this cancer epidemic?

Reduced to a single word, the message of this book is "Enough." We no longer accept that cancer has become a recognized disease of childhood. Or that so many women of all ages wear scarves and turbans awaiting an uncertain fate from breast cancer. Or that more and more young men are diagnosed with testicular cancer. Or that so many workers die "making a living."

May the end of this book mark a beginning for you. There have been many themes, because so many factors contribute to cancer. In turn there are so many ways you can make a difference. "Statistics are people with the tears washed off," the saying goes. We urge you to transform your tears into action.

The challenge to stop the cancer epidemic is huge, but you aren't alone. There are many others who feel the same way, who also want to "do something." All of us *can* make a difference in helping to restore the Earth as a flourishing, fit, sustainable home for everyone — all children, all species, all of us.

Speak up. Use your voice and your vision of a healthy world to create the changes we need. As Audre Lorde wrote in *The Cancer Journals*, "Silence has never brought us anything of worth."

Nourish the strength you have in friends and family, especially those who believe in you and support what you're doing. There will be days when progress seems painfully slow, if there's any at all — that's when to call your loved ones, to share and get things in perspective. It's so much easier when you have special people who are there for you, who understand what you are doing.

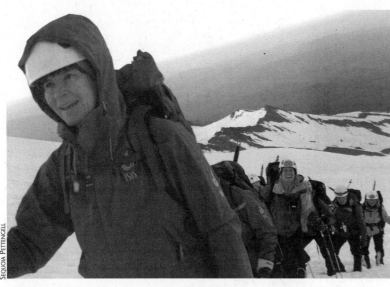

SEQUOIA PETTENGELL

Shasta Lake breast cancer survivor Kay Kobe climbs to the top of California's 14,000 ft. Mt. Shasta in the Breast Cancer Fund's cancer prevention event Climb Against the Odds, July 2006. www.breastcancerfund.org

**Call it a clan, call it a network, call it a tribe, call it a family. Whatever you call it, whoever you are, you need one.**

**— Jane Howard, journalist and author**

Another small piece of advice: Take courage, and remember to laugh. While working to root out the prime causes of this most anguishing of all diseases, share as much love, joy and laughter as possible. Remember the Fifth Law of Sustainability — *If it's not fun, it's not sustainable*.

Keep your spirits up. We humans have created many dire conditions on our planet, but being sad and despondent won't help. The best remedy for depression is positive, life-affirming action.

Our world is changing. There are millions of people whose hearts, like yours, are full of determination. We believe a better world is possible. We can all do something to be the change we want to see.

As the feisty, compassionate, courageous feminist Bella Abzug often said, "We must stop waiting to be rescued by someone else. We are the ones we've been waiting for."

Nobody will give us a world without cancer, war or hunger. We have to claim it. We have to pick up our courage, join with others, and make it happen.

**One person can make all the difference in the world. For the first time in recorded human history, we have the fate of the whole planet in our hands.**

**— Chrissie Hynde, singer and animal rights activist**

**For me it is more interesting to live as a part of the resistance against the forces of death that are destroying life than it is to simply accede to them and say that we can't change them. As a minimum I want to be able to tell my grandchildren that I was part of the resistance; and at the maximum, that the resistance became a peaceful movement that created a sustainable world.**

**— Michael Lerner, founder of Commonweal, and Collaborative for Health and the Environment**

**If you think you are too small to have an impact, try sleeping in a room with a mosquito.**

**— African proverb**

**Twenty years from now you will be more disappointed by the things that you didn't do than by the ones you did do. So throw off the bowlines. Sail away from the safe harbor. Catch the trade winds in your sails. Explore. Dream. Discover.**

**— Mark Twain**

**Another world is not only possible, she is on her way. On a quiet day, I can hear her breathing.**

**— Arundhati Roy, author**

# Appendix 1

## IARC List of Cancer-Causing Agents, Mixtures and Exposures

This is the full list prepared by the International Agency for Research on Cancer, as of December 20, 2006. For the full technical references see http://monographs.iarc.fr/ENG/Classification/crthall.php.

There are other lists, including the California Environmental Protection Agency's list for Proposition 65 (see www.oehha.ca.gov/prop65.html) and the US National Toxicology Program's Report on Carcinogens (see http://ntp.niehs.nih.gov).

### Group 1: Carcinogenic to Humans (100)

AGENTS AND GROUPS OF AGENTS

4-Aminobiphenyl
Arsenic and arsenic compounds
Asbestos
Azathioprine
Benzene
Benzidine
Benzo[a]pyrene
Beryllium and beryllium compounds
N,N-Bis (2-chloroethyl)-2-naphthylamine (Chlornaphazine)
Bis(chloromethyl)ether and chloromethyl methyl ether

1,4-Butanediol dimethanesulfonate (Busulphan; Myleran)
Cadmium and cadmium compounds
Chlorambucil
1-(2-Chloroethyl)-3-(4-methyl-cyclohexyl)-1-nitrosourea (Methyl-CCNU; Semustine)
Ciclosporin
Cyclophosphamide
Diethylstilboestrol
Epstein-Barr virus
Erionite
Estrogen-progestogen menopausal therapy
Estrogen-progestogen oral contraceptives
Estrogens, nonsteroidal
Estrogens, steroidal
Estrogen therapy, postmenopausal
Ethylene oxide
Etoposide in combination with cisplatin and bleomycin
Formaldehyde
Gallium arsenide
*Helicobacter pylori* (infection with)
Hepatitis B virus (chronic infection with)
Hepatitis C virus (chronic infection with)
Human immunodeficiency virus type 1 (infection with)
Human papillomavirus types

Human T-cell lymphotropic virus type I
Melphalan
8-Methoxypsoralen (Methoxsalen) plus ultraviolet A radiation
MOPP and other combined chemotherapy including alkylating agents
Mustard gas (Sulfur mustard))
2-Naphthylamine
Neutrons
Nickel compounds
N'-Nitrosonornicotine (NNN) and 4-(N-Nitrosomethylamino) -1-(3-pyridyl)-1-butanone (NNK)
*isthorchis viverrini* (infection with)
Oral contraceptives, sequential
Phosphorus-32, as phosphate
Plutonium-239 and its decay products (may contain plutonium-240 and other isotopes), as aerosols
Radioiodines, short-lived isotopes, including iodine-131, from atomic reactor accidents and nuclear weapons detonation (exposure during childhood)
Radionuclides, a-particle-emitting, internally deposited
Radionuclides, b-particle-emitting, internally deposited
Radium-224 and its decay products

Radium-226 and its decay
products
Radium-228 and its decay
products
Radon-222 and its decay
products
*Schistosoma haematobium*
(infection with)
Silica crystalline (inhaled in the
form of quartz or cristobalite
from occupational sources)
Solar radiation
Talc containing asbestiform
fibres
Tamoxifen
2,3,7,8-Tetrachlorodibenzo-
*para*-dioxin
Thiotepa
Thorium-232 and its decay
products, administered
intravenously as a colloidal
dispersion of thorium-232
dioxide
Treosulfan
Vinyl chloride
X- and Gamma (g)-Radiation

## MIXTURES

Aflatoxins (naturally
occurring mixtures of)
Alcoholic beverages
Areca nut
Betel quid with and without
tobacco
Coal tar pitches

Coal tars
Herbal remedies containing
plant species of the genus
*Aristolochia*
Household combustion of coal,
indoor emissions from
mineral oils, untreated and
mildly treated
Phenacetin, analgesic mixtures
containing
Salted fish (Chinese-style)
Shale-oils
Soots
Tobacco, smokeless
Wood dust

## EXPOSURE CIRCUMSTANCES

Aluminium production
Arsenic in drinking water
Auramine, manufacture of
Boot and shoe manufacture and
repair
Chimney sweeping
Coal gasification
Coal tar distillation
Coke production
Furniture and cabinet making
Haematite mining (underground)
with exposure to radon
Involuntary smoking (exposure
to second-hand or "environ-
mental" tobacco smoke)
Iron and steel founding
Isopropyl alcohol manufacture
(strong-acid process)

Magenta, manufacture of
Painter (occupational exposure
as a)
Paving and roofing with coal tar
pitch
Rubber industry
Strong-inorganic-acid mists
containing sulfuric acid
(occupational exposure to)
Tobacco smoking and tobacco
smoke

## Group 2A: Probably carcinogenic to humans (68)

### AGENTS AND GROUPS OF AGENTS

Acrylamide
Adriamycin
Androgenic (anabolic) steroids
Aristolochic acids (naturally
occurring mixtures of)
Azacitidine
Benzidine-based dyes
Bischloroethyl nitrosourea
1,3-Butadiene
Captafol
Chloramphenicol
a-Chlorinated toluenes (benzal
chloride, benzotrichloride,
benzyl chloride) and benzoyl
chloride (combined exposures)
1-(2-Chloroethyl)-3-cyclohexyl-
1-nitrosourea (CCNU)
4-Chloro-*ortho*-toluidine
Chlorozotocin

Cisplatin
*Clonorchis sinensis* (infection
  with)
Cyclopenta[*cd*]pyrene
Dibenz[*a,h*]anthracene
Dibenzo[*a,l*]pyrene
Diethyl sulfate
Dimethylcarbamoyl chloride
1,2-Dimethylhydrazine
Dimethyl sulfate
Epichlorohydrin
Ethylene dibromide
*N*-Ethyl-*N*-nitrosourea
Etoposide
Glycidol
Indium phosphide
IQ (2-Amino-3-methylimidazo
  [4,5-*f*]quinoline)
Kaposi's sarcoma
  herpesvirus/human
  herpesvirus 8
Lead compounds, inorganic
5-Methoxypsoralen
4,4´-Methylene bis(2-chloroani-
  line)
Methyl methanesulfonate
*N*-Methyl-*N*´-nitro-*N*-
  nitrosoguanidine(MNNG)
*N*-Methyl-*N*-nitrosourea
Nitrate or nitrite (ingested)
  under conditions that result
  in endogenous nitrosation
*N*-Nitrosodiethylamine
*N*-Nitrosodimethylamine
Phenacetin

Procarbazine hydrochloride
Styrene-7,8-oxide
Teniposide
Tetrachloroethylene
*ortho*-Toluidine
Trichloroethylene
1,2,3-Trichloropropane
Tris(2,3-dibromopropyl)
  phosphate
Ultraviolet radiation A
Ultraviolet radiation B
Ultraviolet radiation C
Vinyl bromide
Vinyl fluoride

**MIXTURES**

Creosotes
Diesel engine exhaust
High-temperature frying,
  emissions from
Hot mate
Household combustion of
  biomass fuel (primarily
  wood), indoor emissions from
Non-arsenical insecticides
  (occupational exposures in
  spraying and application of)
Polychlorinated biphenyls

**EXPOSURE CIRCUMSTANCES**

Art glass, glass containers and
  pressed ware (manufacture of)
Carbon electrode manufacture
Cobalt metal with tungsten
  carbide

Hairdresser or barber (occupational exposure as a)
Petroleum refining (occupational exposures in)
Sunlamps and sunbeds (use of)

**Group 2B: Possibly carcino-
genic to humans (246)**

AGENTS AND GROUPS OF
AGENTS

A-a-C (2-Amino-9*H*-pyrido[2,3-
  *b*]indole)
Acetamide
Acrylonitrile
AF-2 [2-(2-Furyl)-3-(5-nitro-2-
  furyl)acrylamide]
Aflatoxin M1
*para*-Aminoazobenzene
*ortho*-Aminoazotoluene
2-Amino-5-(5-nitro-2-furyl)-
  1,3,4-thiadiazole
Amsacrine
*ortho*-Anisidine
Antimony trioxide
Aramite®
Auramine
Azaserine
Aziridine
Benz[*j*]aceanthrylene
Benz[*a*]anthracene
Benzo[*b*]fluoranthene
Benzo[*j*]fluoranthene
Benzo[*k*]fluoranthene
Benzofuran Benzo[*c*]
  phenanthrene

Benzyl violet 4B

2,2-Bis(bromomethyl)propane-1,3-diol

Bleomycins

Bracken fern

Bromodichloromethane

Butylated hydroxyanisole

b-Butyrolactone

Caffeic acid

Carbon black

Carbon tetrachloride

Catechol

Chlordane

Chlordecone (Kepone)

Chlorendic acid

para-Chloroaniline

3-Chloro-4-(dichloromethyl)-5-hydroxy-2(5H)-furanone

Chloroform

1-Chloro-2-methylpropene

Chlorophenoxy herbicides

4-Chloro-ortho-phenylenediamine

Chloroprene

Chlorothalonil

Chrysene

CI Acid Red 114

CI Basic Red 9

CI Direct Blue 15

Citrus Red No. 2

Cobalt and cobalt compounds

Cobalt sulfate and other soluble cobalt(II) salts

para-Cresidine

Cycasin

Dacarbazine

Dantron (Chrysazin; 1,8-Dihydroxyanthraquinone)

Daunomycin

DDT

N,N'-Diacetylbenzidine

2,4-Diaminoanisole

4,4'-Diaminodiphenyl ether

2,4-Diaminotoluene

Dibenz[a,h]acridine

Dibenz[a,j]acridine

7H-Dibenzo[c,g]carbazole

Dibenzo[a,h]pyrene

Dibenzo[a,i]pyrene

1,2-Dibromo-3-chloropropane

2,3-Dibromopropan-1-ol

Dichloroacetic acid

para-Dichlorobenzene

3,3'-Dichlorobenzidine

3,3'-Dichloro-4,4'-diaminodiphenyl ether

1,2-Dichloroethane

Dichloromethane (methylene chloride)

1,3-Dichloropropene (technical-grade)

Dichlorvos

1,2-Diethylhydrazine

Diglycidyl resorcinol ether

Dihydrosafrole

Diisopropyl sulfate

3,3'-Dimethoxybenzidine (ortho-Dianisidine)

para-Dimethylaminoazobenzene

trans-2-[(Dimethylamino)

methylimino]-5-[2-(5-nitro-2-furyl)-vinyl]-1,3,4-oxadiazole

2,6-Dimethylaniline (2,6-Xylidine)

3,3'-Dimethylbenzidine (ortho-Tolidine)

1,1-Dimethylhydrazine

3,7-Dinitrofluoranthene

3,9-Dinitrofluoranthene

1,6-Dinitropyrene

1,8-Dinitropyrene

2,4-Dinitrotoluene

2,6-Dinitrotoluene

1,4-Dioxane

Disperse Blue 1

1,2-Epoxybutane

Ethyl acrylate

Ethylbenzene

Ethyl methanesulfonate

2-(2-Formylhydrazino)-4-(5-nitro-2-furyl)thiazole

Fumonisin B1

Furan

Glu-P-1 (2-Amino-6-methyldipyrido[1,2-a:3',2'-d]imidazole)

Glu-P-2 (2-Aminodipyrido

Glycidaldehyde

Griseofulvin

HC Blue No. 1

Heptachlor

Hexachlorobenzene

Hexachloroethane

Hexachlorocyclohexanes

Hexamethylphosphoramide

Human immunodeficiency virus type 2 (infection with)
Human papillomavirus types 6 and 11
Human papillomavirus genus beta (some types)
Hydrazine
1-Hydroxyanthraquinone
Indeno[1,2,3-*cd*]pyrene
Iron-dextran complex
Isoprene
Lasiocarpine
Lead
Magenta (containing CI Basic Red 9)
Magnetic fields (extremely low-frequency)
MeA-*a*-C (2-Amino-3-methyl-9*H*-pyrido[2,3-*b*]indole)
Medroxyprogesterone acetate
MeIQ (2-Amino-3,4-dimethylimidazo[4,5-*f*]quinoline)
MeIQx (2-Amino-3,8-dimethylimidazo[4,5-*f*]quinoxaline)
Merphalan
2-Methylaziridine (Propyleneimine)
Methylazoxymethanol acetate
5-Methylchrysene
4,4′-Methylene bis(2-methylaniline)
4,4′-Methylenedianiline
Methylmercury compounds

2-Methyl-1-nitroanthraquinone
*N*-Methyl-*N*-nitrosourethane
Methylthiouracil
Metronidazole
Microcystin-LR
Mirex
Mitomycin C
Mitoxantrone
Monocrotaline
5-(Morpholinomethyl)-3-[(5-nitrofurfurylidene)amino]-2-oxazolidinone
Nafenopin
Naphthalene
Nickel, metallic
Niridazole
Nitrilotriacetic acid and its salts
5-Nitroacenaphthene
2-Nitroanisole
Nitrobenzene
6-Nitrochrysene
Nitrofen
2-Nitrofluorene
1-[(5-Nitrofurfurylidene)amino]-2-imidazolidinone
*N*-[4-(5-Nitro-2-furyl)-2-thiazolyl]acetamide
Nitrogen mustard N-oxide
Nitromethane
2-Nitropropane
1-Nitropyrene
4-Nitropyrene
*N*-Nitrosodi-*n*-butylamine
*N*-Nitrosodiethanolamine
*N*-Nitrosodi-*n*-propylamine

3-(*N*-Nitrosomethylamino) propionitrile
*N*-Nitrosomethylethylamine
*N*-Nitrosomethylvinylamine
*N*-Nitrosomorpholine
*N*-Nitrosopiperidine
*N*-Nitrosopyrrolidine
*N*-Nitrososarcosine
Ochratoxin A
Oil Orange SS
Oxazepam
Palygorskite (attapulgite) (long fibres, > 5 micrometres)
Panfuran S (containing dihydroxymethylfuratrizine)
Phenazopyridine hydrochloride
Phenobarbital
Phenolphthalein
Phenoxybenzamine hydrochloride
Phenyl glycidyl ether
Phenytoin
PhIP (2-Amino-1-methyl-6-phenylimidazo[4,5-*b*]pyridine)
Polychlorophenols and their sodium salts (mixed exposures)
Ponceau MX
Ponceau 3R
Potassium bromate
Progestins
Progestogen-only contraceptives
1,3-Propane sultone
b-Propiolactone
Propylene oxide
Propylthiouracil

Refractory ceramic fibres
Riddelliine
Safrole
*Schistosoma japonicum* (infection with)
Sodium *ortho*-phenylphenate
Special-purpose fibres such as E-glass and '475' glass fibres
Sterigmatocystin
Streptozotocin
Styrene
Sulfallate
Surgical implants and other foreign bodies: Polymeric implants prepared as thin, smooth film (with the exception of poly(glycolic acid)). Metallic implants prepared as thin smooth films. Implanted foreign bodies of metallic cobalt, metallic nickel and an alloy powder containing 66-67% nickel, 13-16% chromium and 7% iron
Tetrafluoroethylene
Tetranitromethane
Thioacetamide
4,4'-Thiodianiline
Titanium dioxide
Thiouracil
Toluene diisocyanates
Trichlormethine (Trimustine hydrochloride)
Trp-P-1 (3-Amino-1,4-dimethyl-5*H*-pyrido[4,3-*b*]indole)

Trp-P-2 (3-Amino-1-methyl-5*H*-pyrido[4,3-*b*]indole)
Trypan blue
Uracil mustard
Urethane
Vanadium pentoxide
Vinyl acetate
4-Vinylcyclohexene
4-Vinylcyclohexene diepoxide
Zalcitabine
Zidovudine

## MIXTURES

Bitumens, extracts of steam-refined and air-refined
Carrageenan, degraded
Chlorinated paraffins of average carbon chain length C12 and average degree of chlorination approximately 60%
Coffee (urinary bladder) NB: There is some evidence of an inverse relationship between coffee drinking and cancer of the large bowel; coffee drinking could not be classified as to its carcinogenicity to other organs
Diesel fuel, marine
Engine exhaust, gasoline
Fuel oils, residual (heavy)
Gasoline
Pickled vegetables (traditional in Asia)
Polybrominated biphenyls

Toxaphene (Polychlorinated camphenes)
Toxins derived from *Fusarium moniliforme*: fumonisin B1 and B2 and fusarin C
Welding fumes

### EXPOSURE CIRCUMSTANCES

Carpentry and joinery
Cobalt metal without tungsten carbide
Dry cleaning (occupational exposures in)
Printing processes (occupational exposures in)
Talc-based body powder (perineal use of)
Textile manufacturing industry (work in)

# Appendix 2

## Glossary

**Age-standardized incidence rate (or age-adjusted rate)**: A statistical procedure used to modify disease rates to a standard population in order to minimize the effects of age differences when comparing different populations. Since cancer is more common in older people, an older average population will have a higher crude incidence rate. The purpose of establishing age-standardized rates is to make comparisons between groups of people from different backgrounds and ages more equitable.

**Cancer**: The uncontrolled growth of abnormal, malignant cells. Cancer can begin in virtually any organ of the body. About 40% of all non-skin cancers will be fatal, usually by spreading through the body in a process called metastasis.

**Carcinogen**: Any substance or process known to cause cancer. The International Association for Research on Cancer (IARC) reports five categories:

1. known human carcinogens
2A. probable human carcinogens
2B. possible human carcinogens
3. not classifiable as carcinogenic to humans
4. probably not carcinogenic to humans

**Chromosome**: A threadlike structure in the nucleus of the cell that carries a body's genetic information. Humans have 23 pairs of chromosomes.

**Dioxins and furans**: The name given to a group of toxic chemicals created by industrial processes that use chlorine, such as the manufacture of bleached paper products or the incineration of polyvinyl chloride (PVC) plastics.

**DNA** (Deoxyribonucleic acid): The genetic material of living organisms; the substance of heredity. DNA is a large, double-stranded, helical molecule that contains genetic instructions for growth, development and replication. The rungs of this double helix are made of base pairs.

**DNA adduct**: A marker of exposure to a particular carcinogen such as those found in PAHs or tobacco smoke, creating an altered form of DNA. If normal repair mechanisms are successful, the DNA returns to its original structure. If incorrectly repaired, the adduct results in a mutation, increasing the risk of cancer.

**Electromagnetic radiation** (EMR): Non-ionizing radiation that includes electrical fields, magnetic fields, radiofrequency transmissions and microwaves.

**Endocrine gland**: A specialized gland in the body that produces a hormone, secreting it directly into the bloodstream. Endocrine glands control many bodily mechanisms for development.

**Endocrine- (or Hormone-) disrupting chemical**: A chemical that disturbs the body's hormonal balance (such as dioxin), interfering with its ability to develop and function normally. Some endocrine disruptors act like the hormone estrogen and may be referred to as "xenoestrogens."

**Environment (and environmental cancers)**: In its broadest sense, "environment" encompasses the full range of physical, chemical, biological, social and cultural factors that influence human life and survival. To many cancer prevention activists, "environmental" carcinogens are toxic substances beyond an individual's control, such as end-of-pipe pollutants; toxic chemicals in air, water and soil; or ionizing radiation from nuclear waste. In this book, "environmental" also embraces natural carcinogens such as asbestos and cosmic radiation as well as all carcinogenic substances we "choose" such as tobacco smoke, x-rays and pharmaceutical drugs. "Environmental" thus describes all causes of cancer that are not hereditary.

**Epidemiology**: The study of the distribution and determinants of disease in human populations. In order for the International Agency for Research on Cancer (IARC) to declare an agent a human carcinogen (Group 1), conclusive epidemiological studies must support a causal relationship.

**Epigenetics**: The study of heritable changes in genome function that occur without changing the sequence of the DNA.

**Hormone**: A substance produced by an endocrine gland that controls key aspects of growth and development, and which is effective at very low concentrations.

**In utero**: Before birth, literally "in the uterus."

**In vitro**: In vitro studies are those conducted in an artificial environment, e.g., on cells in a laboratory dish, rather than in a living organism. From the Latin meaning "in glass."

**In vivo**: Studies conducted in a living organism such as humans or other animals.

**Lipophilic**: Fat-seeking, a term most often applied to chemicals such as DDT and PCBs that enter the fatty tissues of living organisms.

**Organochlorine**: Any hydrocarbon pesticide that contains chlorine. Many organochlorine

pesticides, such as DDT and chlordane, persist in body fat for years. Organochlorines may also be endocrine disruptors and xenoestrogens and are believed to promote the growth of cancer cells.

**Parabens**: Endocrine-disrupting compounds used as preservatives in thousands of cosmetic, food and pharmaceutical products.

**Persistent organic pollutants** (POPs): Organic chemicals that are persistent in the environment and in our bodies, usually in fatty tissues. These include polychlorinated biphenyls (PCBs) and organochlorines.

**Phthalates**: A group of hormone-mimicking chemicals used to render plastics soft and flexible, found in many household products and cosmetics.

**Phytoestrogens**: Plant estrogens that mimic and supplement the body's estrogen hormones, commonly found in whole grains, dried beans, peas, fruits, broccoli, cauliflower and soy products.

**Pineal gland**: A small endocrine gland in the midbrain that secretes many substances including the hormone melatonin, which is only secreted during darkness and appears to have anti-cancer properties.

**Polybrominated dipehnyl ethers** (PBDEs): Flame-retardants used in hundreds of consumer products including furniture, computers, televisions and automobiles.

**Polychlorinated biphenyls** (PCBs): A group of highly toxic, synthetic chemical compounds once used as insulation fluid in electrical transformers, lubricating oil in pipelines, components of plastics and mixed with adhesives, paper, inks, paints and dyes.

**Polycyclic aromatic hydrocarbons** (PAHs): By-products of combustion, including high-temperature cooking of meats and fish, the burning of cigarettes and other tobacco products and the combustion of fuels such as diesel, gasoline and heating oil.

**Polyvinyl chloride** (PVC): A type of plastic also referred to as vinyl used in construction materials, packaging, medical products, appliances, cars, toys, credit cards and rainwear. Contains heavy metals such as lead and cadmium as well as phthalates, all of which can be ingested by children when vinyl toys are sucked or chewed.

**Precautionary principle**: States that when an activity raises the threat of harm to human health or the environment, precautionary measures should be taken even if some cause and effect relationships are not fully established scientifically.[1]

**Prevention**: There are four definitions: *Primordial prevention* refers to preventing the creation of known and suspected causes of cancer. *Primary prevention* generally describes the elimination of risk factors for cancer. *Secondary prevention* aims to discover cancers or its precursors early enough to keep people from dying of the disease, using tools such as Pap smears for cervical cancer and fecal occult blood tests (FOTB) for colon cancer. *Tertiary prevention* is treatment, including prevention and early detection, of second primary cancers in individuals who already have cancer.

**Primary prevention**: Describes strategies that generally fall into two categories — those aimed at changing individual behavior and those aimed at improving environmental conditions. Public health campaigns over the past several decades have tended to favor the former, focused on individuals taking personal responsibility for their health. With relatively few improvements in the mortality rates of some cancers, it is increasingly recognized that the broader environmental approach must also be adopted.

**Radiation**: Energy transmitted in the form of rays, waves or particles. There are two types of radiation: ionizing and non-ionizing. Ionizing radiation can strike genetic material and break off ions, changing the way new cells are formed. Exposure to ionizing radiation occurs during medical procedures such as x-rays and other radiological diagnostic tests, during the mining and processing of uranium and other radioactive ores, from nuclear weapons manufacture and testing, from nuclear accidents such as those at Chernobyl and Three Mile Island, and from hazardous waste produced by nuclear power plants. Non-ionizing radiation is electromagnetic radiation (EMR), which includes electromagnetic fields from power lines and electric appliances, microwaves, and radiofrequency (RF) radiation from cellular phones and transmission towers and antennas.

**Risk**: The chance that a person may eventually develop a particular disease. When comparing two groups, risk can be expressed as a relative risk of disease, or the odds of getting a disease.

**Risk factor**: Anything that increases a person's chance of getting a disease whether as a cause or as a risk marker. Factors associated with decreased risk are known as protective.

**Screening**: The testing of apparently healthy people to separate those who may have a disease from those who probably don't. Positive screening (e.g., with a Pap smear or mammogram) is generally followed up with more complicated diagnostic testing to confirm that the suspected disease is present.

**Synergy, synergistic**: The interaction of two or more elements or forces that results in an effect greater than the sum of the individual effects. This is a key concept in understanding why current regulation of hazardous substances does not take real-world exposures into account. Substances are often regulated as if people were exposed to them one at a time when, in fact, multiple exposures occur every day in our air, water, food and all our environments, such as work and school.

**Xenoestrogens**: Chemicals that mimic the action of estrogen in the body. From the Greek word *xeno* meaning "foreign."

# Notes

## Part One: The Global Epidemic

### THE GLOBAL CANCER CRISIS

1. Rachel Carson. *Silent Spring*. Houghton Mifflin, p. 242, 1962.
2. The button was created by the Women's Community Cancer Project in Cambridge, MA.
3. Rachel Carson's books about the ocean: *Under the Sea Wind* (1941), *The Sea Around Us* (1951), *The Edge of the Sea* (1955). Another book, *The Sense of Wonder*, was published posthumously in 1965. All are still in print.
4. Rachel Carson. *Silent Spring*. Houghton Mifflin, 1994 edition, p. 243.
5. W.C. Heuper and W.D. Conway. *Chemical Carcinogenesis and Cancers*. Springfield: Charles C. Thomas, 1964.
6. *Canadian Cancer Statistics 2006*, p. 13.
7. Because population profiles change over time, it is necessary to "standardize" them: Age-adjusted (or standardized) rates mathematically remove the effects of different population structures that influence overall rates: umanitoba.ca/centres/mchp/concept/thesaurus/thesaurus_references.html (#99-02).
8. Environmental Working Group: chemicalindustryarchives.com/factfiction/facts/4.asp.
9. *Canadian Cancer Statistics 2004*, pp. 40, 42.
10. National Cancer Institute Research on Childhood Cancers: cancer.gov/cancertopics/factsheet/Sites-Types/childhood.
11. *Cancer in Young Adults, Cancer Care Ontario and the Public Health Agency of Canada, 2006*. Highlights, p. 1: cancer.ca.
12. L.X. Clegg, et al. "Impact of Reporting Delay and Reporting Error on Cancer Incidence Rates and Trends." *J Natl Cancer Inst*, 94, pp. 1537-45, 2002.
13. WHO. *Global Cancer Rates Could Increase by 50 Percent to 15 Million by 2020*: who.int/mediacentre/news/releases/2003/pr27/en/index.html.
14. D. Max Parkin, et al. "Global Cancer Statistics, 2002." *CA Cancer J Clin*, 55, pp. 74-108, 2005.

### OUR BODY BURDEN

1. *Body by the Numbers*. UC Davis Health System, 2000.
2. *Body Burden: The Pollution in People*. Environmental Working Group, 2003. For details of these and many other studies, see ewg.org/bodyburden. Accessed Aug. 21, 2006.
3. *Toxic Nation: A Report on Pollution in Canadians*. Environmental Defence Canada, 2005.
4. European Biomonitoring Study, 2004. Accessed Aug. 21, 2006 from WWF: detox.panda.org/the_problem/blood_testing_meps.cfm.
5. *Body Burden: Mother's Milk*. Accessed Aug. 21, 2006 from Environmental Working Group: ewg.org/bodyburden.
6. *Body Burden: Pollution in Newborns*. Accessed Aug. 21, 2006 from Environmental Working Group: ewg.org/bodyburden.
7. C. Charlier, et al. "Analysis of Polychlorinated Biphenyl Residues in Human Plasma by Gas Chromatography-Mass Spectrometry." *Journal of Analytical Toxicology*, 27(2), pp. 74-77(4), March 2003.
8. L. Hardell, et al. "Adipose Tissue Concentrations of Persistent Organic Pollutants and the Risk of Prostate Cancer." *Journal of Occupational & Environmental Medicine*, 48 (7), pp. 700-07, July 2006.

### THE COST OF CANCER

1. Steve Johnson. "Global Sales of Cancer Drugs Are Expected to Double." *Mercury News*, Jan. 30, 2006.
2. Matthew Herper. "Cancer's Cost Crisis." *Forbes*, June 8, 2004.
3. Genentech media statement on Avastin pricing, March 29, 2006.
4. David U. Himmelstein, Elizabeth Warren, Deborah Thorne and Steffie Woolhandler. "Illness and Injury as Contributors to Bankruptcy." *Health Affairs*, Feb. 2, 2005.
5. American Academy of Pediatricians. Accessed Aug. 21, 2006: ww.aap.org/advocacy/washing/Medicaid_today_testimony.htm.

6. Lisa Priest. "Ontario: Cancer Drugs for the Rich." *Globe and Mail*, May 5, 2006.
7. J.S. Bailes. "The Economics of Cancer Care." *Cancer*, 76(suppl), pp. 1886-87, 1995.
8. *Multi-site Cancer Data Collection System.* Accessed Aug. 21, 2006: washington.edu/uif/uif2b/med.html.
9. Public Health Agency of Canada. Accessed Aug. 21, 2006: ebic-femc.hc-sc.gc.ca/figures/table_2_e.pdf.
10. See hanabiosciences.com/pipeline-cb.html. Accessed Aug. 21, 2006.

## WHAT CAUSES CANCER?

1. Richard Clapp, Genevieve Howe and Molly Jacobs. "Environmental and Occupational Causes of Cancer Revisited." *Journal of Public Health Policy*, pp. 61-76, 2006.
2. See note 1.
3. *Child Health and the Environment: A Primer*, p. 30: healthyenvironmentforkids.ca.
4. *Canadian Cancer Statistics 2006*, p. 49.
5. R. Doll and R. Peto. "The Causes of Cancer: Quantitative Estimates of Avoidable Risks of Cancer in the United States Today." *Journal of the National Cancer Institute*, 66, pp. 1191-308, 1981.
6. "Harvard Reports on Cancer Prevention, Vol. I: Human Causes of Cancer." *Cancer Causes & Control*, 7, Nov. 1996: hsph.harvard.edu/cancer/resources_materials/reports/index.htm.
7. R. Doll. "Epidemiological Evidence of the Effects of Behavior and the Environment on the Risk of Human Cancer." *Recent Results in Cancer Research*, 154, pp. 3-21, 1998.
8. R. Clapp, M. Jacobs and G. Howe. *Environmental and Occupational Causes of Cancer: A Review of Recent Scientific Literature*. Lowell Center for Sustainable Production, 2005: healthandenvironment.org.
9. L. Hardell, et al. "Secret Ties to Industry and Conflicting Interests in Cancer Research." *American Journal of Industrial Medicine*, 2006. Accessed Nov. 21, 2006: ourstolenfuture.org/Industry/2006/

2006-1103hardelletal.html. Until 1957 Sir Richard Doll and his wife were members of the Norland branch of the Communist Party in Kensington, London. This allegiance to the cause of social and economic justice fits well with his achievements in public health care and tackling the tobacco industry. With his subsequent allegiance to the agro-chemical industry, he undermined the very same cause by opposing and ignoring evidence that pointed to the environmental causes of cancer, and lending his authority to the conventional explanation of cancer as being caused by "personal lifestyle and diet," with only the smallest of roles being assigned to occupational and environment causes.
10. Martin Walker. "Sir Richard Doll: A Questionable Pillar of the Cancer Establishment." *The Ecologist*, 28(2), March/April 1998.

## WHAT ABOUT AGING, GENETICS AND LIFESTYLE?

1. "Chasing the Cancer Answer," *CBC Marketplace*, March 2006: cbc.ca/consumers/market/files/health/cancer.
2. Canadian Cancer Control Strategy Business Plan: cancer.ca/vgn/images/portal/cit_86751114/35/52/1024277471cw_cscc_business_plan%20_april28_en.pdf.
3. *Canadian Cancer Statistics 2006*, p. 49.
4. American Cancer Society. *Cancer Facts & Figures 2006*, p. 1.
5. Ibid.
6. See note 1.
7. Report Card: Pesticides in Produce: foodnews.org/reportcard.php.
8. Why Organic Bedding? ecobaby.com/cribmattresses.htm.

## THE ENVIRONMENTAL LINKS

1. Obituary of Sir Richard Doll. *Daily Telegraph*, London, July 25, 2005.
2. The American Cancer Society estimated that 162,460 people would die from lung cancer in the US in 2006 (Cancer Facts and Figures 2006. Atlanta, GA: American Cancer Society, 2006); the Canadian

Cancer Society (CCS) estimated 19,300, giving a total of 181,760 (CCS Annual Cancer Statistics). Among men, 80% of the lung cancer is caused by smoking, 75% in women, totaling around 140,000 deaths a year from smoking in North America. Over 50 years, with smaller populations in the earlier years but more people smoking, the total deaths come to around 5 million people.

3. The evidence summarized here is taken from *Environmental and Occupational Causes of Cancer: A Review of Recent Scientific Literature*, by Richard Clapp, Genevieve Howe and Molly Jacobs, University of Massachusetts Lowell Center for Sustainable Production, 2005, which contains 175 footnotes to peer-reviewed scientific papers. See healthandenvironment.org/working_groups/cancer.

CANCER IN CHILDREN

1. In Europe the International Agency for Research on Cancer (IARC) data shows cancer rates rising by 1% a year for children, and 1.5% a year for adolescents. See news.bbc.co.uk/2/hi/health/4079343.stm. See also E. Steliarova-Foucher, C.Stiller, et al., "Geographical Patterns and Time Trends of Cancer Incidence and Survival Among Children and Adolescents in Europe Since the 1970s (the ACCIS project): An Epidemiological Study," *Lancet, 374*, pp. 2097-105, 2004.

2. The US data shows a 27% increase between 1975 and 2002 from 11.5 to 14.6 per 100,000 people. National Cancer Institute Research on Childhood Cancers: cancer.gov/cancertopics/factsheet/Sites-Types/childhood.

3. From 1976 to 2001 the incidence of cancer among Canadian boys and young men up to 19 years old increased by 13.5%. The rate among girls and young women increased by 29.1%. *Canadian Cancer Statistics 2005*, Fig. 8, p. 54.

4. 17% in Canada.

5. "Cancer in Children and Youth." *Canadian Cancer Statistics 2006*, p. 68: cancer.ca.

6. Mary Bachran and Theo Colborn. "Fetal Origins of Cancer Spreadsheet," 2005: healthandenvironment.org/wg_cancer_news/365.

7. Dr. Perera, et al. "Chromosomal Aberrations in Cord Blood Are Associated with Prenatal Exposure to Carcinogenic Polycyclic Aromatic Hydrocarbons." *Epidemiology Biomarkers and Prevention, 14*, pp. 506-11, Columbia University Center for Children's Environmental Health, Feb. 2005.

8. T. Gouveia-Vigeant, J. Tickner and R. Clapp. *Toxic Chemicals and Childhood Cancer: A Review of the Evidence.* Lowell Center for Sustainable Production, 2003.

9. *Body Burden: The Pollution in Newborns.* Environmental Working Group, July 2005: ewg.org.

10. US EPA. *Guidelines for Carcinogen Risk Assessment and Supplemental Guidance for Assessing Susceptibility from Early-Life Exposure to Carcinogens:* cfpub.epa.gov/ncea/cfm/recordisplay.cfm?deid=116283

11. Jack K. Leiss and David A. Savitz. "Home Pesticide Use and Childhood Cancer: A Case-control Study." *Am J Public Health, 85*, pp. 249–52, 1995.

12. R. Lowengart, et al. "Childhood Leukemia and Parents' Occupational and Home Exposures." *Journal of the National Cancer Institute (JNCI)*, pp. 39-46, July 1987.

13. A. Stewart and G.W. Kneale. "Radiation Dose Effects in Relation to Obstetric X rays and Childhood Cancers." *Lancet, 1*, pp. 1185-88, June 6, 1970.

14. G. Draper, T. Vincent, M.E. Kroll and J. Swanson. "Childhood Cancer in Relation to Distance from High Voltage Power Lines in England and Wales: A Case-control Study." *British Medical Journal, 330*, pp. 1290-94, 2005.

15. Twenty-two out of 4,000 is 1 per 181. The normal rate is 15 per 100,000, or 1 per 6,666. When Jean-Dominique persuaded researchers at Hôpital Sainte-Justine in Montreal to compile the official statistics, they found that the cancer rate on Île Bizard was four times that for the entire province of Quebec. See note 15.

16. "A Young Crusader Speaks About Pesticides, Children, and Cancer." Evidence to the Standing Committee on Environment and Sustainable

Development, Ottawa, ON, Sept. 23, 2001:
chebucto.ns.ca/Health/Nsaeha/sep01speak.html.

## CANCER IN ANIMALS AND FISH

1. Daniel Martineau, et al. "Cancer in Wildlife, a Case Study: Beluga from the St. Lawrence Estuary, Québec, Canada." *Environmental Health Perspectives*, *110*(3), pp. 285–92, March 2002.
2. Sandra Steingraber. *Living Downstream*,Vintage Books, p. 139, 1997.
3. Catherine Couillard. *A Multiple Bioindicator Approach to Assess Risk of Liver Cancer in Fish*. Fisheries and Oceans Canada, 2002.
4. Dr. Joseph Gaydos. *Wildlife Are Sentinels of Ocean Health*. Marine Ecosystem Health Program at U.C. Davis Wildlife Health Center. Surfrider: mehp.vetmed.ucdavis.edu/pdfs/SurfriderGaydos.pdf.
5. *Living Downstream*, p. 138.
6. "Study Finds Higher Rates of Bladder Cancer Among Dogs Exposed to Herbicides." *Cleveland Plain Dealer*, March 3, 2005: ewg.org/news/story.php?id=3646.
7. M. Sears, C.R. Walker, R.H.C. van der Jagt and P. Claman. "Pesticide Assessment: Protecting Public Health on the Home Turf." *Pediatrics and Child Health*, *11*(4), pp. 229-34, April 2006: pulsus.com/Paeds/11_04/sear_ed.htm.
8. *Living Downstream*, p. 138.
9. *Tainted Catch: Toxic Fire-retardants in San Francisco Bay Fish – and People*. Environmental Working Group, 2003: ewg.org/reports/taintedcatch.

## RISK ASSESSMENT — THE PRECAUTIONARY PRINCIPLE

1. John Wargo. *Our Children's Toxic Legacy: How Science and Law Fail to Protect Us from Pesticides*. Yale University Press, 1998.
2. Shoe-fitting x-ray devices: mtn.org/quack/devices/shoexray.htm.
3. Dennis J. Paustenbach. *Retrospective on US Health Risk Assessment: How Others Can Benefit*: piercelaw.edu/Risk/Vol6/fall/Pausten.htm.
4. Peter Waldman. "Common Industrial Chemicals in Tiny Doses Raise Health Issue." *Wall Street Journal*, July 25, 2005.

## CHANGING THE CANCER PARADIGM

1. R. Doll and R. Peto. "The Causes of Cancer: Quantitative Estimate of Avoidable Risks of Cancer in the United States Today." *Journal of the National Cancer Institute*, *66*, pp. 1191-308, 1981.
2. Many critics believe that the 1981 Doll and Peto report was the conservative response to the 1978 "Estimates Paper" endorsed by Joseph Califano, then US Secretary of Health, Education and Welfare, which claimed 20% to 40% of all cancers were caused by occupational risks. Robert Proctor's 1995 book, *Cancer Wars: What We Know and Don't Know About Cancer*, provides an excellent overview of this issue and the era.
3. Harvard Center for Cancer Prevention. Accessed Jan. 1, 2007: hsph.harvard.edu/cancer/resources_materials/reports/index.htm.
4. P. Nineis and L. Simonato. *Arch Environ Health*, 1991. The multifactorial approach was used by researchers from the International Agency for Research in Cancer in 1991 who analyzed results of many studies of newly diagnosed lung and bladder cancer.
5. US Federal Chemicals Policy. Accessed Aug. 21, 2006: chemicalspolicy.org/usfederal.shtml.
6. Nancy Trautmann. *The Dose Makes the Poison: Or Does It?* Jan. 2005. Accessed Jan. 1, 2007: actionbioscience.org/environment/trautmann.html.

## IT'S NOT JUST CANCER

1. Sarah Janssen, Gina Solomon and Ted Schettler. *Chemical Contaminants and Human Disease: A Summary of Evidence*. Collaborative on Health and the Environment, 2004: healthandenvironment.org.
2. "Pollutants Cause Huge Rise in Brain Diseases." *Observer*, Aug. 15, 2004.
3. "Hot on Parkinson's Trail." *Los Angeles Times*, Nov. 27, 2005.
4. Sandra Steingraber. "Origins of Dementia." *Rachel's Environment and Health News*, *776* and *777*, Sept. 4, 2003.
5. R.H. Dunstan, et al. *Preliminary Evidence for an Association Between Chlorinated Hydrocarbons and*

*Chronic Fatigue Syndrome*. First World Congress on Chronic Fatigue Syndrome and Related Disorders, Brussels, 1995. Also "Waking Up to Chronic Fatigue," *New Scientist*, May 20, 2006.
6. *Traffic Pollution Shown to Damage Sperm Quality*. Reuters, April 29, 2003.
7. Reported with many other studies in *Infertility and Related Reproductive Disorders* by Ted Schettler, Science Director, Science and Environmental Health Network, 2003.
8. Ibid.
9. Melissa Knopper. "Auto Exposure: Do Immune System Diseases Have an Environmental Cause?"*E-Magazine*, May 1, 2005.
10. Ted Schettler. *Developmental Disabilities. Impairment of Children's Brain Development and Function: The Role of Environmental Factors*. Collaborative on Health and the Environment, 2004: healthandenvironment.org.

### PREVENTION, EARLY DETECTION AND SCREENING

1. Dan Ferber. "Carcinogens: Lashed by Critics, WHO's Cancer Agency Begins a New Regime." *Science*, *301*(5629), p. 36, July 4, 2003.
2. Home page, National Cervical Cancer Coalition. Accessed Dec. 31, 2006: nccc-online.org.
3. Ibid.
4. Canadian Cancer Society. Progress in cancer control: Screening. Accessed Jan. 2, 2007: cancer.ca/ccs/internet/standard/0,3182,3172_ 367655_933585249_langId-en,00.html.
5. Dr. Susan Love Research Foundation. Accessed Jan. 2, 2007: susanlovemd.com/breastcancer/ content.asp?L2=1&SID=119.
6. Breast Cancer Action. *Breast Cancer Screening and "Early Detection"*. Accessed Jan. 8, 2007: bcaction.org/Pages/LearnAboutUs/ BreastCancerScreening.html.
7. "Cancer Prevention and the American Society of Clinical Oncology." Editorial by the Writing Committee of the ASCO Cancer Prevention Committee. *Journal of Clinical Oncology*, *22* (19), pp. 3848-51, 2004: jco.org/cgi/content/full/22/19/3848.

8. L. Tomatis. "Identification of Carcinogenic Agents and Primary Prevention of Cancer." *Ann. N.Y. Acad. Sci.*, *1076* (1–14), p. 1, 2006.
9. See note 1.
10. Tomatis, p. 10.
11. Ibid., p. 12.

### OUR WEAKENED IMMUNITY

1. J. Michael Bishop. "What Causes Cancer: Genetic Sloppiness, the Cellular 'Social Contract,' and Malignancy." *Harvard Magazine*, March/April 2003: harvardmagazine.com/on-line/030392.html.
2. "Emerging Science on the Impacts of Endocrine Disruptors on the Immune System and Disease Resistance." *Our Stolen Future*: ourstolenfuture.org/ NewScience/immune/immune.htm.
3. R. Repetto and S. Baliga. *Pesticides and the Immune System: The Public Health Risks*. World Resources Institute, 1996.
4. "Statement from the Work Session on Chemically Induced Alterations in the Developing Immune System," by a multidisciplinary group of international experts who gathered to evaluate current science on the immune system effects of chemical contaminants in Racine, WI, Feb. 1995. *Environmental Health Perspectives* Suppl. 4, pp. 807-08, 1996. See *Our Stolen Future*, above.
5. F.M. Pottenger, Jr. *Pottenger's Cats: A Study in Nutrition*. Price-Pottenger Nutrition Foundation, 1995. Available from price-pottenger.org.
6. Sandra Steingraber. *Having Faith: An Ecologist's Journey to Motherhood*. Penguin, pp. 230-34, 2001.
7. Andrew Weil. *Spontaneous Healing*. Fawcett Columbine, p. 274, 1995.

### THE CHEMICAL DELUGE

1. *Guide to Less Toxic Products*. Environmental Health Association of Nova Scotia: lesstoxicguide.ca/ index.asp?fetch=usage#synthetic.
2. Ibid.
3. Michael P. Wilson. *Green Chemistry in California*. California Policy Research Center, University of

California, 2006:
ucop.edu/cprc/greenchemistryrpt.pdf.

4. Ibid., p. xii.

5. Ibid., p. 34.

6. James Huff and Ronald Melnick. "What Are the Real Causes of Cancer?" *International Journal of Occupational and Environmental Health, 12* (1), p. 83, January/March 2006.

7. *Everyday Carcinogens: Stopping Cancer Before It Starts,* p. 10: stopcancer.org/pdf/bgpaper.pdf.

8. John Wargo. *Our Children's Toxic Legacy: How Science and Law Fail to Protect Us from Pesticides.* New Haven, CT: Yale University Press, 1996.

9. Scorecard: scorecard.org/chemical-profiles/def/basic_det.html.

## GENDER BENDERS

1. Peter Waldman. "Toxic Traces: New Questions About Old Chemicals." *Wall Street Journal,* A1, July 25, 2005.

2. Paul Goettlich. *What Are Endocrine Disruptors?*: mindfully.org/Pesticide/EDs-PWG-16jun01.htm.

3. "Long-term HRT Doubles Breast Cancer Risk." *New Scientist,* Aug. 8, 2003: newscientist.com/article.ns?id=dn4038.

4. *Our Stolen Future: Are We Threatening Our Fertility, Intelligence and Survival? – A Scientific Detective Story.* Dutton, p. 19, 1996.

5. The "xeno-estrogen" theory advanced by H. Leon Bradlow, Devra Davis and other members of the Breast Cancer Prevention Collaborative Research Group.

6. *Decline in Breast Cancer Cases Likely Linked to Reduced Use of Hormone Replacement.* News release, University of Texas, M.D. Anderson Cancer Center, Dec. 14, 2006.

## CANCER WHERE YOU WORK

1. Larry Stoffman. Personal communication, Feb. 2006.

2. P. Infante. "Cancer and Blue-collar Workers: Who Cares? *New Solutions, 5* (2), 1995.

3. *Take Immediate Action to Protect Communities and Workers.* Background paper for Reform

No. 6 of the Louisville Charter for Safer Chemicals, p. 4.

4. "Burying the Evidence." *Hazards Magazine, 92,* Nov. 2005: hazards.org/cancer/report.htm.

5. "High-Tech Industry Challenges Safety Rules." *Houston Chronicle,* Sept.27, 1998.

## CANCER WHERE YOU LIVE

1. Michael Marmot. *What Are the Social Determinants of Health?* UN Commission on Social Determinants of Health, Feb. 19, 2006.

2. Dimitrios Trichopoulos, Frederick P. Li and David J. Hunter. "What Causes Cancer?" *Scientific American,* Sept. 1996.

3. Peter L. Schnall, Kanan Patel-Coleman and Maritza Jauregui. *Work and Health.* UCLA Center for Occupational and Environmental Health: workhealth.org.

4. "More Blacks Live with Pollution." Chicago AP, Dec. 14, 2005.

5. Tim Montague. "Environmental Justice and Precaution." *Rachel's Democracy & Health News, 770,* May 29, 2003.

6. Athena Thompson. *Homes That Heal (and Those That Don't).* New Society Publishers, p. 102, 2004.

## CANCER FROM CARS, TRUCKS AND BUSES

1. *Injury Chartbook.* World Health Organization, 2002.

2. *Crude Reckoning: The Impact of Petroleum on California's Public Health and Environment.* Center for Energy Efficiency and Renewable Technologies, Sacramento, 2000.

3. *Link Strengthened Between Lung Cancer, Heart Deaths and Tiny Particles of Soot, Dust.* National Institute of Environmental Health Sciences, March 5, 2002.

4. Ami Patel, et al. "Chronic Low Level Exposure to Gasoline Vapors and Risk of Cancer: A Community-Based Study." University of Pittsburgh. *Epidemiology, 15*(4), July 2004.

5. *What Is Benzene?* American Cancer Society website, accessed Dec. 14, 2006.

6. Terry Taminen. *Lives Per Gallon: The True Cost of Our Addiction to Oil*. Island Press, p. 22, 2006.
7. Ibid., p. 19, quoting the study by Gina Solomon, et al., *No Breathing in the Aisles: Diesel Exhaust Inside School Buses*. NRDC and Coalition for Clean Air, Jan. 2001.
8. William C. Hinds. *Southern California Environmental Report Card 2001*, University of California, Los Angeles.
9. *Crude Reckoning: The Impact of Petroleum on California's Public Health and the Environment*. Center for Energy Efficiency and Renewable Technologies, Sacramento CA, Aug. 2000.
10. *Lives Per Gallon*, p. 30.
11. "State of Denial." *Sacramento Bee*, April 27, 2003.
12. *Regulatory Impact Assessment for Petroleum Refineries.* US EPA, Washington DC, 1995.

THE WAY WE FARM

1. *Globe and Mail*, July 5, 2002.
2. Analysis by David Thomas of nutritional values listed in McCance and Widdowson, "The Composition of Foods, UK Food Standards Agency," comparing the 1940 and 2002 editions, published in *Food Magazine*, Feb. 2006.
3. H.D. Foster. "Selenium and Cancer: A Geographical Perspective." *Journal of Orthomolecular Medicine 13* (1), pp. 8-10, 1998. See also papers by Harold Foster: hdfoster.com.
4. UK Food Standards Agency. *Food Surveillance Information Sheet Number 126*. Accessed Nov. 21, 2006: archive.food.gov.uk/maff/archive/food/ infsheet/1997/no126/table2.htm. See also H.D. Foster, "Selenium and Cancer: A Geographical Perspective," *Journal of Orthomolecular Medicine, 13*(1), pp. 8-10, 1998; and papers by Harold Foster: hdfoster.com.
5. G.A. Potter, et al. "The Cancer Preventative Agent Resveratrol Is Converted to the Anticancer Agent Piceatannol by the Cytochrome P450 Enzyme CYP1B1." *British Journal of Cancer, 86*, pp. 774-78, 2002.
6. Charles Benbrook, PhD., chief scientist, Organic Center for Education and Promotion. "Elevating Antioxidant Levels in Food Through Organic Farming and Food Processing." *State of Science Review*, Jan. 2005. Accessed Nov. 21, 2006: organic-center.org/reportfiles/Antioxidant_SSR.pdf.
7. Alyson Mitchell, et al. "Comparison of the Total Phenolic and Ascorbic Acid Content of Freeze-Dried and Air-Dried Marionberry, Strawberry, and Corn Grown Using Conventional, Organic, and Sustainable Agricultural Practices." *Journal of Agricultural and Food Chemistry*, Feb. 26, 2003.
8. V. Worthington. Nutritional Quality of Organic Versus Conventional Fruits, Vegetables, and Grains. *The Journal of Alternative and Complementary Medicine, 7* (2), pp. 161-73, 2001. See also *Organic Farming, Food Quality and Human Health: A Review of the Evidence*. A review of over 400 published papers. Soil Association (UK), 2001.
9. See (e.g.) M.C.R. Alavanja, et al. "Use of Agricultural Pesticides and Prostate Cancer Risk in the Agricultural Health Study Cohort." *American Journal of Epidemiology, 157*, pp. 800-14, 2003.
10. Devra Lee Davis and David Hoel. "Agricultural Exposures and Cancer Trends in Developed Countries." *Environmental Health Perspectives, 100*, pp. 39-44, 1992; Aaron Blair, et al. "Clues to Cancer Etiology from Studies of Farmers." *Scandinavian Journal of Work, Environment and Health, 18*, pp. 209-15, 1992.
11. *Shoppers Guide to Pesticides in Produce*. Environmental Working Group: foodnews.org.
12. Margaret Munro. "Pesticides Discovered in Amniotic Fluid Could Lead to Feminization of Male Fetuses." *National Post*, June 15, 1999.
13. *Healthy Milk, Healthy Baby, Chemical Pollution and Mother's Milk*. Natural Resources Defense Council, 2005.
14. *Environmental Chemicals Implicated in Cancer*. Press release, University of Liverpool, March 21, 2006.
15. Brian Halweil. "Can Organic Farming Feed Us All?" *World Watch Magazine*, May/June 2006.

THE FOOD WE EAT

1. E.E. Calle. "Overweight, Obesity, and Mortality from Cancer in a Prospectively Studied Cohort of

U.S. Adults." *New England Journal of Medicine, 348* (17), April 24, 2003.

2. *Diet, Nutrition, and Cancer.* US National Research Council, 1982.

3. W.E.M. Lands, T. Hamazaki, K. Yamazaki, et al. "Changing Dietary Patterns." *Am J Clin Nutr, 51,* pp. 991-93, 1990.

4. *The China Study II.* Cornell University, Oxford University, Chinese Academy of Preventive Medicine.

5. *Food, Nutrition and the Prevention of Cancer: A Global Perspective.* American Institute for Cancer Research, 1997: aicr.org.

6. A. Trichopoulou, K. Katsouyanni, S. Stuver, et al. "Consumption of Olive Oil and Specific Food Groups in Relation to Breast Cancer Risk in Greece." *J Natl Cancer Inst, 87,* pp. 110-16, 1995.

7. R. Frentzel-Beyne and J. Chang-Claude. "Vegetarian Diets and Colon Cancer: The German Experience." *Am J Clin Nutr, 59* (suppl.), pp. 1143S-52S, 1994.

8. W.E.M. Lands, T. Hamazaki, K. Yamazaki, et al. "Changing Dietary Patterns." *Am J Clin Nutr, 51,* pp. 991-93, 1990.

9. S.A. Bingham. "Are Imprecise Methods Obscuring a Relation Between Fat and Breast Cancer?" *Lancet, 362* (9379), pp. 182-83, July 19, 2003.

10. "Fruit and Vegetable Intake and Risk of Major Chronic Disease." *Journal of the National Cancer Institute, 96*(21), pp. 1577-84, Nov. 3, 2004.

11. *European Prospective Investigation into Cancer and Nutrition.* IARC Press Release 157, Jan. 12, 2005.

12. Ross Prentice, et al. "Low-Fat Dietary Pattern and Risk of Invasive Breast Cancer." *JAMA, 295,* pp. 629-42, Feb. 8, 2006.

13. Winston J. Craig, Professor of Nutrition at Andrews University, Berrien Springs, MI. *Phytochemicals: Guardians of Our Health*: vegetarian-nutrition.info/vn/phytochemicals.htm.

14. Shane Heaton. *Organic Farming, Food Quality and Human Health.* Soil Association, 2001: soilassociation.org.

15. "Perchlorate Found in Produce from Around the World." *Science News,* April 26, 2006.

16. Lu Chensheng. American Association for the Advancement of Science, St. Louis, Feb. 19, 2006: hon.ch/News/HSN/531114.html.

### Awash in Pesticides

1. Charlotte Pomerantz. *The Day They Parachuted Cats on Borneo: A Drama of Ecology.* As told at the Rocky Mountain Institute website: rmi.org/sitepages/pid157.php.

2. John Wargo. *Our Children's Toxic Legacy*, p. ix.

3. Dr. Margaret Sanbord, et al. "Pesticides Literature Review." Ontario College of Family Physicians, April 23, 2004.

4. Ibid.

5. Canadian Association of Physicians for the Environment (CAPE): cape.ca/cancer3.html.

6. Allan Woodburn Associates. "Agrochemicals: Executive Review." Reported in "First Growth in Global Agrochemical Market for a Decade," *Agrow, 466,* p. 17, Feb. 18, 2005.

7. Top Six Agrochemical corporations, 2004: organicconsumers.org/foodsafety/ biotechpesticides080805.cfm.

### For Everyone's Sake, Stop Smoking

1. *Info-tabac.* Newsletter for a Tobacco-Free Quebec: smoke-free.ca/info-tabac/default.htm.

2. Joseph R. DiFranza, et al. "Development of Symptoms of Tobacco Dependence in Youths." Department of Family Medicine and Community Health, University of Massachusetts Medical School, Worcester, MA. *Tobacco Control, 11,* pp. 228-35, 2002.

3. For a list of 599 known additives, see quitsmokingsupport.com/ingredients.htm. See also, cancer.gov/cancertopics/factsheet/ Tobacco/ETS.

4. John R. Polito. *Nicodemon's Lies?*: whyquit.com/whyquit/A_NicodemonsLies.html.

5. US smokers, over 40%: americanheart.org/ presenter.jhtml?identifier=4731; Canadian smokers. "More than half": smoke-free.ca/factsheets/pdf/ Quitting%20Behaviours.pdf.

6. Physicians for a Smoke-Free Canada: smokefree.ca.
7. The Toxicology of Cigarette Smoke and Environmental Tobacco Smoke: csn.ul.ie/~stephen/reports/bc4927.html.
8. P. Reynolds, et al. *Journal of the National Cancer Institute*, Jan. 2004.
9. *Canadian Cancer Statistics 2006*, Cancer Facts & Figures 2006. American Cancer Society.
10. American Cancer Society, 2006: cancer.org/docroot/MED/content/MED_2_1x_Non-Smokers_with_Lung_Cancer_Respond_Better_to_Treatment_than_Smokers.asp.
11. "Blowing Smoke About Tobacco." *Washington Post*: washingtonpost.com/wp-dyn/content/article/2006/05/29/AR2006052900734.html.
12. *The Health Consequences of Involuntary Exposure to Tobacco Smoke: A Report of the Surgeon General*: surgeongeneral.gov/library/secondhandsmoke.
13. Centers for Disease Control ETS Fact Sheet: cdc.gov/tobacco/research_data/environmental/factsheet_ets.htm.
14. ETS and lung cancer in Canada: gov.ns.ca/ohp/tcu/health_effects.htm.
15. American Lung Association. *State of Tobacco Control: 2005*. In 2005 nine smoke-free states prohibited smoking in almost all workplaces, including restaurants and bars: CA, CT, DE, ME, MA, NY, RI, VT and WA.

ELECTROMAGNETIC RADIATION

1. What are EMFs and EMRs?: ecopraxis.co.uk/faq/faq.htm.
2. World Health Organization. *Typical Electromagnetic Fields at Home and in the Environment*: who.int/peh-emf/about/WhatisEMF/en/index3.html.
3. Nancy Wertheimer and Ed·Leeper. "Electrical Wiring Configurations and Childhood Cancer." *American Journal of Epidemiology*, 109 (3), pp. 273-84, 1979.
4. Magda Havas, Trent University faculty. Personal communication, 2004.
5. World Health Organization. *Extremely Low Frequency (ELF) Magnetic Radiation a "Possible Human Carcinogen"*: who.int/mediacentre/factsheets/fs263/en.
6. Louis Slesin. "A Report on Non-Ionizing Radiation." *Microwave News*. Blog, Jan. 21, 2005: microwavenews.com.
7. Ibid.
8. "Is It OK...to Use a Mobile Phone?" *Guardian*, June 27, 2006.
9. Tyler Hamilton and Robert Cribb. "Kids at Risk?" *Toronto Star*, July 9, 2005.

CANCER HAZARD OF IONIZING RADIATION

1. Dr. Rosalie Bertell. Personal communication, Jan. 2003.
2. Radioactive consumer products: orau.org/PTP/collection/consumer%20products/consumer.htm.
3. *Biological Effects of Ionizing Radiation (BEIR) VI Report: The Health Effects of Exposure to Indoor Radon*: epa.gov/iaq/radon/beirvi.html.
4. Radium "girls" and cancer: mun.ca/biology/scarr/Radium_Watch-Dial_Painters.html.

RADIATION AND NUCLEAR POWER

1. *Cancer Risks for Women and Children Due to Radiation Exposure Far Higher Than for Men*. Press release about BEIR VII, Institute for Energy and Environmental Research, July 7, 2005.
2. "All Levels of Radiation Confirmed to Cause Cancer." National Academies of Science BEIR VII Biological Effects of Ionizing Radiation report on *Health Risks from Exposure to Low Levels of Ionizing Radiation*: nirs.org/press/06-30-2005/1.
3. Final Report of the Committee Examining Radiation Risks of Internal Emitters, Oct. 2004: cerrie.org.
4. Joseph J. Mangano. "A Short Latency between Radiation Exposure from Nuclear Plants and Cancer in Young Children." *International Journal of Health Services*, 36 (1), 2006.
5. Quoted in Jay Gould, et al. *The Enemy Within: The High Cost of Living Near Nuclear Reactors*, Four Walls Eight Windows, 1996.
6. Chris Busby. *A Survey of Cancer in the Vicinity of Trawsfynydd Nuclear Power Station in North Wales*.

Green Audit, Aberystwyth, March 2006:
llrc.org/traws.htm.

7. E. Cardis, et al. "Cancer Risk Following Low Doses of Ionizing Radiation: A 15-country Study." *British Medical Journal*, June 29, 2005: iarc.fr/ENG/Units/RCAa1.pdf.

8. Carolyn Stephens and Mike Ahern. *Worker and Community Health Impacts Related to Mining Operations Internationally: A Rapid Review of the Literature.* London School of Hygiene and Tropical Medicine, MMSD Report 25, 2001.

9. "Echoes of the Atomic Age. Cancer Kills Fourteen Aboriginal Uranium Workers." *Calgary Herald*, March 14, 1998.

10. "Risk of Thyroid Cancer after Exposure to 131I in Childhood." *Journal of the National Cancer Institute*, 97, p. 724.

11. "Greenpeace Rejects Chernobyl toll." *BBC News*, April 18, 2006.

12. The US EPA was defeated in court for seeking only 10,000 years safety. The US National Academy of Sciences says 300,000 years. The Swedish government says a million years.

13. "Nuclear Stockpiles Could Create 300,000 Bombs." *New Scientist*, Sept. 7, 2005.

14. Rocky Mountain Institute position on nuclear power. Accessed Aug. 21, 2006: rmi.org/sitepages/pid305.php.

## THE CANCEROUS CORPORATION

1. *Toxic Deception: How the Chemical Industry Manipulates Science, Bends the Law and Endangers Your Health.* Review by Russell Mokhiber, April 21, 1999.

2. Jack Doyle. *Trespass Against Us: Dow Chemical and the Toxic Century.* Common Courage Press, 2004.

3. *BAT's Big Wheeze: The Alternative Report.* Friends of the Earth, UK, April 2004: foe.co.uk.

4. *Multinational Monitor, 10 Worst Corporations of 2005.* W.R. Grace: multinationalmonitor.org.

5. David Egilman and Susanna Rankin Bohme (Guest Eds.). "Over a Barrel: Corporate Corruption of Science and Its Effects on Workers and the Environment. *International Journal of Occupational and Environmental Health*, 11}(4),

Oct./Dec. 2005:
ijoeh.com/pfds/IJOEH_1104_Egilman.pdf.

6. Erika Rosenthal. "Who's Afraid of National Laws? Pesticide Corporations Use Trade Negotiations to Avoid Bans and Undercut Public Health Protections in Central America." *International Journal of Occupational and Environmental Health*, 11 (4), Oct./Dec. 2005.

7. Milton Friedman. "The Social Responsibility of Business Is to Increase Its Profits." *New York Times Magazine*, Sept. 13, 1970.

8. Debra Mayberry. "Just How Many Lobbyists Are There in Washington, Anyway?" *Washington Post*, Jan. 29, 2006.

## THE LIMITS — AND CORRUPTION — OF SCIENCE

1. Austin Bradford Hill. "The Environment and Disease: Association or Causation" in *Report to the Workers' Compensation Board on Lung Cancer in the Hardrock Mining Industry*, Report 12 of Canada Industrial Disease Standards Panel. Toronto, ON: IDSP, March 1994.

2. Devra Davis. *When Smoke Ran Like Water: Tales of Environmental Deception and the Battle Against Pollution.* Basic Books, p. 21, 2002.

3. C.V. Phillips and K.J. Goodman. "The Missed Lessons of Sir Austin Bradford Hill." *Epidemiologic Perspectives and Innovations*, 1(3), 2004, doi:10.1186/1742-5573-1-3.

4. *When Smoke Ran Like Water*, p. 136.

5. David Egilman and Susanna Rankin Bohme. "Over a Barrel: Corporate Corruption of Science and Its Effects on Workers and the Environment." *Int J Occup Environ Health*, 11, pp. 331-37, 2005.

6. Boyce Rensberger. "Science Abuse: Subverting Scientific Knowledge for Short-term Gain." *Scientific American*, Sept. 26, 2005.

7. Dr. Shiv Chopra. *Corrupt to the Core.* KOS Publishing, 2007.

## BIG PHARMA AND THE WAR ON CANCER

1. Ralph W. Moss. *The Cancer Industry.* Equinox Press, Brooklyn, 2002. 1996 edition update, p. vii.

2. Guy Faguet. *The War on Cancer: An Anatomy of a Failure*. Springer, 2005, p. 5. 1997 is the last year for which statistics were available at the time of the book's publication.
3. *The War on Cancer*, pp. xiv, 5.
4. "Chasing the Cancer Answer," *CBC Marketplace*: cbc.ca/consumers/market/files/health/cancer/cashing.html.
5. Thomas J. Moore. *Prescription for Disaster*. Dell, 1998.
6. Ibid., p. 23.
7. Books by Shiv Chopra, Ralph Moss and Samuel Epstein.
8. *Prescription for Disaster*, p. 101.
9. Marcia Angell. *The Truth About the Drug Companies: How They Deceive Us and What to Do About It*. Random House, p. 250, 2005.
10. *The War on Cancer*, p. 123.
11. Ibid., p. 124.
12. From a workshop by Barbara Mintzes, University of Toronto, Nov.1, 2005.
13. *The Truth About the Drug Companies*, p. 252.
14. "CWHN Writes the Minister of Health Re: Diane-35 Drug Ads." Feb. 17, 2004: cwhn.ca.

## WHO IS PROTECTING US?

1. Robert F. Kennedy, Jr. "Crimes Against Nature." *Rolling Stone*, Dec. 11, 2003: commondreams.org/views03/1120-01.htm.
2. "President's Science Advisory Committee Report on Restoring the Quality of the Environment, 1965." Quoted in Edward S. Herman. "Fog Watch: Corporate Sovereignty and (Junk) Science." *Z Magazine*, Nov. 1998: zmag.org/Zmag/articles/nov98herman.htm.
3. For a good analysis of US chemicals policy, see *Background Paper on a Child-Safe US Chemicals Policy*, Children's Environmental Health network, 2005: cehn.org.
4. See note 2.
5. For a good coverage of the legislative status, see *Chemical Regulation: Approaches in the United States, Canada, and the European Union*, United States Government Accountability Office, Nov. 4, 2005: gao.gov/htext/d06217r.html.
6. Peter Montague. "In 2005 the Wheels Came off the US Chemical Regulatory System." *Rachel's Democracy and Health News*, *839*, Jan. 26, 2006.
7. Ibid.
8. Peter Montague. "The Regulatory Box We're In." *Rachel's Precaution Reporter*, *12*, Nov. 16, 2005.

## WHAT ARE CANCER CHARITIES AND HOSPITALS DOING TO PREVENT CANCER?

1. Samuel Epstein. *American Cancer Society: The World's Wealthiest "Nonprofit" Institution*: preventcancer.com/losing/acs/wealthiest_links.htm.
2. 2005 Cash and Cars Lottery: cashandcarslottery.ca/grand2.html.
3. Aptium Oncology: aptiumoncology.com.
4. Rachel Carson. *Silent Spring*. Houghton Mifflin, p. 241, 1962 (1994 edition).
5. *Is the American Cancer Society More Interested in Cancer Profit than Cancer Prevention?*: newstarget.com/010243.html.

## PREVENT CANCER NOW

1. Dr. Ross Hume Hall, Professor Emeritus, McMaster University, former Co-Chair, Human Health Committee, International Joint Commission. *Everyday Carcinogens: Stopping Cancer Before It Starts*, March 29, 1999: stopcancer.org/default2.asp?active_page_id=110.
2. Sweden's Environmental Objectives Portal: miljomal.nu/english/english.php.
3. "Reformers Launch National 'Voters First' Pledge to Build Support for Public Funding of Congressional Campaigns." *Common Cause*, June 21, 2006.

## Part Two: 101 Solutions

### SOLUTION 2

1. Gina Kolata. "But Will It Stop Cancer?" *New York Times*, Nov. 1, 2005.
2. Harvard Center for Cancer Prevention. *Reports on Cancer Prevention, Volume I: Human Causes of Cancer Exercise*, 1996.

3. US Environmental Protection Agency's List of Mobile Source Air Toxics (MSATS): epa.gov.omswww/regs/toxics/msatlist.pdf. Also, "Exercise Keeps Cancer Away", *BBC News*, Oct. 18, 2002: news.bbc.co.uk/1/hi/health/2339787.stm.

4. Caitlin Liu. "Stuck on the Freeway? Here's Something Else to Fume About." *Los Angeles Times*, Nov. 16, 2004.

5. American Cancer Society website: cancer.org. Search "If you drink alcoholic beverages, limit consumption."

6. Carolyn D Runowicz, Sheldon H Cherry and Dianne Lange. *The Answer to Cancer*. Rodale, p. 255, 2004.

7. See cbc.ca/stories/2003/09/29/Consumers/ sunscreen030929.

8. See news.bbc.co.uk/2/hi/health/3226184.stm.

## Solution 3

1. The American Lung Association, among other sources: lungoregon.org/tobacco/companies.html.

2. Philip Morris USA admits smoking is addictive: philipmorrisusa.com/en/health_issues/default.asp.

3. *The Health Benefits of Smoking Cessation*. McGill University: sprojects.mmi.mcgill.ca/ smoking/quittingf/health_benefits.html.

4. "Cigarette Smoking Among Adults: United States, 2000." *Tobacco Information and Prevention Source* (TIPS), *51* (29), National Center for Chronic Disease Prevention and Health Promotion, July 26, 2002: cdc.gov/tobacco/research_data/adults_prev/ mmwr5129_highlights.htm.

5. *Health Harms from Second-hand Smoke*. Campaign for Tobacco-Free Kids: tobaccofreekids.org/ research/factsheets/pdf/0103.pdf.

6. *The Changing Cigarette: Chemical Studies and Bioassays*. National Cancer Institute: dccps.nci.nih.gov/tcrb/monographs/13/m13_5.pdf.

7. *Cancer Facts*. National Cancer Institute: cis.nci.nih.gov/fact/3_14.htm.

8. Donald R, Shopland. *Cigarette Smoking As a Cause of Cancer*: rex.nci.nih.gov/NCI_Pub_Interface/ raterisk/risks67.html.

9. "Active Smoking Associated with Increased Risk of Breast Cancer." *Journal of the National Cancer Institute*: sciencedaily.com/releases/2004/01/ 040107074305.htm.

10. *The Health Benefits of Smoking Cessation*. McGill University: sprojects.mmi.mcgill.ca/ smoking/quittingf/health_benefits.html.

11. *Facts about Lung Cancer*. The American Lung Association: lungusa.org/site/pp.asp?c= dvLUK9O0E&b=35427.

## Solution 4

1. From Dr. Ralph Moss's Cancer Decisions website: cancerdecisions.com/051003_page.html.

2. Virginia Worthington. "Nutritional Quality of Organic Versus Conventional Fruits, Vegetables and Grains." *Journal of Alternative and Complementary Medicine*, 7(2), pp. 161-73, April 2001.

3. The Organic Center for Education and Promotion outlines many of the benefits: organic-center.org.

4. Dr. Charles Benbrook. *Pesticides on Food: 'Almost No' Cancer Danger?*. See also, pmac.net/comments.htm and organic-center.org/about.staff.php?action= detail&bios_id=43.

5. C. Lu, et al. "Biological Monitoring Survey of Organophosphorus Pesticide Exposure Among Preschool Children in the Seattle Metropolitan Area." *Environmental Health Perspectives*, *109* (3), pp. 299-303, March 2001: nutrition4health.org/ NOHAnews/NNSp02PesticideExpChildren.htm.

6. R.H. Fletcher and K.M. Fairfield. "Vitamins for Chronic Disease Prevention in Adults: Clinical Applications." *AMA*, *287* (23), pp. 3128-129, 2002.

7. American Cancer Society. *Well-done Red Meat May Increase Cancer Risk in Some People*. Proceedings of the American Association for Cancer Research, 92nd Annual Meeting, *42*, Abstract No. 201, p. 38.

8. Susan Higginbotham, et al. "Dietary Glycemic Load and Risk of Colorectal Cancer in the Women's Health Study." *Journal of the National Cancer Institute*, *96* (3), pp. 229-33, Feb. 4, 2004.

9. Michael F. Jacobson. *Liquid Candy: How Soft Drinks Are Harming Americans' Health*, Center for Science

in the Public Interest: cspinet.org/sodapop/
liquid_candy.htm.

10. Harvard School of Public Health's Fats and
Cholesterol section: hsph.harvard.edu/
nutritionsource/fats.html.

11. For more on Salvestrol science, see
salvestrolscience.com.

12. Linus Pauling Institute. "Resveratrol": lpi.oregon-
state.edu/infocenter/phytochemicals/resveratrol/.

13. Udo Erasmus. *Fats That Kill, Fats That Heal*. Alive
Books, 1993.

## SOLUTION 5

1. See canada.com/ottawacitizen/news/story.html?
id=9e5a72a9-d392-4516-9c6d-551716cf9964.

2. Executive Summary of *Skin Deep: A Safety
Assessment of Ingredients in Personal Care Products*:
ewg.org/reports/skindeep.

3. Dr. Carolyn Dean. *Hormone Balance: A Woman's
Guide to Restoring Health and Vitality*. Adams Media,
2005.

4. Thomas J. Moore. *Prescription for Disaster*. Dell
Publishing, 1998.

5. L.A. Brinton, et al. "Mortality Among
Augmentation Mammoplasty Patients." *Annals of
Epidemiology, 12*, pp. 321-26, 2001.

6. L.A. Brinton, et al. "Cancer Risks at Sites Other
Than the Breast Following Augmenation
Mammoplasty." *Annals of Epidemiology, 11*, pp. 248-
56, 2001.

7. Sydney Singer and Soma Grismaijer. *Dressed to
Kill: The Link Between Breast Cancer and Bras*. Avery,
1995.

8. J.M. Dixon, et al. "Risk of Breast Cancer in Women
with Palpable Breast Cysts: A Prospective Study."
*Lancet, 353* (9166), pp. 1742-745, May 22, 1999.

9. Ralph L. Reed. *Prevention and Treatment of Fibrocystic
Breast Disease*. Natural Health and Longevity
Resource Center: all-natural.com/fibrocys.html.

## SOLUTION 6

1. Jane Kay. "Homes May Be Hazardous to Your
Health." *San Francisco Chronicle*, May 19, 2004.

2. Debra Lynn Dadd. Home, Safe Home website:
dld123.com/about/about.php?id=A33.

## SOLUTION 8

1. From eartheasy.com/grow_lawn_care.htm.

2. *Grass Cutting Beats Driving in Making Air Pollution*:
mindfully.org/Air/Lawn-Mower-Pollution.htm.

3. Lisa Foderaro. "In a Debate Over Trash Burning, It's
Rural Tradition vs. Health." *New York Times*, March
7, 2005.

4. *Astroturf: This Grass Is Always Greener*: mindfully.org/
Plastic/Nylon/AstroTurf-Always-Greener20apr03.htm.

5. Debra Lynn Dadd's chlorine-free swimming pool:
dld123.com/debraslist/list.php?topic=
Water%20#L00297.

## SOLUTION 9

1. Catherine Caulfield. *Multiple Exposures: Chronicles of
the Radiation Age*. Stoddart, p. 224, 1988.

2. Ibid., p. 202.

3. *Full Body CT Screening Found to Be Risky*. Columbia
University: cumc.columbia.edu/news/
in-vivo/Vol13_Iss10_sept_04/radiology.html.

4. Eric J. Hall. "Lessons We Have Learned from Our
Children: Cancer Risks from Diagnostic Radiology."
*Pediatric Radiology, 32* (10), Oct. 2002.

5. For more information about the ongoing mammography debate, see Breast Cancer Action's
website: bcaction.org/Pages/GetInformed/
MammographyAndNewTech.html.

6. Few realize that form of EMR from digital cordless
phones is likely to exceed exposure to
radio frequency (RF) energy from local cellphone
antennas and intermittent cellphone use. Personal
communication with Magda Havas, Trent
University, Jan. 4, 2007.

## SOLUTION 11

1. Sat Dharam Kaur. *The Complete Natural Guide to
Women's Health*. Robert Rose, Toronto, 2005.

2. National Cancer Institute Division of Cancer
Prevention: www.cancer.gov/prevention/
epigenetics/summary.html.

3. International Labour Organization. *Your Health and Safety at Work: Male and Female Reproductive Health Hazards in the Workplace*: itcilo.it/english/actrav/telearn/osh/rep/prod.htm#Appendix%20I.
4. Thousands of thalidomide babies were born with flipper-like hands sprouting from their shoulders, and numerous daughters of DES mothers later contracted a rare and sometimes fatal form of vaginal cancer.
5. *Body Burden: The Pollution in Newborns*. Executive Summary, Environmental Working Group, ewg.org.
6. Sandra Steingraber. *Having Faith: An Ecologist's Journey to Motherhood*. Berkley Publishing Group, 2003.

## SOLUTION 12

1. The editors of *E/The Environmental Magazine*. *Green Living, The E Magazine Handbook for Living Lightly on the Earth*. Penguin, New York, p. 175, 2005.

## SOLUTION 13

1. M.K. Davis, D.A. Savitz and B.I. Graubard. "Infant Feeding and Childhood Cancer." *Lancet, 2*, pp. 365-68, 1998.
2. *Mothers' Milk*. From sidebar, Executive Summary, a study by the Environmental Working Group, Sept. 2003, p. 1: ewg.org/reports/mothersmilk.
3. Canadian Partnership for Children's Health & Environment. *Child Health and the Environment: A Primer*, p. 63: healthyenvironmentforkids.ca.
4. Ibid., *Concerns with Infant Formulas*.
5. See checnet.org/healthehouse/chemicals/chemicals-detail-print.asp?Main_ID=275.

## SOLUTION 14

1. *Broadcasting Bad Health: Why Food Marketing to Children Needs to Be Controlled*. International Association of Consumer Food Organizations (IACFO), p. 5, July 2003.
2. *Healthy Eating, Part III: The Five Greatest Motivators for Pre-School Children to Eat Healthy Foods*: drgreene.com.

3. *Eating Organic for Less Than Processed Food*: mercola.com/2005/feb/16/organic_food.htm.
4. Environmental Working Group: foodnews.org.
5. Chensheng Lu, et al. "Organic Diets Significantly Lower Children's Dietary Exposure to Organophosphorus Pesticides." *Environmental Health Perspectives, 114* (2), Feb. 2006: ehponline.org/members/2005/8418/8418.pdf.
6. "Parental Exposure to Pesticides and Risk of Wilm's Tumor in Brazil." *American Journal of Epidemiology, 141* (3), pp. 210-17, 1995.

## SOLUTION 15

1. EPA, quoted by Coalition for Healthier Schools: healthyschools.org/documents/CHS_2006_Position_Statement.pdf.
2. "Girl's Illness Traced to 'Toxic' School: Some Doctors Alarmed by Hidden Chemicals at Schools." *Good Morning America*, ABC News, Oct.11, 2005.
3. "The ABCs of Healthy Schools." From the program BE SAFE, coordinated by the Center for Health, Environment & Justice, Falls Church, VA: besafenet.com.
4. "School Location Matters: Preventing School Siting Disasters": childproofing.org; and Clearinghouse REVIEW *Journal of Poverty Law and Policy*, May-June 2005.

## SOLUTION 16

1. *International Journal of Advertising & Marketing to Children*, pp. 49–50, July/Sept., 2002: kidstuff.com/info/facts.html.
2. Youth spending and the planet: newdream.org/buy/buydifferent.php.

## SOLUTION 17

1. Marketing cigarettes to children: ash.org.uk/html/conduct/html/tobexpld3.html.
2. StatsCanada: statcan.ca/Daily/English/040615/d040615b.htm.
3. "Cigarette Smoking Among American Teens Continues to Decline, But More Slowly Than in the Past." Dec. 21, 2004, monitoringthefuture.org.

4. Chris Lackner. "Smoking Among Teens Plummets." *Globe and Mail*, Aug. 10, 2004.
5. For the full commentary, go to womensenews.org/ article.cfm/dyn/aid/2025/context/archive. For information on smoking as a women's health issue, see "Issue Brief," National Research Center for Women and Families: center4research.org/ibrief-05-04smoking.html.
6. From googolplex.cuna.org/15378/ajsmall/ story.html?doc_id=889.
7. See frostillustrated.com/news/2005/0518/ Arts_And_Entertainment/023.html.
8. News-Medical.net: news-medical.net/?id=5374.
9. *The Global Impact of Tobacco*. June 30, 1997: corpwatch.org.

## SOLUTION 18

1. "Nalgene Water Bottles Appear to Be Unsafe": mercola.com/2004/apr/7/nalgene_water.htm. For Nalgene's perspective, see nalgene-outdoor.com/technical/bpainfo.html.
2. Paul Goettleich. *Get Plastics Out of Your Diet*: mindfully.org/Plastic/Plasticizers/ Out-of-DietPG5nov03.htm.
3. *The Green Guide Product Report: Sunscreen*: thegreenguide.com/reports/product.mhtml?id=27.
4. Ibid.
5. "New Evidence That Vitamin D Fights Cancer." *The Moss Reports*, June 12, 2005: cancerdecisions.com/061205.html.
6. "The Case Against Indoor Tanning": skincancer.org/artificial.
7. *MicroWave News* carries and comments on print media reports about cellular phones, including a 2005 series from the *Toronto Star*: microwavenews.com/fromthefield.html#tstar.
8. "Children and Mobile Phones ... Is There a Health Risk? The Case for Extra Precautions." *Journal of Australasian College of Nutritional & Environmental Medicine*, 22 (2), Aug. 2003.

## SOLUTION 19

1. Gary Ruskin, Executive Director, Commercial Alert. *Smoking Class: How Schools and Channel One Promote Tobacco to Students*. Sept. 2005: commercialalert.org/smokingclass.pdf.
2. "The Next Niche: School Bus Ads." *Washington Post*, June 4, 2006: commercialexploitation.org/news/busradio.htm.

## SOLUTION 20

1. Illai Kenney, quoted at the Earth Island Institute: earthisland.org/project/viewProject.cfm?subSiteID= 40.
2. Elizabeth May, quoted in *Vue* magazine (Edmonton, AB): vueweekly.com/articles/default.aspx?i=180.

## SOLUTION 27

1. 17 Principles of Environmental Justice, First National People of Color Environmental Leadership Summit, Washington DC, Oct. 1991.

## SOLUTION 31

1. Thomas Milne, Executive Director, National Association of County and City Health Officials. Quoted in "Public Health Professionals Afraid to Speak Out," *Rachel's Environment & Health Weekly*, *814*, March 31, 2005: rachel.org.
2. See extensive footnotes in *Rachel's Environment & Health Weekly*, *814*, March 2005: rachel.org.
3. Dr. Carolyn Bennett, Minister of Public Health. Speech to the Toronto Board of Trade, April 30, 2004.
4. *Rachel's Environment & Health Weekly*, *814*: rachel.org.
5. *Ensuring Risk Reduction in Communities with Multiple Stressors: Environmental Justice and Cumulative Risks/Impacts*: epa.gov/compliance/resources/publications/ej/nejac_publications.html.
6. The National Environmental Education & Training Foundation. *Position Statement, Health Professionals and Environmental Health Education*, Jan. 2004: neetf.org/Health/PositionStatement2.pdf.

## SOLUTION 32

1. Dr. Lieberman. Quoted on his website at the Center for Occupational & Environmental

Medicine, *Preconception Care*:
coem.com/preconception.asp.

2. T. Gouveia-Vigeant, J. Tickner and R. Clapp. *Toxic Chemicals and Childhood Cancer: A Review of the Evidence*, 2003: sustainableproduction.org/downloads/Child%20Canc%20Exec%20Summary.pdf.

3. Ted Schettler, Science Director, Science and Environmental Health Network. *Infertility and Related Reproductive Disorders*: healthandenvironment.org/infertility/peer_reviewed.

4. Sat Dharam Kaur. *The Complete Natural Medicine Guide to Women's Health*. Robert Rose, Oct. 2005.

5. Ted Schettler. *Infertility and Related Reproductive Disorders*: healthandenvironment.org/infertility/peer_reviewed.

## Solution 33

1. *Environmental Health Perspectives*, Dec. 2004: ehp.niehs.nih.gov/docs/2004/7166/abstract.html.

2. *Pediatric Environmental Health*, p. 559.

## Solution 34

1. Personal communication, 2005.

2. More information on the wider investigation of young African-American women's high incidence of breast cancer is available on the center's Environmental Exposure Links to Breast Cancer website: upci.upmc.edu/ceo/activities.html.

3. Dr. Margaret Sanborn, et al. *Pesticides Literature Review*, Ontario College of Family Physicians, April 2004.

4. CCS website: cancer.ca/ccs/internet/standard/0,2939,3172_335253__langId-en,00.html.

## Solution 35

1. "Health Care Without Harm": noharm.org/us/healthybuilding/issue.

2. Andrew Jameton and Jessica Pierce. "Environment and Health: 8. Sustainable Health Care and Emerging Ethical Responsibilities." *CMAJ*, Feb. 6, 2001, *164* (3): cmaj.ca/cgi/content/full/164/3/365.

3. "Hospitals: Green Revelation." Jan. 1, 2005: noharm.org/details.cfm?type=news&ID=88.

4. Continuum Center for Health and Healing Environmental Health & Design: healthandhealingny.org/center/environ.asp.

5. "Sick Children's Hospital Waste Reduction": c2p2online.com/documents/SickChildrenHospital.pdf.

6. Karen Olson. "The Greening of Health Care." *Utne Reader*, Nov./Dec. 2002.

7. Dominican Hospital organic food program: organicconsumers.org/hospitals21705.cfm.

## Solution 36

1. *New Internationalist* magazine *313*: newint.org/issue313/contents.htm.

2. *Innovative Solutions Create Urban Sustainability*: usinfo.state.gov/journals/itgic/0300/ijge/gj-04a.htm.

3. "Urban Health: Is the City Infected?" Lecture by Victor G. Rodwin, Director, World Cities Project, 2000: nyu.edu/projects/rodwin/urbanhealth.html.

## Solution 37

1. Vanessa Bird. "Green Cities." *New Internationalist*, *313*, June 1999: newint.org/issue313/keynote.htm.

2. From Johnson's presentation to Everyday Carcinogens: Stopping Cancer Before It Starts, McMaster University, March 1999. Conference transcripts, published by the Canadian Environmental Law Association, Toronto.

3. Text of San Francisco's Precautionary Principle Policy: greenaction.org/cancer/alert061803.shtml.

## Solution 38

1. *When Smoke Ran Like Water: Tales of Environmental Deception and the Battle Against Pollution*, Basic Books, p. 8, 2002.

2. Charlene Porter. "It Takes Us All, It Takes Forever." "Green Cities: Urban Environmental Solutions." *Global Issues*, an electronic journal of the US Department of State, *5* (1), March 2000: usinfo.state.gov/journals/itgic/0300/ijge/gj-08.htm.

## SOLUTION 39

1. From a keynote presentation to the conference, Everyday Carcinogens: Stopping Cancer Before It Starts, McMaster University, March 1999: stopcancer.org/default2.asp?active_page_id=112.
2. Jim Motavalli. "Zero Waste." *E/The Environmental Magazine*, March 2001.

## SOLUTION 40

1. For the full text of "Winterize Your Lawn" (by Anonymous), see achievebalance.com/think/lawn.htm.
2. Robert Fulford. "The Lawn: North America's Magnificent Obsession." *Azure*, July/Aug. 1998: robertfulford.com/lawn.html.
3. Joan Lowy. "More Lawns Go Green, Organically." *KnoxNews National*, Aug. 10, 2004.
4. *Pesticides and Human Health: A Resource for Health Care Professionals*. Physicians for Social Responsibility: pesticidereform.org; Ontario College of Family Physicians: ocfp.on.ca/English/OCFP/Communications/CurrentIssues/Pesticides/default.asp?s=1.
5. *CBC News*. "Pesticide Timeline": cbc.ca/news/background/pesticides/timeline/html.
6. Holden Frith. "Urban Farms: Oasis in the Inner City." *Conscious Choice*, Oct. 2003.
7. "Urban Agriculture and Community Food Security in the United States: Farming from the City Center to the Urban Fringe." Report from the Community Food Security Coalition, Feb. 2002: foodsecurity.org/urbanag.html.

## SOLUTION 41

1. Coalition for Healthier Schools. "Position Statement: 2004" (Background on Issues: Improving Education, Child Health and Learning, and the Environment). Accessed July 2006: pollutionfreeschools.org/coalition/ncps.
2. Division of the State Architect of California Sustainable Schools Resource. Accessed July 2006: sustainableschools.dgs.ca.gov/sustainableschools.
3. Coalition for Healthier Schools. "Position Statement: 2004" (Background on Issues: Improving Education, Child Health and Learning, and the Environment). Accessed July 2006: pollutionfreeschools.org/coalition/ncps.
4. Toronto School Ground Greening Initiative. Accessed July 2006: evergreen.ca/en/lg/trsb.html.

## SOLUTION 42

1. *European Heart Journal*: eurheartj.oxfordjournals.org/cgi/content/full/27/20/2385.
2. Americans for Non-Smokers Rights: no-smoke.org.
3. Microwave News.com: Louis Slesin blog for Feb. 16, 2005.

## SOLUTION 43

1. E.B. Bassin. "Age-specific Fluoride Exposure in Drinking Water and Osteosarcoma (United States)." *Cancer Causes and Control*, 17, pp. 421-28, May 2006.
2. *Harvard Study: Strong Link Between Fluoridated Water and Bone Cancer in Boys*. Environmental Working Group, April 5, 2006: ewg.org/issues/fluoride/20060405/index.php.
3. Natural Resources Defense Council. "Urban Stormwater Pollution, Fact and Fiction." Accessed July 2006: nrdc.org/water/pollution/q2storm.asp.
4. Dana W. Kolpin, et al. "Pharmaceuticals, Hormones and Other Organic Wastewater Contaminants in U.S. Streams, 1999-2000: A National Reconnaissance." *Environmental Science & Technology*, March 15, 2002: sciencenews.org/articles/20020323/fob6ref.asp.
5. Canadian Cancer Society statement on chlorinated water. Accessed July 2006: cancer.ca/ccs/internet/standard/0,3182,3172_372124_langId-en,00.html.
6. *Biosolids Applied to Land: Advancing Standards and Practices*. The National Academies Press, 2002: nap.edu/books/0309084865/html.
7. Accessed July 2006: organicconsumers.org/foodsafety/sludge101403.cfm.

8. Santa Monica Urban Runoff Recycling Facility. Accessed July 2006: santa-monica.org/epwm/smurrf/smurrf.html.

## SOLUTION 44

1. L.Tomatis. "Poverty and Cancer." *Cancer Epidemiol Biomark Prev, 1*, pp. 1992.
2. Harvard Center for Public Health. *Report on Cancer Prevention*, 1996: hsph.harvard.edu/cancer/publications/reports/vol1_full_text/vol1_ses.html.
3. Eugenia E. Calle and Rudolf Kaaks. "Overweight, Obesity and Cancer: Epidemiological Evidence and Proposed Mechanisms." *Nature Reviews Cancer, 4*, pp. 579-91, 2004; doi:10.1038/nrc1408.
4. Sierra Club. *Highway Health Hazards*. Aug. 2004: sierraclub.org.
5. "The Greening of Regent Park." *Globe and Mail*: theglobeandmail.com/servlet/story/LAC.20060225.GREEN25/TPStory/Environment.
6. RUAF Foundation. Accessed July 2006: ruaf.org/node/513.
7. Alan Durning. *The Car and the City*. Executive Summary: carsharing.net/library/carandcityexecsummary.html.

## SOLUTION 45

1. From the host city (San Francisco) invitation to World Environment Day meetings, 2005: wed2005.org/6.0.php.
2. Interview with former Bogota Mayor Enrique Penalosa. May 2006: downtoearth.org.in/full6.asp?foldername=20030515&filename=Anal&sec_id=7&sid=4.

## SOLUTION 46

1. Peter Montague. "The Emperor of Risk Assessment Isn't Wearing Any Clothes." *Rachel's Democracy & Health News, 831*, Dec. 1, 2005.
2. Canadian Auto Workers. *Devil of a Poison*: caw.ca/whatwedo/health&safety/pdf/cawcancer.pdf.
3. Only 13% of American workers belonged to unions in 2005, down from a high of 35% in the 1950s.

The strength of Canada's public sector unions has helped keep Canadian unionization rates higher at 31%, but there has been a decline of 9% since the early 1980s.

## SOLUTION 47

1. *Hazards, 67*, July/Sept. 1999.
2. *Hazards, 88*, Dec. 2004.

## SOLUTION 48

1. In Canada WHMIS was the successful product of hard negotiating by the Canadian Labour Congress and its affiliates.
2. European Commission. *Employment and Social Affairs, Health & Safety At Work*: europa.eu.int/comm/employment_social/health_safety/chemicals_en.htm.
3. Section 5.57 of the British Columbia Workers Compensation Board Regulation: www2.worksafebc.com/Publications/OHSRegulation/Part5.asp#SectionNumber:5.57.
4. *Prevention of Occupational and Environmental Cancers in Canada: A Best Practices Review and Recommendations*. Canadian Strategy for Cancer Control, May 2005, p. 44. To download the full report, see 209.217.127.72/cscc/pdf/BestPractieReview.pdf.
5. Windsor Occupational Health Clinic for Ontario Worker's CROME program (Computerized Recording of Occupations Made Easy): ohcow.on.ca/services/research.html and ohcow.on.ca/clinics/sarnia/docs/Oct.Brophy.pdf.

## SOLUTION 49

1. Union Networks International (UNI). *Unions Urge Governments to Join World "Asbestos Ban."* Media release, June 8, 2005: union-network.org/uniindep.nsf/0/06e992ddb85a35f5c125701a00477190? OpenDocument.
2. Personal communication, Dec. 2006.

## SOLUTION 50

1. Personal communication, July 2005.

2. Best Practises review:
209.217.127.72/cscc/pdf/BestProactiseReview.pdf.
3. Canadian Cancer Society's 2005 Occupational Exposure Statement:
cancer.ca/ccs/internet/standard/0,3182,3172_335253_372253_langId-en,00.html.

## SOLUTION 53

1. "UMass Lowell's Toxics Use Reduction Institute Five Chemicals Study Reveals Practical Alternatives for Massachusetts Industry and Consumers." Toxics Use Reduction Institute, July 6, 2006:
turi.org/content/content/view/full/3811/.
2. "Chemical Strategies Partnership, Tools for Optimizing Chemical Management," 2004:
chemicalstrategies.org.

## SOLUTION 54

1. Terry Collins. "Toward Sustainable Chemistry." *Science Magazine*, Jan. 2001:
sciencemag.org/cgi/content/full/291/5501/48.
2. Referenced in *Green Chemistry in California* report.

## SOLUTION 56

1. International Joint Commission. *Sixth Biennial Report on Great Lakes Water Quality*, 1992, p. 29.

## SOLUTION 57

1. Corporate Knights. *The 2002 Green Machines*: corporateknights.ca/greenmachines/profile_Husky.asp.
2. WHO. *Occupational Health: Ethically Correct, Economically Sound*. Geneva, 1999:
who.int/inf-fs/en/fact084.html.
3. There has been very little research into the health risks in women's trades and professions, which needs doing because so many women work outside the home.

## SOLUTION 59

1. In 1989 the Chemical Manufacturers Association (CMA) spent $298,000 to fight a Massachusetts toxics use reduction initiative that never reached the ballot. See chemicalindustryarchives.org/dirtysecrets/RtK/6.asp.
2. In 1990 the CMA contributed $800,000 to fight the "Big Green" omnibus environmental initiative in California, which was defeated by a margin of almost 2 to 1 after a total expenditure by the corporate sector of $15 million. Big Green would have been the most far-reaching environmental law ever passed, phasing out carcinogenic pesticides, banning oil drilling in coastal areas, promoting tree-planting and cutting emissions of $CO_2$ by 40% within 20 years.
3. In 1992 the CMA contributed $720,000 to successfully oppose a right to know initiative in Ohio.
4. In 1994 the CMA contributed $800,000 to oppose a Massachusetts Public Interest Research Group initiative prohibiting corporate contributions to ballot campaigns; it was soundly defeated.
5. In 2006 Bill H.R. 4591, to modify the Toxic Substances Control Act, would pre-empt and invalidate state standards on chemicals added to the global POPs treaty once they become binding for the US, jeopardizing the progress made in many states.

## SOLUTION 60

1. George D. Thurston, et al. "Lung Cancer, Cardiopulmonary Mortality, and Long-term Exposure to Fine Particulate Air Pollution." *Journal of the American Medical Association*, March 6, 2002.
2. Amir Sapkota and Timothy J. Buckley. *The Mobile Source Effect on Curbside 1,3 butadiene, Benzene and Particle-Bound Polycyclic Aromatic Hydrocarbons Assessed at a Tollbooth*. John Hopkins Bloomberg School of Public Health, June 2003.
3. Robert L. Pearson, et al. "Distance-Weighted Traffic Density in Proximity to a Home Is a Risk Factor for Leukemia and Other Childhood Cancers." *Journal of Air and Waste Management Association*, Feb. 2000.

## SOLUTION 61

1. "New Global Wind Map May Lead to Cheaper Power Supply." *Stanford Report*, May 20, 2005:
news-service.stanford.edu/news/2005/may25/wind-052505.html.

2. See bettermines.org/paddocks.cfm.
3. Carolyn Stephens and Mike Ahern. "Worker and Community Health Impacts Related to Mining Operations Internationally: A Rapid Review of the Literature." *MMSD Report 25*, London School of Hygiene & Tropical Medicine, 2001.
4. "EPA's Toxics Release Inventory": epa.gov/triexplorer.
5. "Improving Safety and Health in Mines: A Long and Winding Road?" *MMSD Report 54*. Norman S. Jennings International Labour Office, 2001.

## SOLUTION 62

1. Joseph LaDou. "The Asbestos Cancer Epidemic." *Environmental Health Perspectives, 112*, March 3, 2004: caut.ca/en/issues/asbestos/art_epidemic.pdf.
2. *The Poisonwood Rivals: High Levels of Arsenic Found in Lumber from Home Depot & Lowe's.* Environmental Working Group, Nov. 2001: ewg.org/reports/poisonwoodrivals/pr.html.
3. Formaldehyde: see World Health Organization data: who.dk/document/aiq/5_8formaldehyde.pdf; US government data: atsdr.cdc.gov/toxprofiles/tp111.pdf.

## SOLUTION 63

1. *Organic Farming, Food Quality and Human Health: A Review of the Evidence.* Soil Association, 2001.
2. Kori Flower, et al. "Cancer Risk and Parental Pesticide Application in Children of Agricultural Health Study Participants." *Environmental Health Perspectives*, April 2004.
3. A. Abell, E. Ernst and J.P. Bonde. "High Sperm Density Amongst Members of Organic Farmers' Association." *Lancet, 343*, p. 1498, 1994.
4. T.K. Jensen, et al. "Semen Quality Among Members of the Organic Food Associations in Zealand, Denmark." *Lancet, 347*, p. 1844, 1996.
5. "The World of Organic Agriculture: Statistics and Emerging Trends, 2006." IFOAM. Accessed Nov. 20, 2006: orgprints.org/5161/01/yussefi-2006-overview.pdf.
6. "Are Fizzy Drinks Doing This to Our Children?" *Guardian Weekly*. Jan. 23, 2003.

7. E.g., H.R. 4167, the National Uniformity of Foods Act 2005.
8. See www2.marksandspencer.com/thecompany/trustyour_mands.

## SOLUTION 64

1. A hundred million products: blog.commerce.net/archives/2004/10/how_many_produc.html.
2. Obesity: see cdc.gov/nccdphp/dnpa/obesity.
3. Plastic wrap: see ecologycenter.org/iptf/toxicity/seventhgrade.html. This is not an urban myth, even though the plastics industry is trying to make it so.
4. Paul Goettlich. "Get Plastic Out of Your Diet." *Living Nutrition*, April 2004.
5. Beatrice Trum Hunter. "Dangers of Packaging Chemicals Getting into Food." *Consumers' Research Magazine, 76* (12), p. 8(2), Dec. 1993: mindfully.org/Plastic/Packaging-Chemicals-Food-Dec93.htm.

## SOLUTION 65

1. Cathy Flanders. *Candles, Toxic Emissions & Property Damage*: ameliaww.com/fpin/candles.htm.
2. For a summary of the medical evidence, see inchem.org/documents/iarc/vol63/dry-cleaning.html.
3. "Cancer Risk Seen in 'Green Earth' Dry Cleaning." *NPR Morning Edition*, Jan. 10, 2005: npr.org/templates/story/story.php?storyId=4256304.
4. Michael Wilson. *Green Chemistry in California.* California Policy Research Center, 2006.
5. *Millennium Ecosystem Assessment, 2000*: greenfacts.org/ecosystems.

## SOLUTION 66

1. European Environment and Health Committee, Sweden: euro.who.int/eehc/implementation/20051019_2.
2. Michael P. Wilson, et al. *Green Chemistry in California: A Framework for Leadership in Chemicals Policy and Innovation.* California Policy Research Center, University of California, 2006: coeh.berkeley.edu/FINALgreenchemistryrpt.pdf.

## Solution 67

1. Anne Platt McGinn. *Why Poison Ourselves? A Precautionary Approach to Synthetic Chemicals.* Worldwatch Institute Report: 2000 worldwatch.org/pubs/paper/153.
2. *Late Lessons from Early Warnings: The Precautionary Principle 1896-2000*: reports.eea.eu.int/ environmental_issue_report_2001_22/en.

## Solution 68

1. Finland's ASA Register: riskobservatory.osha.eu.int/systems/osm/reports/finnish_system_007.stm.
2. Canada's National Dose Registry: hc-sc.gc.ca/ ewh-semt/occup-travail/radiation/regist/index_e.html.

## Solution 69

1. *The Toxic Lobby: How the Chemicals Industry Is Trying to Kill REACH.* Greenpeace International, May 2006: greenpeace.org.

## Solution 70

1. "Provincial Papers Inc. Found Guilty of Environmental Offence and Must Pay $200,000." Environment Canada, Nov. 24, 2000.
2. "Polluters' Fines Help Buy Park Land." *Philadelphia Enquirer*, Jan. 20, 2003.

## Solution 71

1. "Government Spending on Canada's Oil and Gas Industry: Undermining Canada's Kyoto Commitment." News release, Pembina Institute, Jan. 2005.
2. Recommendations for Budget 2006, Green Budget Coalition: greenbudget.ca.
3. "Canada Lags on Air Pollution Cleanup Compared to the US." *Environmental Defence.* Nov. 2005.
4. Beverley Thorpe. "A Citizens' Guide to Clean Production." *Clean Production Network.* Aug. 1999, p. 34.

## Solution 73

1. Sect. 34:5A-2, New Jersey Worker and Community Right to Know Act PL 1983, c.315, as amended July 1, 2003.

2. Environment Canada. *Pollution Prevention Success Stories*: ec.gc.ca/pp/en/storyoutput.cfm? storyid=106
3. British Columbia Workers' Compensation Act: www2.worksafebc.com/publications/ OHSRegulation/Part5.asp?ReportID=18044.

## Solution 74

1. United Nations. *The State of the Planet Is Getting Worse But for Many It's Still "Business As Usual".* United Nations Environment Program, May 15, 2002.
2. *The Big Deal.* Friends of the Earth, UK.
3. M. Graham. "Regulation by Shaming." *Atlantic Monthly, 285,* pp. 36-40, April 2000.
4. J. Hamilton. "Exercising Property Rights to Pollute: Do Cancer Risks and Politics Affect Plant Emission Reductions?" *Journal of Risk and Uncertainty, 18,* pp. 105-24, 1999.
5. *Green Industry and New Roles for Communities, Markets and Government.* World Bank, Ch. 3.

## Solution 75

1. D. Michaels. "Doubt Is Their Product." *Scientific American, 292* (6), June 2005.
2. Buzzflash interview with Bev Harris, Sept. 30, 2003: workingforchange.com.

## Solution 76

1. Volvo: volvocars.us/_Tier2/WhyVolvo/Environment/ EnvironmentProductDeclaration.htm.
2. Electrolux: electrolux-zanussi.com/node476.asp.

## Solution 77

1. Heschong Mahone Group. *Daylighting in Schools.* Prepared for the California Board for Energy Efficiency, Aug. 20, 1999.
2. Daniel Strait. "A Shrimp Spawns Partnerships." *Endangered Species Bulletin, 21* (1), Jan/Feb. 1996.
3. J. Michael Murphy. *Findings from the Evaluation Study of the Edible Schoolyard.* Harvard Medical School, Center for Ecoliteracy, April 2003.
4. Angela Murrills. "Lessons Rooted in the Soil." *Best Eating*, May 25, 2006.

5. Frank M. Torti, Jr., et al. "Survey of Nutrition Education in U.S. Medical Schools." *Medical Education Online*, 6, 2001.

### SOLUTION 78

1. Interview in *Grist Magazine*, July 13, 2004.
2. L. Budnick. "Cancer and Birth Defects Near the Drake Superfund Site, Pennsylvania." *Archives of Environmental Health*, 39 (6), Nov./Dec. 1984, pp. 409-13.
3. Michael P.Wilson. *Green Chemistry in California*, 2006.
4. Besafenet.com/Superfund.htm.
5. "The Legacy of Federal Contaminated Sites." Office of the Auditor General of Canada, 2002: oag-bvg.gc.ca/domino/reports.nsf/html/c20021002ce.html.

### SOLUTION 79

1. Prabhat Jha and Frank J. Chaloupka, eds. *Tobacco Control in Developing Countries*. World Health Organization and World Bank Tobacco Study. Oxford: Oxford University Press, 2000.
2. *Smoking Rates in Canada Lowest Ever*. Health Canada, Aug. 11, 2005.
3. "Declines in Lung Cancer Rates: California, 1988-1997." *JAMA*, 284, pp. 3121-22, 2000.
4. Karen Friend and David T. Levy. "Reductions in Smoking Prevalence and Cigarette Campaign Associated with Mass-Media Campaigns." *Health Education Research*, 17 (1), pp. 85-98, Feb. 2002.

### SOLUTION 81

1. "Scientists Warn Parents on Pesticides and Plastics." *Guardian*, March 21, 2006.
2. Chensheng Lu, et al. "Organic Diets Significantly Lower Children's Dietary Exposure to Organophosphorus Pesticides." *Environmental Health Perspectives*, 114 (2), Feb. 2006.

### SOLUTION 82

1. *Cancer: Coal's Hidden Cost*. Earthjustice, reporting on a draft EPA report, March 6, 2007.
2. Hydrogen is a possible future energy carrier, as long as the hydrogen is made from a sustainable feedstock, not natural gas, and uses sustainable energy to separate it from the molecules it clings to. "Clean coal" is also a possibility, provided all the mercury, sulfur dioxide and heavy metals are captured, and the coal companies capture and store 100% of the $CO_2$. Cold fusion is probably a distant pipe dream that will come far too late to make a difference, if it works at all.

### SOLUTION 83

1. "Cancer Risk from Industrial Chemical Rises, Study Finds." *Los Angeles Times*, July 27, 2006.
2. "Toms River Still Asking a Question: Why Us?" *New York Times*, Dec. 24, 2001.
3. City of Toronto Sewer Use Bylaw: city.toronto.on.ca/water/protecting_quality/pollution_prevention/iwcu.htm.

### SOLUTION 84

1. Military Toxics White Paper: ccaej.org/projects/whitpaper/milittoxics.htm.
2. Military Toxics Project. *Communities in the Line of Fire*. June 2002.
3. Center for Community Action and Environmental Justice, Communities at Risk. *Military Toxics: Our Own Worst Environmental Enemy*: ww.ccaej.org/projects/whitpaper/milittoxics.htm.
4. Ibid.
5. Carmelo Ruiz. *Puerto Rico: Bombs Away, Vieques Unearths Toxic Navy Trash*. Interpress Service News Agency, Dec. 30, 2003.
6. Lisa Stiffler. "Hanford Water Cleanup Not Working, Report Says." *Seattle Post Intelligencer*, July 28, 2004.
7. Barry Yeoman. "Deadly Dependence." *Creative Loafing*. Atlanta, GA, Aug. 25, 2004.
8. ATSDR. *ATSDR Releases Survey of Childhood Cancers and Birth Defects at USMC Camp Lejeune, NC, 1968-85*. July 16, 2003: atsdr.cdc.gov/sites/lejeune/index.html.
9. Peter Eisler. "Military Tries to Exempt Acres from Environmental Laws." *USA Today*, Nov. 13, 2004.
10. Julius Strauss. "A Toxic Legacy in the Heart of the Wilderness." *Globe and Mail*, Nov. 21, 2005.

## Solution 85

1. UK Working Group on the Primary Prevention of Breast Cancer. *Breast Cancer: An Environmental Disease, The Case for Primary Prevention*: nomorebreastcancer.org.
2. *Clemenceau: A Victory for the International Law and Environmental Justice*. Basel Action Network, Feb. 15, 2006.
3. Office of Pollution Prevention and Toxics. *Chemical Hazard Data Availability Study*. US Environmental Protection Agency, April 1998.
4. Simon Pickvance, et al. *Final Report: Further Assessment of the Impact of REACH on Occupational Health with a Focus on Skin and Respiratory Diseases*. University of Sheffield, UK, prepared for the European Trade Union Institute, Sept. 2005.

## Solution 86

1. Global Cancer Statistics, 2002: caonline.amcancersoc.org/cgi/content/full/55/2/74.
2. "Scandal of Child Cancer Deaths." *Scotsman*, Feb. 15, 2004.
3. See sciencenews.org/articles/20050115/bob10.asp. For scientific references on betel chewing, see forsyth.org/marianas/bib_betel.htm.

## Solution 87

1. G. Yang, et al. "Smoking in China: Findings of the 1996 National Prevalence Survey." *JAMA*, *282*, pp. 1247-53, 1999.
2. Asian Harm Reduction Network. Accessed Dec. 8, 2006: ahrn.net.
3. Tobacco causes poverty for 1.3 million. VietnamNetBridge: english.vietnamnet.vn/social/2005/12/524005/.
4. For a summary of the Islamic ruling on smoking by Sheikh Mahdi Abdul-Hamid Mustafa, Director of Information, Al-Azhar, Member of the Higher Council for Islamic Affairs, see emro.who.int/Publications/HealthEdReligion/Smoking/Summary.htm.

## Solution 88

1. Anil Agarwal. *My Story Today, Your Story Tomorrow*. Centre for Science and Environment, Delhi: cseindia.org/html/au/anilji/mystory.htm.
2. Anil Agarwal. *When Will India Be Able to Control Pollution?*: cseindia.org/aboutus/anilji/airpollution.htm.
3. *Pollution Is Causing Havoc in New Delhi*. Chittaranjan National Cancer Institute, Oct. 24, 2004: terradaily.com/2004/041025114342.t6gp34nz.html.
4. Robert Pearson, Howard Wachtel and Kristie Ebi. "New Study Links High Traffic Streets to Childhood Leukemia, Other Cancers." *Journal of Air and Waste Management Association*, Feb. 2000: colorado.edu/news/releases/2000/91.html.
5. *Air Pollution Cancer Fears Grow*. BBC, March 6, 2002: news.bbc.co.uk/1/low/health/1853675.stm.
6. *Scientists Find Structures That May Cause Mutations Leading to Cancers*. Oak Ridge Laboratory, 1995: sdsc.edu/GatherScatter/GSsummer96/broyde.html.
7. "The Filthy Truth About Diesel Mules." *New Scientist*, May 7, 2005.
8. Hugh Warwick and Alison Doig. *Smoke: The Killer in the Kitchen*. Intermediate Technology Development Group, 2004: itdg.org/html/smoke/smoke_index.htm.

## Solution 89

1. "Farmers Persist with Organics, See Results." *India Together Punjab Diary*, October 22, 2005: indiatogether.org/2005/oct/agr-organicmv.htm.
2. Brian Halweil. "Can Organic Farming Feed Us All?" *WorldWatch Magazine*, May/June 2006.
3. *The Real Green Revolution*. Greenpeace, 2002. Accessed Dec. 8, 2006: greenpeace.org.uk/MultimediaFiles/Live/FullReport/4526.pdf.
4. Ibid.
5. C. Mundt, et al. "Genetic Diversity and Disease Control in Rice." Letters to *Nature*, *Nature Journal*, Aug. 2000.
6. Kunda Dixit. "The Miracle It's No Miracle." *Nepali Times*, 256, 2003: nepalitimes.com/issue256/nation.htm. And see ciifad.cornell.edu/sri.

7. J. Pretty. "Can Sustainable Agriculture Feed Africa?" *Environment, Development and Sustainability, 1,* pp. 253-74, 2000.
8. Bill McKibben. "Cuba: What Will You Be Eating When the Revolution Comes?" *Harpers Magazine,* April 2005.
9. Vandana Shiva. *Poverty and Globalization.* 2000 BBC Reith Lecture: news.bbc.co.uk/hi/english/static/events/reith_2000/lecture5.stm.
10. Guy Dauncey. *The Sekem Initiative, Egypt.* LEDIS, Glasgow, 2005: earthfuture.com/economy/sekemegypt.asp.

### SOLUTION 90

1. Guy Dauncey. *The Sekem Initiative*: earthfuture.com/economy/sekemegypt.asp.

### SOLUTION 92

1. Devra Davis. *When Smoke Ran Like Water.* Basic Books, pp. 141-42, 2002.

### SOLUTION 93

1. John Buccini. *The Global Pursuit of the Sound Management of Chemicals.* World Bank, 2004.
2. The incineration of chemicals at sea ended in 1991, but Japan, North Korea and the Philippines still dump sewage sludge (often full of toxic chemicals) at sea. Since 1996 no permits to dump industrial wastes at sea have been issued.
3. ILO Convention #139.
4. ILO Convention #162.
5. ILO Convention #170.
6. ILO Convention #170

### SOLUTION 94

1. Jack Wienberg. *IPEN Calls for Immediate SAICM Actions.* IPEN, Feb. 7, 2006.

### SOLUTION 95

1. *The Basel Ban: A Triumph for Global Environmental Justice.* Briefing paper 1, Basel Action Network, Oct. 2004.
2. Laurence Summers. Memo, Dec. 12, 1991: tech.mit.edu/V121/N16/col16guest.16c.html.

3. These nations have either ratified, acceded to, accepted or approved the ban, depending on the stage at which they entered the treaty process.
4. *Exporting Harm: The High-Tech Trashing of Asia — The Canadian Story.* Basel Action Network, Oct. 2002.

### SOLUTION 96

1. Jock McCulloch. "Mining and Mendacity or How to Keep a Toxic Product in the Marketplace." *International Journal of Occupational and Environmental Health, 11,* pp. 398-403, 2005.
2. David Gee and Morris Greenberg. "Asbestos: From 'Magic' to Malevolent Mineral." *Late Lessons from Early Warnings: The Precautionary Principle 1896-2000.* European Environment Agency Environmental Issue Report No. 22, 2001.
3. International Metalworkers' Federation. "The Deadly Asbestos Legacy." April 12, 2005: imfmetal.org.
4. Laurie Kazan-Allen. "The Asbestos War." *International Journal of Occupational and Environmental Health, 9,* pp. 173-93, 2003.

### SOLUTION 97

1. Frank R. de Gruijl. "Impacts of a Projected Depletion of the Ozone Layer." *Consequences, 1* (2), Summer 1995.
2. GLOBOCAN 2002 database: www-dep.iarc.fr.
3. Dale Hurst. *New Measurements of Ozone Depleting Substances from the US and Canada.* NOAA Global Monitoring Division, Earth System Research Laboratory, Boulder, CO: American Geophysical Union, Dec. 2005.
4. Neil Finley. *Severe High Altitude Ozone Depletion at the 43 km, 2 mbar Isoline: Are There New Causes to Consider?* Private unpublished paper. Aug. 9, 2005. See also William Broad, "Blasting Through the Ozone Layer," NY Times News Service, *Vancouver Sun,* May 18, 1991; and *NOAA Scientific Assessment of Ozone Depletion,* 1998, 12.3.2.1 ("Shuttle and Rocket Launches") where "minuscule effects" are noted, but not amplification to far more dangerous levels of ozone destruction by stratospheric thinness.

## SOLUTION 98

1. Over 940,000 30-millimeter uranium-tipped bullets and "more than 14,000 large-caliber DU rounds were consumed during Operation Desert Storm/Desert Shield." (US Army Environmental Policy Institute) Statement by Ramsey Clark, former US Attorney General: iacenter.org/depleted/appeal.htm.
2. Douglas Westerman. "The Real WMDs in Iraq: Ours." Quote by Dr. Jawad Al-Ali, head oncologist at the largest hospital in Basra. *American Chronicle*, April 17, 2006. See also Doug Westerman, *Depleted Uranium: Far Worse Than 9/11*, Vital Truths and Information Clearing House, May 3, 2006: informationclearinghouse.info/article12903.htm.
3. James Denver. "Horrors of USA's Depleted Uranium in Iraq Threatens World." *Vive le Canada*, April 29, 2005: vivelecanada.ca/article.php/ 20050429121615724.
4. *Lancet*, *351* (9103), Feb. 1998.
5. David Rose. "Weapons of Self-Destruction." *Vanity Fair*, Nov. 2004: vanityfair.com/commentary/ content/printables/041115roco04.
6. Leuren Moret (international radiation specialist). *Depleted Uranium Is WMD*: commondreams.org/views05/0809-33.htm.
7. "Who Suppressed Scientific Study into Depleted Uranium Cancer Fears in Iraq." *Sunday Herald*, Feb. 22, 2004.
8. "UK Radiation Jump Blamed on Iraq Shells." *Sunday Times*, Feb. 19, 2006.
9. See note 6.

## SOLUTION 99

1. "Eco-Islam Hits Zanzibar Fishermen." *BBC News*, Feb. 17, 2005.
2. Verses 40:57.
3. Midrash Ecclesiastes Rabbah, ch. 7.
4. "Policy Statement on Ecology." General Board of the American Baptist Churches, June 1989.

## APPENDIX 2

1. Wingspread Statement. Accessed January 1, 2007: www.sehn.org/wing.html.

# Index

Centers for Disease Control, 5, 111, 202, 225
CEP. *See* Energy and Chemical Workers
cervical cancer, 2, 26, 70, 73, 238
*Channel One*, 105
"Chasing the Cancer Answer," 11, 63
Chattanooga, 142
chemical industry, 9, 17, 20, 30, 54, 56-57, 61,
　　122, 123, 183, 185, 252
chemicals, 4-5, 14, 32, 34-35, 61, 195, 206
　　substitution, 172-73, 204-05, 208, 261. *See also*
　　green chemistry; and chemicals by name
chemical service programs, 173
chemotherapy, 6, 34, 58, 59
Chicago, 38, 143, 147, 149
children, 2-3, 130-33, 134-35
　　as activists, 98-99, 106-07. *See also* by name
　　and environmental health, 15, 52
　　as fetuses, 14, 33, 45, 88
　　and healthy homes, 90-91
　　as infants, 14, 50, 88, 92-93
　　and legislation, 201
　　as newborns, 5, 119, 185
　　and organic food, 94-95, 229
　　and pesticides, 5, 8, 51, 95
　　and x-rays, 50, 51. *See also* breast milk;
　　leukemia
Children's Health Environmental Coalition
　　(CHEC), 37, 81, 83, 89, 90
China, 42, 230, 240, 242-43, 244, 246-47.
　　*See also* Baima
chlorine, 74, 77, 79, 178-79
　　by-products, 19, 93, 178
　　industry, 178, 179
　　replacements, 83, 91, 105, 114, 153, 174
chlorinated fluorocarbons (CFCs), 260, 261

Chopra, Dr. Shiv, 57
chronic fatigue syndrome, 6, 24, 25, 78
cities, 36, 138-57
　　greening, 142-43, 146-47
　　and housing, 155
　　and sustainability, 140-41. *See also* mayors;
　　poverty; smart growth; and cities by name
*Citizens' Agenda for Zero Waste*, 144
Citizens Environmental Coalition, 122
Clapp, Dr. Richard, 8, 12
Clarke, Bob, 160-61
Clean Air Act, 207
cleaning products, 4, 25, 80-81, 125, 136,
　　140, 166
　　anti-bacterial, 90
clean production, 165, 226-27
Clean Production Action, 195
Clean Water Act, 232
climate change, 156-57, 188, 189, 231
clinical trials, 40, 58
closed-loop system, 153, 172
clothing, 71, 77, 104. *See also* bras
Coalition for Healthier Schools, 148, 149
coalitions, 122-23. *See also* action groups; and
　　groups by name
Colborn, Theo, 14, 32-33, 86, 204
Collaborative on Health and the Environment
　　(CHE), 12, 116, 123, 135
collective agreements, 163
colon cancer, 6, 13, 43, 71
colorectal cancer, 3, 34, 43, 154
　　screening, 26
Coming Clean, 89, 122-23
Compact for Safe Cosmetics, 125, 194
Company Law Reform Bill, 215

trade, 256-57. *See also* depleted uranium; sewage treatment; Superfund; zero waste

Waste from Electrical and Electronic Equipment Directive (WEEE), 226

water, 83, 152-53
   drinking, 79, 140, 148, 208, 232-33
   fluoridation, 152
   pollution, 18, 170, 172, 178, 234, 246

*When Smoke Ran Like Water: Tales of Environmental Deception and the Battle Against Pollution*, 56

whistleblower protection, 163, 181

wireless fidelity (Wi-Fi), 49, 151

wildlife, 16, 33. *See also* by animal's name

Women's Voices for the Earth (WVE), 110-11

wood, 78, 190

Work Environment Council (WEC), 166-67

Workers' Compensation, 158, 198

Workers' Health & Safety Centre, 159

workplace exposure, 18, 22, 30, 34-35, 158-63, 203, 208, 258, 262
   farmers, 41, 163
   miners, 34, 53, 188-99, 200

protection, 158-59, 180-81. *See also* asbestos; firefighters

Workplace Hazardous Materials Information System (WHMIS), 162

World Bank, 225, 238, 249, 256

World Cancer Research Fund, 42

World Health Assembly, 192

World Health Organization, 15, 44, 94, 180, 224, 240, 250, 251

World Summit on Sustainable Development, 254

World Trade Organization, 249, 258

Worldwatch Institute, 244

World Wildlife Fund (WWF), 118-20, 168

W.R. Grace mine, 54, 190

**X**

x-ray, 15, 20, 50-51, 84

**Z**

zero emissions, 162, 172-73, 255

zero energy, 155, 191

zero exposure, 162

zero waste, 144-45, 172, 174, 227

# About the Authors

**L**iz **Armstrong** co-wrote *Whitewash* (HarperCollins, 1992), which focused on the problems of chlorine bleached paper products. She is principal author of *Everyday Carcinogens: Stopping Cancer Before It Starts* (background paper for the 1999 McMaster Conference: www.stop-cancer.org). She was co-founder of both the Women's Environmental Health Network and the Breast Cancer Prevention Coalition and is Co-Chair of Prevent Cancer Now. She lives in Erin, Ontario.

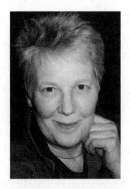

**Guy Dauncey** is an author, speaker and organizer who works to develop a positive vision of a sustainable future and to translate that vision into action. He is author of *Stormy Weather: 101 Solutions to Global Climate Change* (New Society Publishers, 2001) and other titles, and publisher of *EcoNews*, a monthly newsletter that serves the vision of a sustainable Vancouver Island. He is founder and series editor of The Solutions Project, President of the BC Sustainable Energy Association and Co-Chair with Liz of Prevent Cancer Now. He lives in Victoria, British Columbia. His website is www.earthfuture.com.

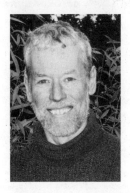

**Anne Wordsworth** is an environmental researcher and writer and a former producer for CBC's *Health Show*. She is author of *Best Practices Review: Primary Prevention of Exposures to Occupational and Environmental Carcinogens* for the Canadian Strategy for Cancer Control (2005).

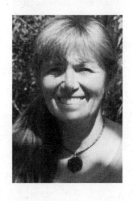

If you have enjoyed *Cancer: 101 Solutions to a Preventable Epidemic*
you might also enjoy other

# BOOKS TO BUILD A NEW SOCIETY

Our books provide positive solutions for people who want to
make a difference. We specialize in:

**Sustainable Living • Green Building • Peak Oil • Renewable Energy**
**Environment & Economy • Natural Building & Appropriate Technology**
**Progressive Leadership • Resistance and Community**
**Educational and Parenting Resources**

## New Society Publishers

### ENVIRONMENTAL BENEFITS STATEMENT

New Society Publishers has chosen to produce this book on Enviro 100, recycled
paper made with **100% post consumer waste**, processed chlorine free, and old
growth free.

For every 5,000 books printed, New Society saves the following resources:[1]

| | |
|---:|---|
| 44 | Trees |
| 3,969 | Pounds of Solid Waste |
| 4,367 | Gallons of Water |
| 5,696 | Kilowatt Hours of Electricity |
| 7,214 | Pounds of Greenhouse Gases |
| 31 | Pounds of HAPs, VOCs, and AOX Combined |
| 11 | Cubic Yards of Landfill Space |

[1]Environmental benefits are calculated based on research done by the Environmental Defense Fund and
other members of the Paper Task Force who study the environmental impacts of the paper industry.

*For a full list of NSP's titles, please call* **1-800-567-6772** *or check out our website at:*

**www.newsociety.com**

NEW SOCIETY PUBLISHERS